HUMAN TROPHOBLAST NEOPLASMS

ADVANCES IN EXPERIMENTAL MEDICINE AND BIOLOGY

Recent Volumes in this Series

Volume 169
OXYGEN TRANSPORT TO TISSUE – V
Edited by D. W. Lübbers, H. Acker, E. Leniger-Follert, and T. K. Goldstick

Volume 170
CONTRACTILE MECHANISMS IN MUSCLE
Edited by Gerald H. Pollack and Haruo Sugi

Volume 171
GLUCOCORTICOID EFFECTS AND THEIR BIOLOGICAL CONSEQUENCES
Edited by Louis V. Avioli, Carlo Gennari, and Bruno Imbimbo

Volume 172
EUKARYOTIC CELL CULTURES: Basics and Applications
Edited by Ronald T. Acton and J. Daniel Lynn

Volume 173
MOLECULAR BIOLOGY AND PATHOGENESIS OF CORONAVIRUSES
Edited by P. J. M. Rottier, B. A. M. van der Zeijst, W. J. M. Spaan, and M. C. Horzinek

Volume 174
GANGLIOSIDE STRUCTURE, FUNCTION AND BIOMEDICAL POTENTIAL
Edited by Robert W. Ledeen, Robert K. Yu, Maurice M. Rapport, and Kunihiko Suzuki

Volume 175
NEUROTRANSMITTER RECEPTORS: Mechanisms of Action and Regulation
Edited by Shozo Kito, Tomio Segawa, Kinya Kuriyama, Henry I. Yamamura, and Richard W. Olsen

Volume 176
HUMAN TROPHOBLAST NEOPLASMS
Edited by Roland A. Pattillo and Robert O. Hussa

A Continuation Order Plan is available for this series. A continuation order will bring delivery of each new volume immediately upon publication. Volumes are billed only upon actual shipment. For further information please contact the publisher.

HUMAN TROPHOBLAST NEOPLASMS

Edited by

Roland A. Pattillo

and

Robert O. Hussa

The Medical College of Wisconsin
Milwaukee, Wisconsin

PLENUM PRESS • NEW YORK AND LONDON

Library of Congress Cataloging in Publication Data

World Congress on Trophoblast Neoplasms (1st: 1982: Nairobi, Kenya)
Human trophoblast neoplasms.

(Advances in experimental medicine and biology; v. 176)
"Proceedings of the First World Congress on Trophoblast Neoplasms, held October 25-27, 1982, in Nairobi, Kenya"—T.p. verso.
Includes bibliographical references and index.
1. Trophoblastic tumors—Congresses. 2. Trophoblastic tumors—Chemotherapy—Congresses. I. Pattillo, Roland A. II. Hussa, Robert O. III. Title. IV. Series. [DNLM: 1. Throphoblastic Tumor—congresses. 2. Uterine Neoplasms—congresses. W1 AD559 v.176 / WP 465 W927 1982h]
RC280.P6W67 1982 616.99'2 84-11367

ISBN-13: 978-1-4684-4813-9 e-ISBN-13: 978-1-4684-4811-5
DOI: 10.1007/978-1-4684-4811-5

Proceedings of the First World Congress on Trophoblast Neoplasms, held October 25-27, 1982, in Nairobi, Kenya

A Division of Plenum Publishing Corporation
233 Spring Street, New York, N.Y. 10013

FOREWORD

This book addresses neoplasms of the human trophoblast. The scant literature available on the epidemiology of trophoblast neoplasms suggests that they are as much as ten times more common in Africa, Asia, India, and much of the developing world than in Western countries. The stimulus for the book evolved out of a common interest to combine Western technology with the clinical experience in the developing world in a common pursuit of the study and eradication of trophoblast neoplasia. There is substantial evidence to contend that gene derepression as seen in trophoblastic disease may be a universal prerequisite to neoplastic transformation in general. The recent discovery that the tumor markers, human chorionic gonadotropin (hCG) or its subunits, are identifiable in over 90 percent of all extracted neoplasms suggests a critical role for this common denominator of gene derepression in neoplasia. This gene derepression concept in reproductive biology and neoplasia spans many of the basic parameters of human cell replication as related to endocrinology, immunology, biochemistry, electrophysiology, genetics, and pharmacology.

The International Society for the Study of Trophoblastic Disease focuses on the global aspects of trophoblast neoplasms. These global aspects include epidemiology and etiology of the disease, regional variations in treatment of trophoblastic neoplasms, and potential ways to adapt and apply Western technology to effective use in developing countries. It was this perspective that formed the basis for the First World Congress on Trophoblast Neoplasms, which convened in Nairobi in October, 1982. Through the cooperation of the University of Nairobi Medical School and Kenyatta National Hospital, the International Society for the Study of Trophoblast Disease brought together scientists and clinicians from all continents to discuss epidemiology, etiology, immunobiology, clinical diagnosis, and chemotherapy of trophoblast neoplasms.

The intent of this book is to provide a broad perspective to neoplasms of the human trophoblast. Since the majority of the chapters contain data presented at the First World Congress in Nairobi, there is clear emphasis on epidemiology and clinical treatment of trophoblast disease around the world. While these two topics are probably the highlights of the book, there has been a deliberate effort to include chapters on etiology, genetic origin, and immunology of trophoblast disease. Furthermore, since the detection and treatment of trophoblast disease relies on the monitoring of hCG, an understanding of hCG becomes prerequisite to having the clinical expertise in trophoblast neoplasms. Accordingly, there is emphasis in this book, as in the Congress, on immunochemistry, molecular biology, biosynthesis, and clinical chemistry of hCG.

Roland A. Pattillo
Robert O. Hussa
Milwaukee
January, 1984

CONTENTS

PREGNANCY AND NEOPLASIA 1

On the Nature of Gestational Trophoblastic Disease 3
Roy Hertz

Exposure to Chemical Carcinogens During Pregnancy: Consequences for Mother and Conceptus 13
Jerry M. Rice

IMMUNOLOGY, GESTATION, AND NEOPLASIA 51

Genetic Origin, Immunobiology, and Gonadotropin Expression in Trophoblast and Nontrophoblast Neoplasms 53
Roland A. Pattillo

Immunology in Genesis of Partial and Total Hydatidiform Mole 81
Shoshichi Takeuchi

Complement System in Abnormal Pregnancy and Chorionic Neoplasia: Immunotherapy and Chemotherapy of Chorionic Neoplasia 111
Ryoki Ohkawa, Kimiyasu Ohkawa, Norio Tosaka, Toshikatsu Ohhashi, Akira Hatano, and Tsutomu Ohkawa

Placental Senescence 127
Tim Parmley

GENETIC ORIGIN OF TROPHOBLAST NEOPLASMS 133

Complete and Partial Hydatidiform Moles: Cytogenetic and Morphological Aspects 135
A. E. Szulman and Urvashi Surti

Genetic Studies on Hydatidiform Moles 147
Sylvia D. Lawler

EPIDEMIOLOGIC ASPECTS OF TROPHOBLASTIC NEOPLASMS . . 163

Epidemiology of Gestational Trophoblastic Neoplasm at the Dr. Cipto Mangunkusumo Hospital, Jakarta, Indonesia 165
M. Farid Aziz, Nugroho Kampono, Endy Muhardin Moegni, Sjahrul Sjamsuddin, Budianto Barnas, and Ratna Suprapti Samil

Epidemiologic Aspects of Gestational Trophoblastic Diseases in Ibadan, Nigeria 177
T. A. Junaid

Epidemiology of Trophoblast Disease in Africa - Lagos . . . 187
Akin Agboola and O. O. Abudu

HUMAN CHORIONIC GONADOTROPIN 197

Immunochemistry of Human Chorionic Gonadotropin 199
R. E. Canfield, S. Birken, P. Ehrlich, and G. Armstrong

New Horizons in hCG Detection 217
Robert Hussa and Laurence A. Cole

The Carbohydrate on Human Chorionic Gonadotropin Produced by Cancer Cells 245
Laurence A. Cole and Robert O. Hussa

Paradoxical Effect of Antibodies Against Chorionic Gonadotropin on BeWo Choriocarcinoma Cells In Vitro and In Vivo: Evidence for Heterogeneity of Cell Types 271
S. K. Gupta and G. P. Talwar

The Surface Charge of Cells Producing hCG 289
Lawrence L. Hause, Norio Tosaka, and R. A. Pattillo

The Role of Trophoblast Differentiation in the Control of the hCG and hPL Genes 299
Makoto Hoshina, Robert Hussa, Roland Pattillo, H. Marvin Camel, and Irving Boime

Clinical Applications of hCG 313
K. D. Bagshawe

CLINICAL STAGING 325

A Proposal on the Clinical Staging of Malignant Trophoblastic Neoplasms Based on the Study of Process of Development of the Disease 327
Hung-Chao Sung, Pao-Chen Wu, Yuan-E Wang, Ming-Yi Tang, and Hsiou-Yu Yang

CHEMOTHERAPY AND CLINICAL MANAGEMENT 341

The Role of Methotrexate in the Chemotherapy of Gestational Trophoblastic Neoplasms 343
Alberto Sobrero and Joseph R. Bertino

Re-Evaluation of 5-Fluorouracil as a Single Agent for Gestational Malignant Trophoblastic Neoplasms 355
Hung-Chao Sung, Pao-Chen Wu, and Yuan-Bh Wang

Management of Patients with Gestational Trophoblastic Neoplasia: Experience of the Southeastern Regional Center 369
Charles B. Hammond, Daniel L. Clarke-Pearson, and John T. Soper

The Role of Regional Centers for Gestational Trophoblastic Disease 383
Donald P. Goldstein and Ross S. Berkowitz

The Study and Treatment of Gestational Trophoblastic Diseases at the Brewer Trophoblastic Disease Center, 1962 - 1979 401
John R. Lurain and John I. Brewer

Pitfalls in the Management of Trophoblastic Disease in Africa 409
J. K. G. Mati and C. Sekade Kigondu

The Problems of Management of Gestational Trophoblastic Neoplasms at the University of Benin Teaching Hospital, Benin City, Nigeria 417
F. M. E. Diejomaoh, A. E. Omu, E. E. Okpere, M. Ezimokhai, O. Tabowei, and L. N. Ajabor

Ten Years' Experience with Trophoblastic Tumors in Portugal 429
Luis Wandschneider, José Rueff, and João Branco

ABSTRACTS
FIRST WORLD CONGRESS ON TROPHOBLAST NEOPLASMS
October 25-27, 1982
University of Nairobi Medical School
Nairobi, Kenya 435

CONTRIBUTORS 465

INDEX 471

PREGNANCY AND NEOPLASIA

According to the available literature, the apparent difference in incidence in trophoblast neoplasms in the developing world, compared to the developed world, is an order of magnitude, ranging from 1 in 100-200 pregnancies in Asia and Africa, to 1 in 1,000-2,000 pregnancies in the United States. It is well known that pregnancy represents a vulnerable period of rapid growth, metabolism, and DNA synthesis. It is a period of immunosuppression, during which the foreign allograft proliferates in the maternal host, who rejects skin grafts from the paternal source only in a delayed fashion. Carcinogenic exposure in the maternal host includes a spectrum of known and unknown stimuli, including potentially carcinogenic chemicals, oncogenic viruses, and environmental ionizing radiation. All of these are capable of inducing malignancy in experimental systems. Oncogene and proto-oncogene theories of cancer have been supported by the findings of group specific antigen expression in murine and avian species which have been shown to be regulated by endogenous, dominant Mendelian genes. In addition, histocompatibility transplantation antigens influence leukemia and sarcoma expression in certain viral RNA-induced tumors, leading to the conclusion that genes for the RNA tumor virus might also be important as gene determinants in the developing placenta and embryo. The mutation and switching on of oncogene expression by various means may explain a number of cancers, including trophoblast malignancies possibly induced by chemical, hormonal, physical, or viral agents. It is known that DNA from tumors can be extracted and can subsequently transform normal cells to the same tumor state. A proto-oncogene is a gene embedded in normal DNA, as has been shown in certain bladder carcinomas which may lead to the production of human bladder tumors. Temin proposed the genetic hypothesis for cancer, which stated that the germ line in its chromosomes contains only the "potential" for genetic evolution by the somatic cells, that may lead to the formation of the information for cancer. This concept portrays vertical transmission of the information for cancer, even though the germ line does not contain this cancer-causing information until mutations or translocations have induced them. These are mechanisms of RNA-to-DNA information transfer and may play a normal role in cellular differentiation by providing a mechanism for variability in the genome of somatic cells without disturbing the stability of the germ line. Since only DNA-to-DNA, DNA-to-RNA, and RNA-to-protein modes of information transfer occur in the germ line, variability of DNA is permitted only by mutation and random selection. A normal means of permitting variability without mutation may result through formation of new sequences of DNA, from RNA-to-DNA information transfer. This is accomplished using the normal cellular RNA-dependent DNA polymerase enzyme system (reverse transcriptase) which is found in normal cells. In 1973, the first editor proposed the designation of the genetic information for cancer in trophoblast cells as proto-germ DNA. Current knowledge has identified this genetic information as the proto-oncogene. The first section of this book focuses upon chemical carcinogens in trophoblastic cancers which may permit the expression of a cancer-producing proto-oncogene.

ON THE NATURE OF GESTATIONAL TROPHOBLASTIC DISEASE

Roy Hertz

The George Washington University Medical Center
2300 Eye Street, NW
Washington, D.C. 20037

It is for me most gratifying to be called upon to serve as your Honorary President for this First World Congress of Trophoblastic Disease. Your kindness in providing me with this acknowledgement is most satisfying reward for over three decades of effort toward the resolution of some of the problems we shall review.

May I ask your indulgence in opening these sessions by showing you (Fig. 1) a portrait of my late colleague, Dr. Min Chiu Li, who played such a major role in the initial phases of our studies in this field. Fate has deprived us of Dr. Li's participation in the Congress because of his untimely death just a few years ago.

On such occasions as this it has become a senior investigator's privilege, and also his obligation, to wax historical. Hence I show you in Fig. 2 the title page of the embryological study by the renowned Dutch embryologist, Hubrecht, in 1895, in which he first used the term "trophoblast" to refer to that portion of the developing zygote which is not destined to be involved in the genesis of any of the definitive organs of the embryo. Accordingly, he considered this first histogenetic product of the embryo as providing only nourishment or sustenance for the embryo, and he coined the term, "trophoblast." The use of this term in the sense first employed by Hubrecht has proven useful to this day (1).

The application of the term "trophoblastic disease" to that clinical complex of lesions containing cells having morphogenetic and biochemical properties related to normal trophoblast was introduced simply to have a generic handle on these syndromes taken collectively. To further define our special concern for these lesions arising in relation to an antecedent pregnancy, we also

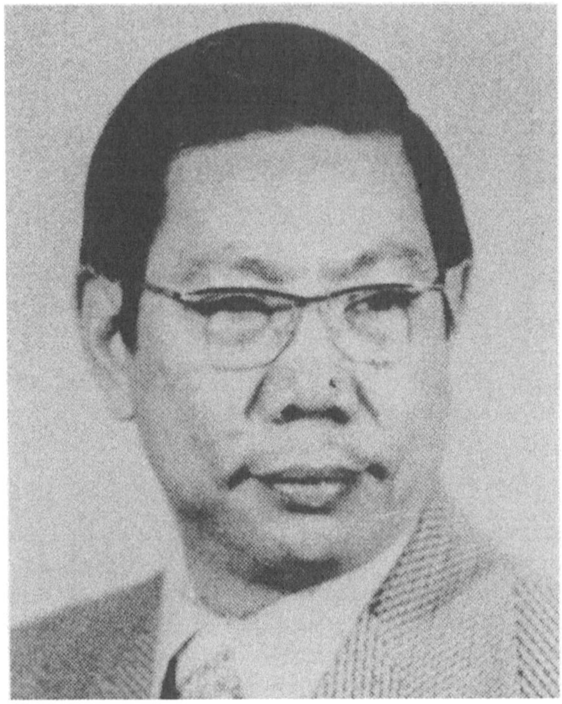

Fig. 1. Photograph of M. C. Li (1972).

began the use of the term, "gestational trophoblastic disease" (2).

In this sense the term "gestational" can only be considered to refer to a temporal rather than to a more fundamental qualitative difference from other lesions containing trophoblast. For, actually, all of us are products of an antecedent gestation and we, of necessity, will remain so until we die. In this respect, then, all of our somatic tumors are products of conception and so are all of our somatic tissues. In the case of our so-called "gestational trophoblastic tumors," the essential distinction is a purely chronological one, since we can somewhat more readily envision the temporal relationships involved.

However, our "gestational trophoblastic tumors" are also potentially distinguished by the fact that they involve elements genetically derived from both parental and fetal origin. But this distinction may also be challenged by asking which of our normal somatic or tumor cells are not also endowed with genetic elements from two parents, with the possible exception of our germ cells in

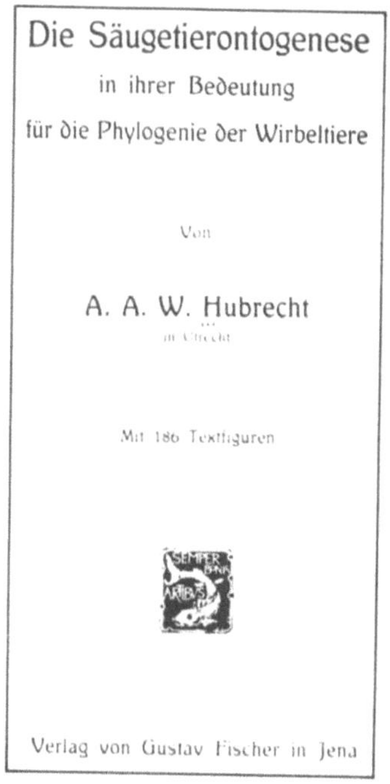
Die Säugetierontogenese
in ihrer Bedeutung
für die Phylogenie der Wirbeltiere

Von

A. A. W. Hubrecht

Mit 186 Textfiguren

Verlag von Gustav Fischer in Jena

Fig. 2. Hubrecht's thesis, title page.

the haploid state. Hence our earlier designation of "gestational trophoblastic tumors" as a "cancer à deux" may prove to be more descriptive than specific (3).

These considerations bear directly upon some of the more recent exciting findings concerning the cytogenetic distinction between complete moles and partial moles. In such discussions we understand the term "complete mole" to refer to those lesions containing no persisting fetal structures other than hydropic villi with compromised vasculatures. Such lesions are almost always exclusively of paternal cytogenetic makeup, although rare exceptions are noted in almost all series. In contrast, the partial mole, which is characterized by the presence of partially hydropic villi lacking substantial vascular abnormality, is accompanied by a wide variety of fetal parts presenting varying dyskaryotic patterns, including trisomy and other chromosomal derangements.

These distinctions are highly correlated with the propensity for persistent trophoblastic disease, in that the complete mole appears to be the almost exclusive source of persistent disease. I say "almost," because exceptions are well documented in the original series of Lawler and associates, and in many others (4-6).

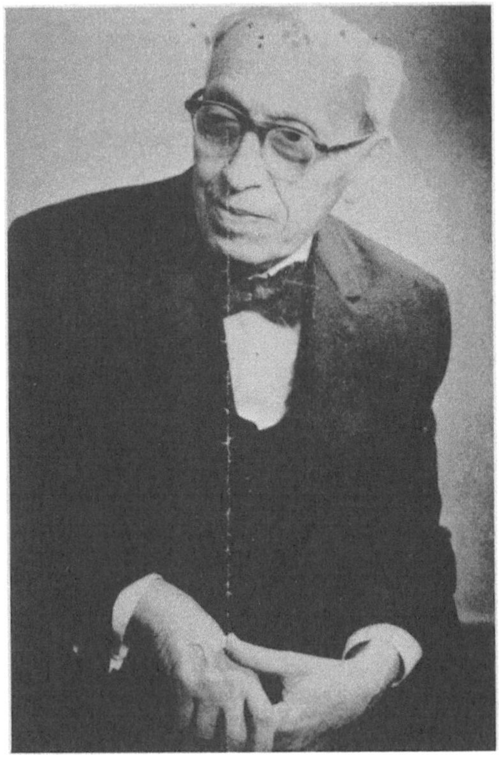

Fig. 3. Dr. Herman Zondek.

Nevertheless, these cytogenetic data have important implications in considering etiology, pathogenesis, epidemiology, and even therapy and prophylaxis of gestational trophoblastic disease. However, until the cytogenetic techniques required for such differential diagnosis are more generally available, I know of no more readily applicable criterion for management than the accurately determined gonadotropin titer.

This brings us, then, to a consideration of Dr. Herman Zondek's (Fig. 3) monumental identification in 1926 of "human chorionic gonadotropin" in the urine of not only normally pregnant women, but also of women with choriocarcinoma and with a variety of ovarian tumors (7). It is interesting that Hirose, in Japan, had also shown that implants of placental tissue, especially from early pregnancy, would induce extensive luteinization of the rabbit ovary (8). The elegant elucidation of the chemical constitution and the biosynthesis of hCG will be a most welcome contribution of later speakers. However, certain biological aspects of hCG are appropriately treated here.

At the outset, we should recall the biological Law of Biogenesis, which states that "Ontogeny repeats phylogeny. In other words, the individual in its development must pass through the stages experienced in evolution by its species. Since in ontogenetic development hCG is a readily identifiable product of the very early trophoblast, this substance must be regarded as one deriving from our most primeval cells. Small wonder, then, that it is now clear that hCG is not only to be found in such primitive cells as bacteria and sperm, but also in a wide variety of malignant tumor cells having no immediate or apparent relationship to trophoblast (9-11).

In this connection, it is interesting that as long ago as 1877, Cohnheim, a distinguished German pathologist, was led on morphological grounds to infer that all malignant tumors may, indeed, represent reactivation of embryonal foci remaining dormant for prolonged periods in the host organism, or, in modern terms, a derepression (12). Perhaps hCG provides us with a biochemical verification of Dr. Cohnheim's thesis.

There are several aspects of the behavior of hCG in the course of modern management which merit our discussion. Chief among these is the widely held belief that the continuing presence of detectable hCG in the plasma of the patient with trophoblastic disease represents the persistence of viable trophoblastic cells. While this is generally true, one noteworthy exception has repeatedly impressed us. This circumstance we have termed the "intramural syndrome." We have repeatedly noted that in numerous resistant cases, intramural uterine lesions which are complegely necrotized will provide readily bioassayable hCG which completely disappears from the patient's blood and urine promptly after hysterectomy. One wonders how often other sources of hormone from nonviable tissue may arise during therapy.

Another striking feature of the behavior of hCG is the fact that, irrespective of how high the original titer may be, the development of resistance to single drug therapy - whether with methotrexate or actinomycin D - will be accompanied by a fairly fixed level of hCG production reflected in a titer of from 2,000 to 5,000 IU per 24 hours of urinary excretion as determined by bioassay (3). This phenomenon suggests a selection of a fairly constant cell population capable of secreting a form of hCG with a limited capacity for renal clearance, an inference capable of experimental analysis.

Another endocrinological puzzle arises when we try to rationalize the occurrence of spectacular cystic ovarian enlargement in about one third of cases of molar pregnancy and its failure to occur in the remaining cases. We know that the titer of hCG is not a quantitative determinant of this ovarian effect. We also know that whereas hCG alone can prolong the life of the normal corpus luteum, it has by itself little other gonadotropic effect on the human ovary. However, when given in sequence with FSH, hCG will in some cases induce a hyperstimulation syndrome resembling that seen in mole patients. Also, we know that by some as yet unidentified mechanism, FSH is markedly reduced if not absent in early human pregnancy. Can it be, then, that the cystic ovarian enlargement seen in the mole cases reflects failure of the normal repression of FSH and essentially an augmentation phenomenon? With modern techniques of differential assays for FSH and the β-subunit of hCG, this hypothesis can be put to test. Moreover, because of the data from several series now showing that ovarian enlargement connotes a bad prognostic sign with respect to the persistence of trophoblastic disease, this consideration becomes of practical as well as theoretical importance (13).

The special quality of gestational trophoblastic disease raises a host of questions regarding the materno-fetal relationships involved. A noteworthy feature is the capacity of the maternal organism to reject both normal as well as malignant trophoblast. This rejection ability is manifested (a) in the frequency of spontaneous abortion, (b) the resolution of normal trophoblastic nodules when deported to the lungs, (c) the delivery of normal placenta at term with its antecedent infarction and necrosis, and (d) even the rejection seen in rare cases of proven highly malignant metastatic choriocarcinoma. This maternal capacity to reject trophoblast without help may lie at the root of our favorable experience in treating gestational trophoblastic disease. This may also account for the fact that even in the most malignant form of advancing choriocarcinoma, autopsy frequently reveals a totally absent primary, a phenomenon unique in all the gamut of malignant diseases.

The materno-fetal relationship has been widely characterized as the equivalent of an allograft. However, this relationship differs from the usual graft-host relationship in one basic feature. A graft derives its vasculature from the host, whereas the fetus forms its own vasculature by an altogether distinctly different process of angiogenesis. This differentiates the materno-fetal relationship from a graft-host relationship in a most fundamental way even though in normal pregnancy there does develop transport of such fetal elements as red cells, leukocytes, and trophoblast cells. However, unlike the case of the tissue graft, such exchanges are mediated through the escape of the elements of the fetus from its own vasculature and not by direct vascular continuity as in the case of a graft.

This leads to my favorite speculation as to why gestational trophoblastic tumors respond so readily to chemotherapy. I would like to offer the suggestion that this susceptibility is due to the singularly high vascularity of gestational trophoblastic tumors, thereby providing a uniquely elevated tissue drug uptake. Support

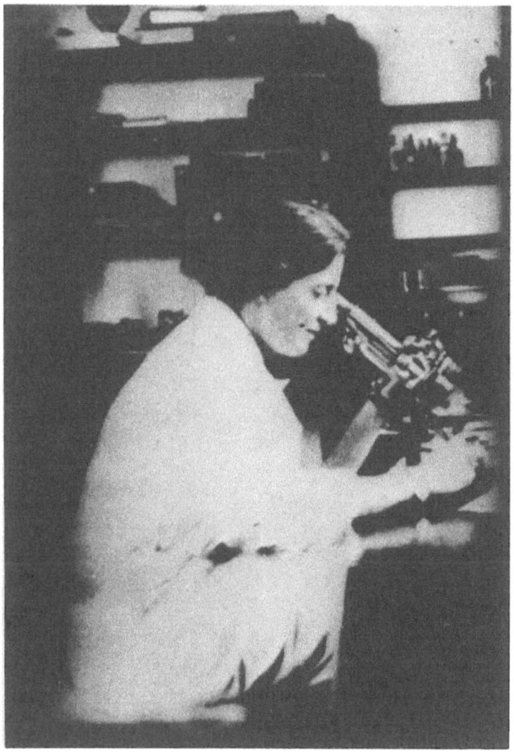

Fig. 4. Dr. Helen Wills.

of this view is indicated by the relative resistance to chemotherapy of some peripheral metastatic lesions as opposed to the highly vascular vaginal or pulmonary metastases. Brain metastases are, of course, a special case because of the blood-brain barrier.

I will now briefly dwell on the genesis of the scientific developments upon which certain of our modern therapeutic approaches are based. We begin with Dr. Helen Wills (Fig. 4), who as a missionary physician in a small village in India in the early 1900s noted that when her patients became pregnant they developed a highly characteristic megaloblastic anemia. This was readily cured by the addition of leafy vegetables to the diet. The nutritional factor provided by this supplement, through a prolonged series of investigations of the properties of a substance abundant in leafy vegetables became appropriately termed, "folic acid," from the term, *folia*.

The actual determination of the chemical structure of folic acid was greatly facilitated by the prior studies by Dr. Gowland-Hopkins (Fig. 5), on the chemistry of the pigment in the wings of the common yellow butterfly (Fig. 6), a class of substance which he

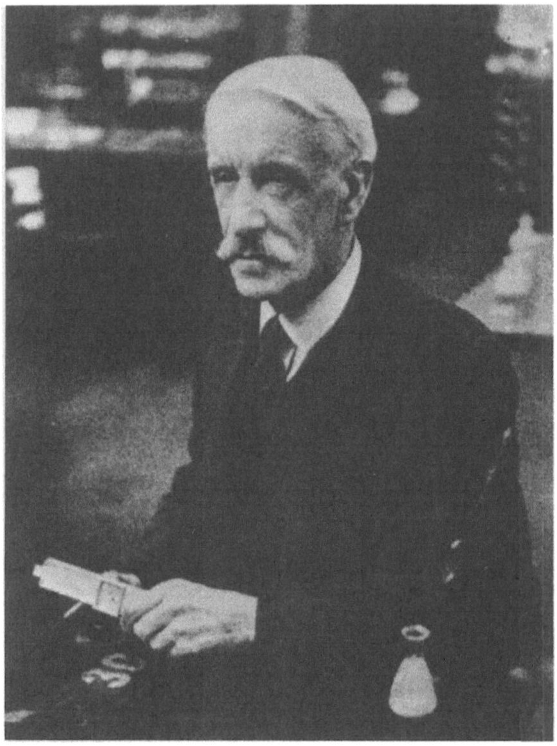

Fig. 5. Dr. F. Gowland-Hopkins.

termed, "pteridins," from the Greek term, *pterygium*, for "wing." When pure folic acid proved to be of this same yellow color despite its original isolation from spinach, Stokstadt's proof of its structure as consisting of a pterin plus glutamic acid was facilitated and the compound was named, "pteroylglutamic acid" (Fig. 7).

Meanwhile, Dr. Hans Krebs had observed that malic acid is capable of blocking succinic acid in certain *in vivo* metabolic tissue functions. With great insight he inferred that this antagonism depends upon the close similarity in chemical structure between these two compounds, and he postulated what we now know as the antagonist principle.

This approach ultimately led to the synthesis of a broad range of folic acid antagonists, also bearing evidence of their winged ancestry in the names, "aminopterin" and "amethopterin," the latter now known as methotrexate. Thus, we flutter toward a cancer cure, not knowing on what wings we fly.

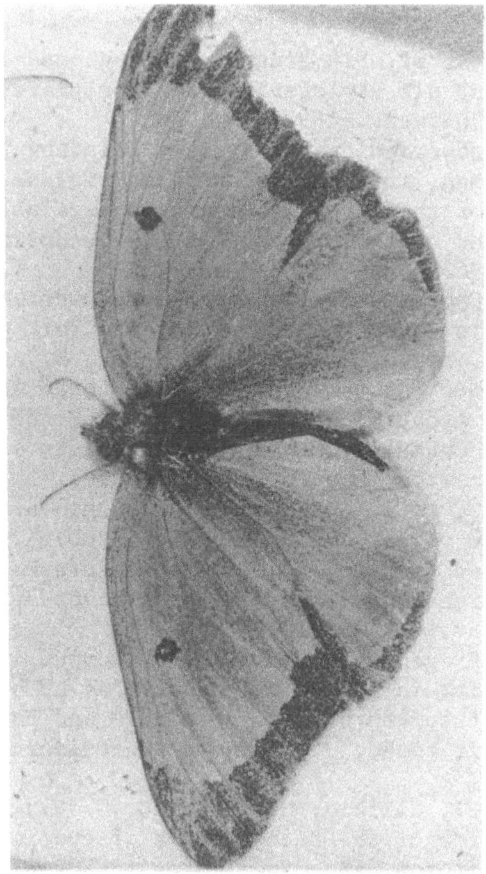

Fig. 6. Yellow butterfly.

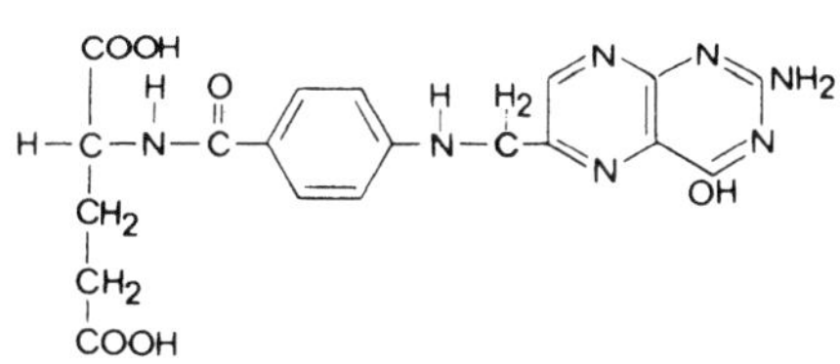

Fig. 7. Structure of folic acid (pteroylglutamic acid).

In closing, may I again express to all my warmest appreciation of your kindness in permitting me to open these sessions which I am sure will prove most stimulating and rewarding to us all. For it is such kind salutations from my junior colleagues which so greatly enhance for me what Browning termed, "the last of life for which the first was made."

REFERENCES

1. Hubrecht, A. A. W., Die Säugetiereontogenese in ihrer Bedeutung für die Phylogenie der Wirbeltiere, Verlag von G. Fischer, Utrecht (1895).
2. Hertz, R., Endocrinological studies relating to trophoblastic disease in man, in: "Choriocarcinoma: Transactions of a Conference of the International Union Against Cancer," J. F. Holland and M. Hreschyshyn, eds., Springer, Berlin (1967), p. 94.
3. Hertz, R., "Choriocarcinoma and Related Gestational Trophoblastic Tumors in Women," Raven Press, New York (1978).
4. Lawler, S. D., Pickthall, V. J., Fisher, R. A., Povey, S., Wyn-Evans, M., and Szulman, A. E., Genetic studies of complete and partial hydatidiform moles, Lancet 2:580 (1979).
5. Kajü, T. and Ohama, K., Androgenetic origin of complete hydatidiform mole, Nature 268:633 (1977).
6. Jacobs, P. A., *et al.*, Mechanism of origin of complete hydatidiform moles, Nature 286:714 (1980).
7. Zondek, B. and Ascheim, S., Die Schwangerschafts Diagnose aus men Harn durch Nachweis des Hypophysenvorderlappen hormone, Klin. Wchschr. 7:1404 (1928).
8. Hirose, T., Exogenous stimulation of corpus luteum formation in the rabbit; influence of extracts of human placenta, decidua, fetus, and hydatidiform mole and bovine corpus luteum on the rabbit gonad, J. Japanese Gynecological Society 16: 1055 (1920).
9. Acevedo, H. F., Slifkin, M., Pouchet, G. R., and Rakhshan, M., Identification of the beta subunit of choriogonadotropin in human spermatozoa, in: "The Testes in Normal and Infertile Men," P. Troen and H. R. Nankin, eds., Raven Press, New York (1977), p. 185.
10. Braunstein, G. D., Rasor, J., and Wade, M. E., Presence of chorionic gonadotropin-like substance in normal testes, New Engl. J. Med. 293:1339 (1975).
11. Koide, S. S., Maruo, T., Cohen, H., and Segal, S. J., Gonadotropin produced by a microorganism, in: "Chorionic Gonadotropin," S. J. Segal, ed., Plenum Press, New York (1980), p. 421.
12. Cohnheim, J., "Vorlesungen über Alleemeine Pathologie; ein Handbuch für Aertzte und Studierende," Ersterband, Verlag von August Hirschwald, Berlin (1877).
13. Curry, S. L., Hammond, C. B., Tyrey, L., Creasman, W., and Parker, R. T., Hydatidiform mole; diagnosis, management, and long term follow-up of 347 patients, Obstet. Gynecol. 45:1 (1975).

EXPOSURE TO CHEMICAL CARCINOGENS DURING PREGNANCY: CONSEQUENCES FOR MOTHER AND CONCEPTUS*

Jerry M. Rice

Laboratory of Comparative Carcinogenesis
National Cancer Institute
Frederick Cancer Research Facility
Frederick, Maryland 21701 USA

INTRODUCTION

The causes of the overwhelming majority of human neoplasms, including gestational choriocarcinoma, remain unknown. However, an increasing body of evidence has shown that at least some human cancers have resulted from exposure to non-infectious agents in the human environment. These agents include both ultraviolet and ionizing radiation, and diverse and in some cases as yet poorly characterized group of both organic and inorganic substances and industrial processes. The International Agency for Research on Cancer has recently concluded that at least 7 such industrial processes and 23 chemicals and groups of chemicals are causally associated with certain cancers in humans (1). A few of these agents are listed in Table 1; ironically, a significant number are used clinically as anti-neoplastic drugs. An additional 61 chemicals, groups of chemicals, or industrial processes are considered probably carcinogenic to humans by the International Agency for Research on Cancer. Hundreds more have been shown to cause tumors in experimental animals, and by inference must be considered hazardous to humans. While inorganic substances, including minerals such as asbestos and elements such as arsenic, chromium, and their salts are included in this list, the overwhelming majority of substances known to cause cancer when applied experimentally to animals and to have caused cancer in humans either as a result of

*Presented at the First World Congress on Trophoblast Neoplasms, Nairobi, Kenya, October 25-27, 1982.

Table 1. A Partial List of Chemicals that are Causally Associated with Cancer in Humans (from Ref. 1).

Organic compounds	
4-Aminobiphenyl	Bis(chloromethyl)ether
2-Aminonaphthalene	Myleran [1,4-butanediol dimethanesulfonate] [a]
Benzidine	Benzene
Chlornaphthazine [N,N-bis(2-chloroethyl)-2-aminonaphthalene] [a]	Vinyl chloride
	Diethylstilbestrol
Inorganic substances	
Asbestos	
Arsenic and arsenic compounds [b]	
Chromium and chromium compounds [b]	

[a] Antineoplastic drug.
[b] The compound(s) responsible for the carcinogenic effect in humans cannot be specified.

industrial exposure or as a consequence of anti-tumor chemotherapy are organic compounds of low molecular weight, and it is exclusively with the latter that this overview will be concerned.

Exposure of experimental animals to chemical carcinogens during pregnancy results in the development of tumors in their offspring. This phenomenon is known as transplacental carcinogenesis. Approximately 50 organic chemical carcinogens, known from experiments in adult animals and, in some cases, also from human experience to cause tumors by direct exposure during postnatal life, have been found in experimental systems to cause tumors in offspring as a consequence of exposure during an appropriate period of intrauterine life. Transplacental carcinogenesis has been demonstrated experimentally in the mouse, rat, rabbit, two species of hamster, the pig, and both the patas (*Erythrocebus patas*) and rhesus (*Macaca mulatta*) monkeys, and has occurred in humans exposed to diethylstilbestrol *in utero*. Representative studies and a partial list of transplacental chemical carcinogens are listed in Tables 2 and 3. The subject of transplacental carcinogenesis has been extensively

Table 2. Representative Transplacental Carcinogens: Direct-Acting Alkylating Agents

Compound	Test species	Principal target organs	References
Sulfate and sulfonate esters			
Dimethyl sulfate	Rat	Nervous system	2
Diethyl sulfate	Rat	Nervous system	2
Methyl methanesulfonate	Rat	Nervous system	3
Propane sultone	Rat	Nervous system	4
N-Nitrosoalkylureas			
N-Nitrosomethylurea	Rat	Nervous system	5
N-Nitrosoethylurea	Rat	Nervous system	5-10
	Mouse	Lung, liver	11-13
	Rabbit	Kidney	14, 15
	Rabbit	Nervous system	16
	Patas monkey	Connective tissues	17
Other			
Ethylurea and	Rat	Nervous system	18
sodium nitrite	Rabbit	Kidney	19

reviewed, most recently by Kleihues (38) and by Rice (39), and has been the subject of several international scientific meetings, the proceedings of which have been published (40-42).

Recent laboratory studies have provided evidence that in gravid females of at least one nonhuman primate species, exposure to chemical carcinogens early in pregnancy leads to gestational choriocarcinoma, as well as to nontrophoblastic tumors in their offspring. These studies, which provide an animal model for gestational choriocarcinoma, are summarized in the contexts of current understanding of the mechanisms of chemical carcinogenesis; existing data on the phenomenon of transplacental carcinogenesis as it occurs in nonhuman species; and their possible relevance to etiology of gestational choriocarcinoma in humans.

Table 3. Representative Transplacental Carcinogens: Metabolism-Dependent Compounds

Compound	Test species	Principal target organs	References
N-Nitrosodialkylamines			
N-Nitrosodimethylamine	Rat	Kidney	20
N-Nitrosodiethylamine	Rat	Kidney	21
	Mouse	Lung, liver	22
	Syrian hamster	Trachea	23, 24
Polynuclear aromatic hydrocarbons			
Benzo[*a*]pyrene	Mouse	Lung, skin[a]	25, 26[a]
Methylcholanthrene	Mouse	Lung	27
7,12-Dimethylbenz[*a*]-anthracene	Rat	Nervous system, kidney	30, 31
Natural products of plant and fungal origin			
Aflatoxin	Rat	Liver	32
Cycasin (methylazoxy-methyl-β-*D*-glucopyranoside	Rat	Nervous system, intestine	33
Safrole	Mouse	Kidney	34
Drugs			
Urethane (ethyl carbamate)	Mouse	Lung, skin	28[a], 29[a], 35
Procarbazine (N-(1-methylethyl)-4-[(2-methylhydrazino) methyl]benzamide	Rat	Nervous system	36
Miscellaneous			
Vinyl chloride	Rat	Blood vessels, kidney	37

[a]Skin tumors developed in mice only after postnatal topical application of croton oil or phorbol ester promoting agents.

Mechanisms of Chemical Carcinogenesis

The term, chemical carcinogen, is a phenomenological one, referring with equal validity to agents that can increase the incidence of tumors, or increase the multiplicity of tumors, or shorten the latency period for tumor development in an experimental animal or in humans, irrespective of the mechanism by which these phenomena occur. Even within the restricted category of organic compounds of low molecular weight, it is now clear that a variety of mechanisms is operative in bringing about the development of tumors. Of the substances that have been found to be carcinogenic in man, and of those that have been shown to be transplacental carcinogens in animals, all with the possible exception of the estrogen, diethylstilbestrol, exert their carcinogenic effects as a result of chemical reactivity within the target cell, by acting as an electrophile in nucleophilic substitution reactions with such components of target cells as DNA (43). A minority of such compounds are chemically reactive without metabolic modification, and are termed direct-acting carcinogens. Most of these are alkylating agents, including sulphate and sulphonate esters, N-nitrosoalkylureas, and the human carcinogens bis(chloromethyl)ether and myleran. These react by either unimolecular, S_N1 mechanisms, as in the case of N-nitrosoethylurea (Fig. 1), or by bimolecular reactions (S_N2), as in the case of bis(chloromethyl)ether (Fig. 1). Far more common are the metabolism-dependent agents which undergo enzyme-mediated metabolism to chemically reactive intermediates that in turn participate as reactive electrophiles in reactions like those of the direct-acting alkylating agents. As a consequence of chemical reactivity, the carcinogens or their reactive metabolites form covalent bonds with both purine and pyrimidine bases in DNA (43). Predictably, such agents can frequently be shown to be potent mutagens in both bacterial and mammalian cell systems. For this reason, as a class, carcinogens that act by participation in reactions of this kind are described as "genotoxic."

The enzymes responsible for conversion of metabolism-dependent carcinogens into their reactive intermediates are most commonly the mixed function oxidases that are widely distributed in animal tissues, and require molecular oxygen and reduced nucleotide coenzymes, generally NADPH, as cofactors. A single enzyme-catalyzed reaction may be sufficient to achieve formation of a chemically reactive intermediate, as in the case of vinyl chloride (Fig. 2) or N-nitrosodimethylamine (Fig. 2). Alternatively, a sequence of oxidation and conjugation reactions may be necessary. As many as three successive steps are known to be necessary for transformation of some carcinogens to their most reactive mutagenic and carcinogenic derivatives, such as the successive transformation of the polynuclear aromatic hydrocarbon, benzo[*a*]pyrene, to the 7,8-oxide, followed by hydrolysis to the 7,8-dihydrodiol and, finally, oxidation to the 7,8-dihydrodiol-9,10-oxide (44).

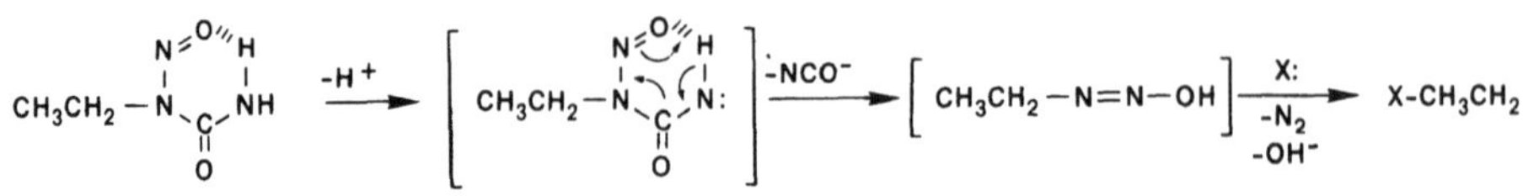

S_N1 : N-Nitrosoethylurea : $T_{1/2}$ (pH 7.25, 37°) = 7.7 min, X = H_2O

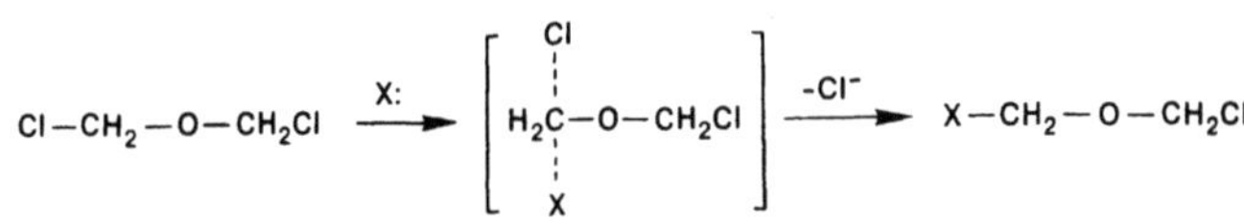

S_N2 : Bis(chloromethyl)ether : $T_{1/2}$ (pH 7, 0°) ≤ 2 min, X = H_2O

Fig. 1. Metabolism-independent carcinogens. Metabolism-independent carcinogens, such as N-nitrosoethylurea, spontaneously form highly reactive, electropositive intermediates that form covalent bonds with virtually any electron-rich molecules in the vicinity; the rate-determining step is generation of the reactive intermediates (*brackets*), and the mechanism of product formation is described as unimolecular nucleophilic substitution (S_N1). The rate-determining step in reactions of other metabolism-independent carcinogens, such as bis(chloromethyl)ether, involves molecular collision with a reactant to form an activated complex (*brackets*); such reactions are termed bimolecular nucleophilic substitution (S_N2).

The effects of chemical carcinogens, both direct acting and metabolism-dependent agents, typically display a high degree of selectivity for the tissues they affect, in some cases causing tumors of only a single cell type, or in only one organ. A variety of mechanisms account for these selective effects, including the kinetics of transport and delivery of the carcinogen to target tissue, metabolism of the carcinogen within target and nontarget tissues, and -- especially important but least understood -- intrinsic susceptibility factors characteristic of specific cell types and often unique to or at least highly characteristic of a given species. These mechanisms have been recently discussed in detail in the proceedings of a major symposium on the subject of organ specificity and interspecies differences in chemical carcinogenesis (45). It is commonly found that metabolism-dependent carcinogens or their metabolites form covalent bonds with DNA in the cells of tissues in which exposure to these agents gives rise to neoplasms, although there is no strict correlation demonstrable between extent of DNA binding in target tissues and relative susceptibility of one target cell over another, except in

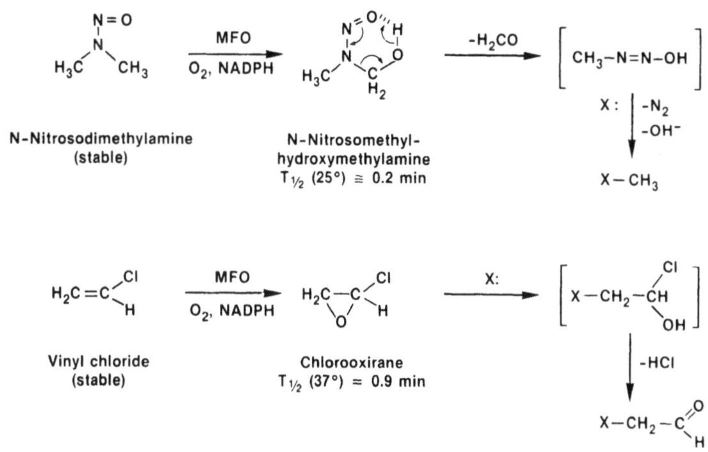

Fig. 2. Metabolism-dependent carcinogens. Metabolism-dependent carcinogens require enzyme-mediated catalysis, often by cytochrome-containing mixed-function oxidases (MFO), to generate reactive intermediates that may then react with tissue components (X) by either S_N1 (N-nitroso-dimethylamine) of S_N2 (vinyl chloride) mechanisms. The examples illustrated are both characterized by short-lived reactive intermediates ($T_{1/2}$<1 minute).

relatively restricted contexts. Metabolism-dependent agents are often, but not invariably, metabolized to reactive intermediates within the cells that are the precursors of neoplasms. Whether it is essential that metabolism occur in a target tissue is in part determined by the stability of the reactive metabolite. The carcinogenic effects of an agent are essentially restricted to the cells in which its metabolism occurs in cases where metabolites are very short-lived. It is extremely unlikely, due to their intrinsic chemical reactivity in aqueous medium, that such metabolites may diffuse outside the cell in which they are formed and be transported into a different, and perhaps remote, target cell. The short-chain N-nitrosodialkylamines (Fig. 2) are good examples of metabolism-dependent carcinogens with short-lived reactive metabolites (46). N-nitrosodiethylamine in rats, for example, is metabolized chiefly in the liver and is primarily carcinogenic for hepatocytes. This agent also induces tumors in the rat kidney or olfactory epithelium when given as a single large dose, under which conditions metabolism occurs primarily in extrahepatic tissues (47). In contrast, some agents are metabolized to reactive intermediates that are relatively more stable, with a chemical and biological half-life that is on the order of a minute or longer under *in vivo* conditions. These may diffuse outside the cells in which they are formed and efficiently induce neoplasms at distant sites. Vinyl chloride (Fig. 2), which is best known for its ability to produce tumors in vascular endothelium, especially in the liver, also in experimental animals is effective at inducing tumors in a wide variety of extrahepatic sites, presumably at least in part due to the stability and consequent mobility of the reactive intermediate, chlorooxirane (48, 49). Obviously, metabolic determinants of organ specificity for chemical carcinogens become increasingly complex when alternate pathways of metabolism are possible, and as conjugation reactions subsequent to oxidations become involved. This is the case with most carcinogens containing an aromatic ring.

There are cases in which the metabolism of chemical carcinogens, at least those possessing certain chemically distinct structures, can occur outside the tissues of the victim. This most commonly occurs as a result of metabolic activities of the microflora of the gut. A notable case is that of the natural product, cycasin, which is found in nature as a nontoxic glycoside of the toxic and carcinogenic hydrazine derivative, methylazoxymethanol (50). Cleavage of the β-glycosidic bond between the hydrazine and sugar moieties of this compound liberates the intrinsically reactive methylazoxymethanol, which is sufficiently stable to be absorbed through the lining of the gut and to be widely distributed in distant tissues, in which both toxic effects and carcinogenesis can occur.

The enzymes that are involved in metabolism of chemical carcinogens, notably the oxidative enzymes of the mixed-function oxidase or cytochrome category, can be induced in mammalian cells by exposure to both substrates and, in some cases, to other chemical agents. Induction of these enzymes, which increases metabolic capacity for certain chemicals including chemical carcinogens, is under genetic control and is not possible in all individuals (51). It is a peculiar fact that increased levels of the oxidase enzymes necessary for metabolic activation of chemical carcinogens as a result of such chemical induction generally reduces, rather than increases, the carcinogenic risk of subsequent exposure to one of the chemical carcinogens that is a substrate for the enzymes induced (52). The mechanisms of this effect are not well understood and are currently an object of research. An obvious mechanism in the case of carcinogens for which a variety of pathways of metabolism are possible is selective increase in detoxification pathways over activation pathways, as in the generation of noncarcinogenic phenols rather than the highly carcinogenic diol-epoxides in metabolism of polynuclear aromatic hydrocarbons, or of phenols in preference to hydroxylamine derivatives in the metabolism of carcinogenic aromatic amines. In other cases, as in the metabolism of simple agents like N-nitrosodimethylamine, for which such a variety of metabolic pathways does not exist, it is not clear how enhanced intracellular generation of the putative reactive metabolites required for the initiation of the carcinogenic process actually reduces the risk of carcinogenesis.

There is at least one category of chemical carcinogen in the general class of organic compounds of low molecular weight that appear to act by mechanisms completely distinct from those of the metabolism-dependent or direct acting genotoxic agents. These substances generally yield positive results in bioassays in animals for suspected carcinogenic activity, but as a group cannot be shown to have genotoxic activity, and are being increasingly referred to as acting through non-genetic, or epigenetic, mechanisms. A major subclass of this group comprise the agents known as promoters of carcinogenesis.

The essence of the phenomenon of promotion is that it is sequential. Typically, exposure to a promoter must, in order to be maximally effective, follow previous exposure to a genotoxic agent. It must be continuous over a period of time, and must occur at relatively frequent intervals during the period of sustained exposure. The biologically observable effect is a significant increase in the incidence of tumors that would be expected from exposure to the carcinogen alone. In its most extreme form, sequential initiation/promotion exposures may reveal the presence of latent, potentially neoplastic cells in tissues that, in the absence of exposure to a promoter, would not have been suspected of being affected by the initial exposure to a genotoxic agent. Mouse skin is the most extreme example of this phenomenon. A single exposure to a very low dose of a potent chemical carcinogen will not yield tumors on the skin of a mouse; very large numbers of squamous papillomas in each animal thus exposed may result from subsequent exposure to an appropriate promoting agent (53). Because promoting agents may also be inducers of the enzymes of carcinogen metabolism, simultaneous exposure to a carcinogen and a promoter may reduce, rather than increase, the risk of carcinogenesis to be expected from exposure to the carcinogen alone (54).

Promoting agents that have been identified to date include the small molecules phenobarbital, saccharin, a variety of chlorinated hydrocarbons, and certain esters of phorbol, a natural product of the Asian plant, *Croton tiglium*. These agents are weakly carcinogenic or noncarcinogenic when administered to experimental animals, are essentially without genotoxic effects in mammalian cells, and are very highly tissue specific in their promoting effects. Phenobarbital and the chlorinated hydrocarbons affect hepatocytes (55), saccharin is specific for the urinary bladder (56), and the phorbol esters are specific for squamous epithelium or for epithelium readily subject to squamous metaplasia (57). The mechanism by which these compounds exert their promoting effects is not understood. The promoting process has been divided experimentally into at least two stages, one of "conversion" of latent, potentially neoplastic cells to a state in which the second phase, "propagation", consisting essentially of response to a proliferative stimulus, can occur (58). Carcinogen-damaged cells undergoing promotion expand into a population of neoplastic precursor cells that may then, under favorable conditions, continue to proliferate autonomously to generate a tumor. While promotion phenomena have been well characterized in rodent systems, especially in rats and mice, and the process is anticipated to be of significance for humans, the phenomenon of tumor promotion has not been established unequivocally in humans or in nonhuman primate species. Preliminary experiments in nonhuman primates, however, suggest that at least some agents which are capable of tumor promotion in rodents will do so under comparable conditions in primate species, and presumably in human beings as well (59). A working hypothesis, currently under active investigation, is that the process of conversion involves a reduction in the efficiency of cell-cell communication, possibly between adjacent cells in an epithelium containing potentially neoplastic cells capable of promotion, or possibly between those cells and their adjacent mesenchymal stroma (60). Only epithelium has so far been shown clearly to be susceptible to tumor promotion, although tumor promoters can have profound metabolic effects in cells of nonepithelial origin. The relation of such a process of interference in cell-cell communication to tumor promotion, if in fact this is a correct interpretation of the phenomenon, at the present time lacks clear definition and remains tentative.

TRANSPLACENTAL CARCINOGENESIS

The effects of chemical carcinogens during pregnancy have been largely focused on the consequences for offspring, rather than for the mother. This is because of profound, quantitatively increased susceptibility of the fetus relative to that of the adult in certain tissues of experimental animals subjected to chemical carcinogens, especially those of the direct acting variety, during specific stages of prenatal development. In some tissues, such as the developing nervous system of the rat, the fetal/maternal risk ratio for chemical carcinogenesis may approach two decimal orders of magnitude.

The results of an experiment illustrating this effect are summarized in Table 4. When N-nitrosoethylurea (Fig. 1) is given as a single injection, or as multiple sequential exposures, to a gravid rat at any time during the second half of the period of gestation, if the dose is chosen so that the offspring survive they will be at increased risk for tumor development after birth. This risk first becomes apparent in the rat at approximately the twelfth day of gestation, and increases exponentially thereafter. Exposure prior to this time generally does not result in an increased risk of tumors in surviving offspring. High doses administered between the day of implantation (approximately day 6-7) and approximately day 10 may be severely teratogenic, resulting in a wide variety of skeletal, central nervous system, and visceral developmental anomalies. Exposure prior to implantation will either be without effect or

Table 4. Neurogenic Tumors in Rats after Exposure to a Total of 0.50 Millimole N-Nitrosoethylurea Per Kg Body Weight[a] at Different Stages of Development

Route and timing	Rats at risk	% With tumors	Tumors per rat
Transplacental, single dose, day 24	13	100	2.5
Transplacental, single dose, day 21	15	100	2.4
Transplacental, single dose, day 18	3	100	2.7
Transplacental, single dose, day 15	51	100	1.6
Transplacental, single dose, day 12	25	8	0.1
Transplacental, single dose, before day 12	66	0	0
Transplacental, 8 divided doses, days 16-23	13	92	2.5
Transplacental, 8 divided doses, days 8-16	22	91	1.7
Transplacental, 8 divided doses, days 1-8	10	0	0
Intravenous, adults, single dose	66	10	0.1

Data from ref. 7.
[a]Based on combined body weight of gravid female and conceptus for transplacental exposures.

embryocidal. Carcinogenic effects of this compound in the rat are, to a very large extent, limited to the central and peripheral nervous systems, and the neoplasms that develop evolve from glial elements of the central nervous system or from Schwann cells of the cranial and peripheral nerves. The latency for tumor development is inversely proportional to the magnitude of exposure, as is commonly seen in experiments in chemical carcinogenesis, and may vary from a few months to the natural life span of the animals (approximately 2½ years for rats). The tumors seen are generally not embryonal in nature. Rather, they evolve from differentiated structures and have the properties associated with differentiated

Schwann cells, oligodendrocytes or, less commonly, other glial or neuroepithelial cells. Tumors of largely the same kind may occur in the mothers, but in the case of the nervous system the adult females are at lower risk than their offspring. The mothers may, in addition, develop tumors of other tissues, including some such as the mammary gland that are relatively uncommon in the offspring. In the case of the rat, there are no distinctive neoplasms induced in the females that are characteristically associated with a state of pregnancy at the time of exposure to the chemical carcinogen, although an increased incidence of genital tract tumors has been observed (61).

When the same experiment is carried out at the same dosage level in different but closely related species, such as the mouse, hamster, or rabbit, quantitative points of similarity are immediately evident in comparison with results seen in rats. In mice, neoplasms are also inducible at comparable doses of N-nitrosoethylurea administered during comparable periods of gestation (11-13). Furthermore, as in rats, the fetus is quantitatively more susceptible than the adult, and neoplasms are seen in offspring exposed after approximately day 12 of gestation. However, there is a radical difference in the nature and location of tumors in these two species. While tumors are rare outside the nervous system in the rat, the nervous system is rarely the site of tumor development in the mouse. Mice, in response to single or multiple transplacental exposures to N-nitrosoethylurea, develop principally multiple tumors of the peripheral lung (derived from type II pneumocytes and Clara cells of the terminal bronchioles) and from hepatocytes. Neoplasms also occur in other tissues, but much more rarely. If the experiment is performed with rabbits, exposure late in gestation gives rise exclusively to tumors of the kidney, with characteristic nephroblastic morphology (14, 15). Exposure slightly earlier in gestation, but at a stage of development comparable to that of the earlier portions of the period of susceptibility in the rat or mouse, gives rise to tumors of the nervous system in offspring (16).

The same general pattern is seen with other kinds of direct acting alkylating agents (1-5, 8), although the most intensively studied to date is N-nitrosoethylurea (5-7, 9-16). From these studies it is evident that the nature of the neoplastic response is largely determined by the species subjected to a given agent. It is not an intrinsic property of the agent administered. In fact, the nervous system alone, of all the tissues of the body, appears uniformly, although highly variably, to be at greater risk for carcinogenesis by chemicals during prenatal development in all species. Furthermore, in experimental animals, at least those of the rodent and rabbit families, there is a definite tendency for transplacental exposure, even during periods where target tissues are in a highly undifferentiated state, to elicit development during subsequent postnatal life of kinds of tumors that develop characteristically from differentiated adult epithelium and other tissue elements, and are analogous to neoplasms characteristic of maturity or even of old age in man. Selective induction of embryonal tumors, which one might tend to expect as a consequence of prenatal exposure during periods of organogenesis, is in fact relatively uncommon. It is reasonable to predict *a priori* that the sustaining of a carcinogenic lesion by an undifferentiated cell might arrest the further differentiation of that cell. This does not seem to be the case for most tissues in most experimental species. Embryonal tumors are characteristically induced by direct acting agents only in certain tissues of certain species, most notably the nervous system and kidney of the opossum (62), which as a marsupial is used not in transplacental studies, but as an animal that can be directly manipulated outside the mother's body during stages of development comparable to those of intrauterine life in placental mammals, including man.

Many metabolism-dependent agents are also powerfully carcinogenic to rodents by transplacental exposure. Many enzymes on which the metabolism of such agents depends, including the mixed-function oxidases, are present at extremely low and, in some cases, undetectable levels in fetal rodent tissues during most of the period of intrauterine development (63). These tend to increase to detectable levels that are much lower than those found in comparable tissues of adults very late in gestation. Chiefly for this reason, carcinogens that act through short-lived reactive metabolites tend to be relatively weak transplacental carcinogens, although the same agents may be extremely potent for adults. An example of such an agent is N-nitrosodimethylamine (Fig. 2), which is a potent carcinogen for the kidney in the rat. When given to pregnant rats, however, it can be seen by inspection of the data in Table 5 that as a transplacental carcinogen, it has a detectable effect only when administered during the final week of gestation. Furthermore, the effects in offspring are proportionately much less than those in their mothers. A major contributor to this phenomenon, as well as to the relatively narrow organ specificity of this particular agent, is doubtless the dependence of N-nitrosodimethylamine (DMN) on metabolic transformation to a reactive intermediate (Fig. 2) whose chemical half-life is on the order of seconds (46). Such an agent cannot survive transport from metabolically competent maternal tissues in which it might be formed through the maternal bloodstream and across the placenta in quantities sufficient for significant effects in fetal target tissues. Rather, it must be formed within fetal target tissues, and as this process is exceedingly ineffective due to the low levels of enzymes present, its effects are minimal in the fetus. Even agents of this kind, however, may be comparably carcinogenic to selected tissues in both fetus and adult in some species, presumably because the low rate of generation of the reactive metabolite in fetal tissues is compensated by the intrinsically greater vulnerability to the carcinogen of rapidly proliferating fetal
Data from ref. 20.

Table 5. Renal Tumors in Rats after Exposure to a Total of 0.67 Millimole N-Nitrosodimethylamine Per Kg Body Weight at Different Stages of Development

Route and timing	Rats at risk	Rats with tumors	% With tumors
Transplacental, 7 divided doses, days 15-21	92	4	4
Transplacental, 7 divided doses, days 8-14	85	0	0
Transplacental, 7 divided doses, days 1-7	29	0	0
Oral, adults, 7 divided doses at 1-day intervals	38	30	79

target tissue. The next higher homologue of DMN, N-nitrosodiethylamine, is selectively carcinogenic for the upper respiratory tract in the adult Syrian hamster, and when given as single exposures to pregnant animals, is comparably effective both in mothers and in offspring exposed by the transplacental route during any of the last two to four days of pregnancy (23, 24). Metabolism-dependent agents that act through long-lived reactive metabolites may, however, be extremely effective transplacental carcinogens. An example is 7,12-dimethylbenz[*a*]anthracene (DMBA), which on transplacental administration to rats not only is exceedingly effective as an inducer of tumors of the central and peripheral nervous system, like N-nitrosoethylurea (ENU), but in addition is a potent carcinogen for the kidney and for the blood vascular system (30, 31). This metabolism-dependent agent is thus comparable in potency to some of the direct acting carcinogens, and actually has a broader spectrum of target tissues than the direct acting agents. Also, like the direct acting agents, DMBA is an effective teratogen, especially when given early in gestation. DMBA effectively destroys the small neurons of the internal granular layer of the developing cerebellum, resulting in a kuru-like syndrome in the offspring. As the chemical half-life for reactive intermediates increases, the probability increases that such agents can be metabolically activated not only in fetal tissues, but in placental and maternal tissues as well. Contributions of nonfetal metabolism to the transplacental carcinogenic effectiveness of agents such as DMBA are highly likely.

It is highly characteristic of certain tissues in the more commonly used experimental rodents that neoplasms do not develop in these tissues after exposure to relatively low levels of a chemical carcinogen *except* when, subsequent to exposure to the carcinogen, a second exposure to a non-genotoxic tumor promoter occurs. As a result of the sequential exposure to two different agents, neoplasms develop in such tissues that otherwise would not have appeared during the lifetime of the animal as a result of exposure to the carcinogen alone. Transplacental exposure to a variety of agents, followed by postnatal exposure to the tumor promoter, tetradecanoyl phorbol acetate (TPA), results in mice in the development of epidermoid papillomas and carcinomas of the skin (26, 28, 29), which otherwise would rarely or never be seen as a consequence solely of transplacental exposure to a carcinogen. Since transplacental exposures are likely to be of relatively low intensity, due not only to the low levels of fetal metabolism that are possible for many agents but also to the limiting effect of the relatively short duration of intrauterine life, the phenomenon of prenatal initiation followed by postnatal promotion may be more significant for humans than prenatal exposure to carcinogens alone. This area of research is expanding at the present time.

Extrapolation of transplacental carcinogenesis studies in rodents to prediction of human risks is difficult. Diethylstilbestrol (DES) remains the only chemical agent unequivocally demonstrated to be a transplacental carcinogen in humans (64). Despite intensive investigation, which has produced some evidence that a genotoxic intermediate may be formed enzymatically from DES and could be involved in carcinogenesis (65), the fact remains that DES is completely selective for the female reproductive tract in humans. The estrogenic activity of the agent is therefore probably at least a major contributor to the net carcinogenic effect of DES in humans. In this respect, the estrogen is significantly different from other transplacental carcinogens, and appears to have more in common with the nongenotoxic carcinogens, including tumor promotors, than with the genotoxic agents, both metabolism-dependent and metabolism-independent, described here.

With respect to the genotoxic agents well characterized in rodents, the relevant conclusions appear to be, first, that the fetus is often significantly more susceptible than the mother and, second, that susceptibility tends to increase dramatically toward the end of gestation. Simple extrapolation of these conclusions to man, without consideration for the importance of comparable stages of prenatal development, initially led to the assumption that for humans, accustomed to regarding the first trimester of pregnancy as the period of greatest risk for teratogenic damage, the third trimester might in contrast be predicted to be the period of greatest risk for transplacental carcinogenesis.

Table 6. Physical Characteristics and Reproductive Parameters of Patas and Rhesus Monkeys

Common name	Rhesus monkey	Patas monkey
Genus-species	*Macaca mulatta*	*Erythrocebus patas*
Adult weight		
Female	6 - 8 Kg	8 Kg
Male	12 - 15 Kg	14 Kg
Estrous cycle	28 Days	30 Days
Menses	Heavy	Slight
Pregnancy		
Detection by palpation	30 Days	30 Days
Placentation	Usually bidiscoidal	Usually bidiscoidal
Duration	160 ± 5 Days	167 ± 5 Days
Number offspring	1 (Twins rarely)	1 (Twins rarely)
Age (in captivity) at		
Weaning	6 Months	6 Months
Sexual maturiey		
Female	3 - 4 Years	3 Years
Male	4 - 5 Years	4 Years
Life span (captivity)	35 Years	>20 Years

In part to test the validity of these predictions in a nonhuman experimental system as comparable as possible to man, studies were initiated in two species of nonhuman primates with some of the same carcinogens studied in rodents. Similar studies were performed first in the patas monkey, *Erythrocebus patas*, an Old World species indigenous to sub-Saharan Africa, and later in the rhesus, *Macaca mulatta*, indigenous to the Indian subcontinent. Pertinent features of these species are summarized in Table 6. Preliminary results from studies that have been in progress at the National Cancer Institute since 1973 have now shown that only part of the extrapolated predictions are valid (17, 66, 67). In the patas monkey, fetal susceptibility, like that in rodents, does indeed appear to be significantly greater than maternal susceptibility to the effects of the direct acting transplacental carcinogen ENU, administered by protocols diagrammed in Fig. 3 and summarized in Table 7 (17, 66). The kinds of tumors induced have some similarities with those seen in rodents, in that tumors of the central nervous system and its meninges occur only in animals treated prenatally, and differ in

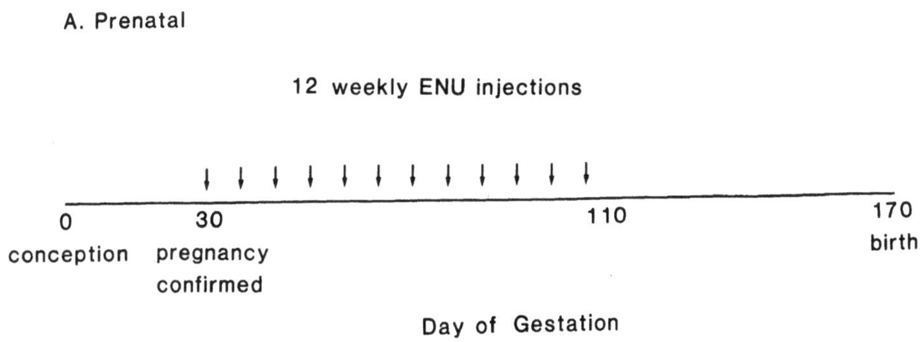

B. Postnatal

natural birth

infant nursed by mother

offspring and parent observed for carcinogenesis

surgical removal of tumors whenever possible

Fig. 3. Experimental protocol for administration of the direct acting transplacental carcinogen, N-nitrosoethylurea (ENU), to patas monkeys. Temporal relationships among timing of conception, palpable swelling of gravid uterus by which pregnancy is confirmed, intravenous injections of carcinogen (*arrows*), and parturition in investigations on the effects of ENU on patas monkeys during gestation are indicated. Multiple sequential injections were continued at one-week intervals until parturition in some studies.

Table 7. Protocols for and Preliminary Results of Administration of ENU to Patas Monkeys, Either by Direct Intravenous Injection (Juveniles) or Transplacentally by Intravenous Injection of the Gravid Female (Rice *et al.*, in Preparation)

Protocol	Monkeys with tumors	Monkeys at risk
Juveniles		
0.1 mMole/kg, 1x/2 weeks x 52	12	13[a]
0.1 mMole/kg, 1x/week x 18	0	6
Transplacental		
0.1 mMole/kg, 1x/2weeks, days 60-170	0	15[a]
0.1 mMole/kg, 1x/week, days 60-170	1	4
0.1 mMole/kg, 1x/week, day 30-170	9	16
0.05 mMole/kg, 1x/week, day 30-170	1	10
0.2 mMole/kg, 1x/week, day 30-110	3	10
0.1 mMole/kg, 1x/week, day 30-110	6	11

[a]Protocol terminated

that the patas monkey is most susceptible to induction by ENU of tumors of the blood vascular system, rather than the nervous system, in both fetus and adult (Table 8). The greatest and most significant difference between the patas monkey and rodent species is in the period of gestation when susceptibility appears greatest. In the monkey, in contrast to rat, mouse, and other experimental rodents, the period of maximum susceptibility is greatest in the first month of gestation, which in the patas has an average duration of 167 days. Fetal susceptibility consequently is greatest in the first trimester and is coincident roughly with the period of greatest teratogenic susceptibility. Exposure late in gestation to comparable doses of ENU elicits a very much lower incidence of neoplasia.

To confirm that these results in patas monkeys might be considered representative of primates in general, similar experiments were then performed in the unrelated rhesus monkey (67). Using the same experimental protocol, it has been found to date that exposures to

Table 8. Preliminary Survey[a] of Primary Neoplasms of Major Tissues and Organ Systems in Juvenile/Adult Patas Monkeys Given ENU by Repeated Intravenous Injection, and in the Offspring of Females Given Lower Total Dosages of the Same Agent During Gestation

	Number of tumors: local (disseminated)	
Location	13 Juveniles (52 x 0.1 mmole/kg)[b]	42 Transplacentals (10-20x0.1-0.2 mmole/kg)[b]
Blood vessels	7 (3)	9
Other connective tissues	3	3
Intestine	8 (4)	1
Lymphoreticular	2 (1)	1 (1)
Reproductive	3 (2)	--
Liver	--	2
Lung	--	5
Kidney	1	2 (1)
Central nervous system	--	4
Other	2 (1)	1
Total	26 (11)	27 (2)

[a]Experiments are still in progress.
[b]Number of injections x dosage per injection.

ENU which have failed to elecit tumors in gravid females have proved potently carcinogenic in the offspring, giving rise to neoplasms of lung, liver, and lymphoreticular system in a high proportion of rhesus infants during the first few years of postnatal life subsequent to intrauterine exposure to ENU. The high susceptibility early in gestation observed in patas monkeys is recapitulated in the rhesus, and in the rhesus, as in the patas and in rodents, susceptibility of the fetus is demonstrably much greater than that of the parent. Only in one respect is there a difference in transplacental carcinogenesis by ENU in these two primate species: a number of distinctive types of tumors are observed in the rhesus that have not occurred in the patas, and vice versa. These include embryonal tumors of the lung in rhesus, and tumors of the nervous system and its meninges, as well as nephroblastomas in the patas. This result is reminiscent of the difference between rats and mice in the nature and location of neoplasms transplacentally induced by ENU, and reinforces the generalization that the kinds of tumors that result from exposure to ENU or another carcinogen may be expected to be those characteristic of a given species, and therefore unpredictable by extrapolation in any species, including man, from results obtained in a second species, however closely related. It is significant that an earlier attempt to demonstrate transplacental carcinogenesis with ENU in rhesus monkeys failed (68), almost certainly because the carcinogen was only given toward the end of pregnancy.

CARCINOGENESIS IN GRAVID FEMALES: GESTATIONAL CHORIOCARCINOMA

In general, tumors observed in gravid female rodents given either direct acting or metabolism-dependent carcinogens have differed insignificantly in numbers, location, or kind from those in nonpregnant adults given the same agents. There have been reports of a higher incidence of neoplasms of the female reproductive system in rats exposed to chemical carcinogens during pregnancy, but none of these has been uniquely associated with exposure to a carcinogen during pregnancy (61).

A striking departure from this finding in rodent species was observed in experiments in which pregnant patas monkeys were given ENU. In the course of studies described above on transplacental carcinogenesis, a rapidly fatal neoplasm with biological and histological features of gestational choriocarcinoma was observed in 7 adult female patas monkeys given ENU intravenously during early pregnancy (69, 70). The histopathology of this neoplasm has been described, and is summarized here. This tumor has not been observed in males, in untreated control females, in nonpregnant females exposed to ENU or in exposed or control offspring of either sex.

Female patas were given ENU during pregnancy at doses ranging from 0.1 to 0.4 mmoles per kilogram body weight per injection, the injections given at weekly or fortnightly intervals and continued either throughout pregnancy (a maximum of 20 injections) or limited to a maximum of 12 weekly injections beginning at 30 days gestation (Fig. 3, Table 7). A total of more than 70 females have been used in these experiments, and seven cases of the same disease have been

Table 9. Preliminary Dose/Effect Relationships for Induction of Choriocarcinoma in Patas Monkeys Given ENU During Pregnancy and for Transplacental Induction of Nontrophoblastic Neoplasms in Their Offspring

ENU Dose	Pregnant females		Live offspring	
(mmole/kg/injection)	Treated	Choriocarcinoma	At birth	With tumor
0.4[a]	13	5	0	--
0.2[a]	15	1	10	3
0.1[b]	30	1	24	10
0.05[b]	15	0	10	0
Buffer	20	0	15	0

[a]Maximum of 12 injections
[a]Maximum of 18 injections

observed (Table 9). These seven animals died or were euthanized with a widely disseminated neoplasm within six months after receiving their last injection. Four of these were among 12 monkeys that had been subjected to the highest dosage, 0.4 mmoles per kilogram per injection for a total of 12 weekly injections, all of which had aborted their pregnancies. Of the other three, one had aborted, one had died of vaginal hemorrhage during delivery of a full term stillborn infant, and one had delivered a live full term infant that was normal at birth. The last died suddenly and quite unexpectedly of massive exsanguinating pulmonary hemorrhage approximately two months postpartum. At necropsy, multiple hemorrhagic nodules were observed in the lungs of all seven affected monkeys (Figs. 4 and 5). Random sections of grossly normal lung frequently contained microscopic emboli in veins (Fig. 4), which consisted chiefly of cytotrophoblast-like cells, some of them in mitosis. Grossly visible nodules 2 to 10 millimeters in diameter were fully established metastases, actively invading pulmonary parenchyma (Fig. 5). Metastases generally presented a pattern of sheets of extremely pleomorphic cells, divided into nests by connective tissue septa. Many of these pleomorphic cells contained glycogen, revealed by the PAS stain as multiple diastase-digestible, PAS-positive, intracytoplasmic granules. Similar metastases were less frequently observed in abdominal viscera, especially the spleen and kidneys. No exophytic tumor mass was ever seen within the uterus. Sections of that organ were grossly unremarkable except for the frequent presence of clotted blood within the cavity (Fig. 6). Microscopically, diffuse or well-demarcated foci of tumor tissue resembling that of the pulmonary metastases was frequently identified, characteristically infiltrating the endometrial stroma (Fig. 7) and

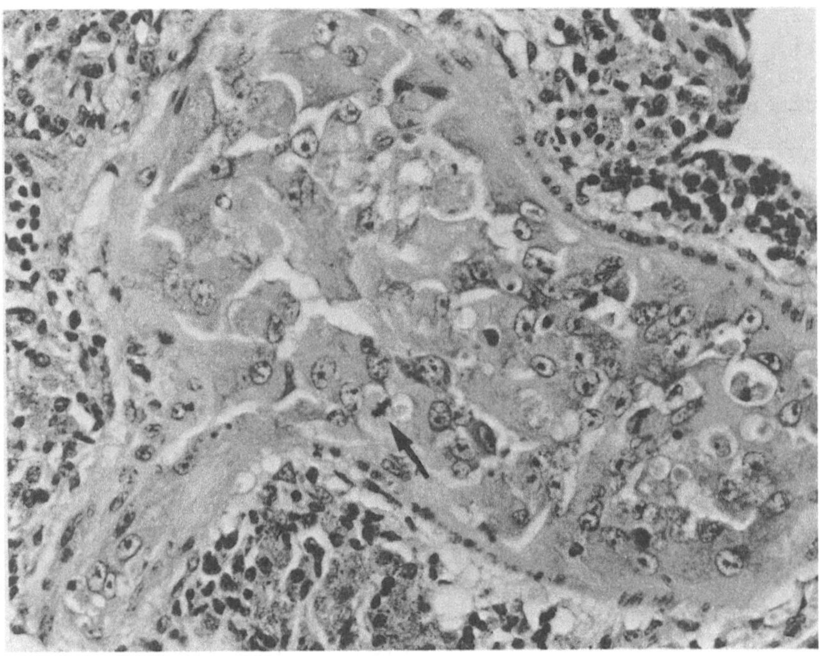

Fig. 4. Section of grossly normal lung of female patas monkey given N-nitrosoethylurea during pregnancy, showing an intravenous tumor embolus consisting of large, extremely pleomorphic cells, one of them in mitosis (*arrow*). A leukocytic infiltrate surrounds the tumor deposit. X 300. Reproduced from (70), by permission.

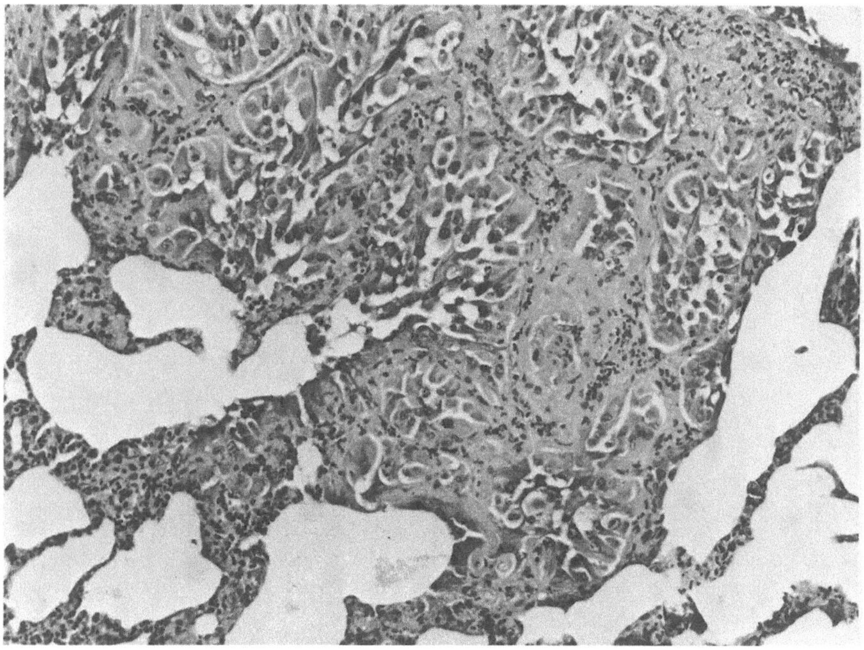

Fig. 5. Periphery of a grossly visible nodule from the same lung of Fig. 4, showing invasive features of metastatic tumor. X 130. Reproduced from (70), by permission.

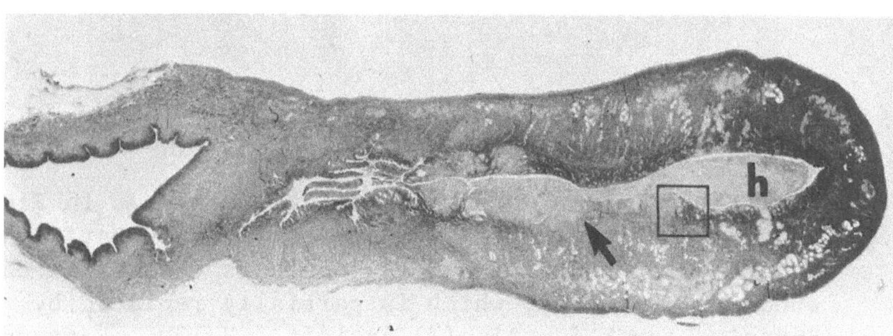

Fig. 6. Section of uterus, showing hemorrhagic deposit (*h*) within the cavity. The deposit is continuous with areas in which less basophilic tissue appears to replace the endometrial lining (*arrow, box*). X 2.5. Reproduced from (70), by permission.

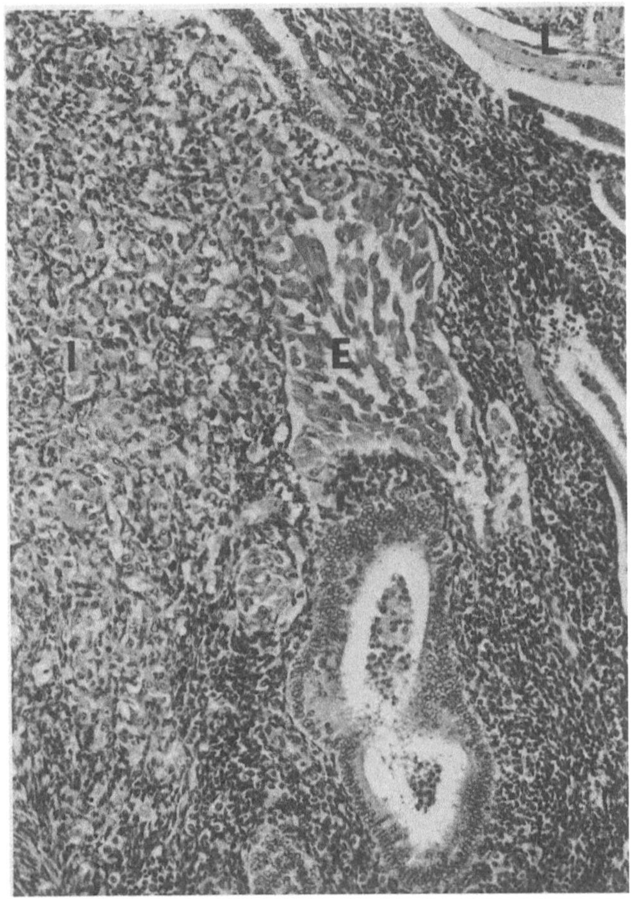

Fig. 7. Higher magnification of area delimited by *box* in Fig. 6. The lumen of the uterine cavity (*L*) is at upper right. Endovascular tumor tissue (*E*) occludes vessels in the endometrial stroma, which is partially replaced by invasive tumor deposit (*I*) at left. X 130. Reproduced from (70), by permission.

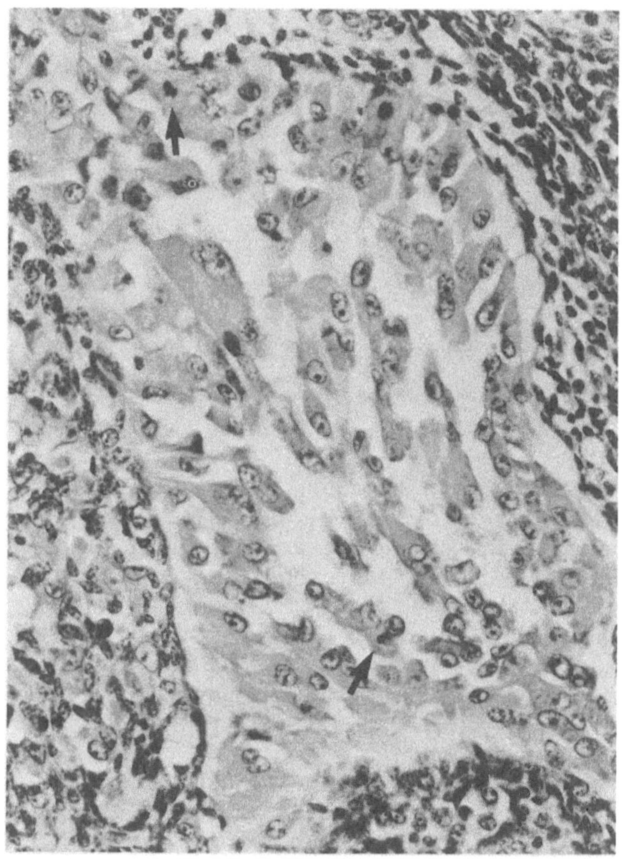

Fig. 8. Endovascular tumor deposit (*E* in Fig. 7) in the endometrium consisting of tissue like that in pulmonary emboli and metastases. Mitoses are readily found (*arrows*). X 330. Reproduced from (70), by permission.

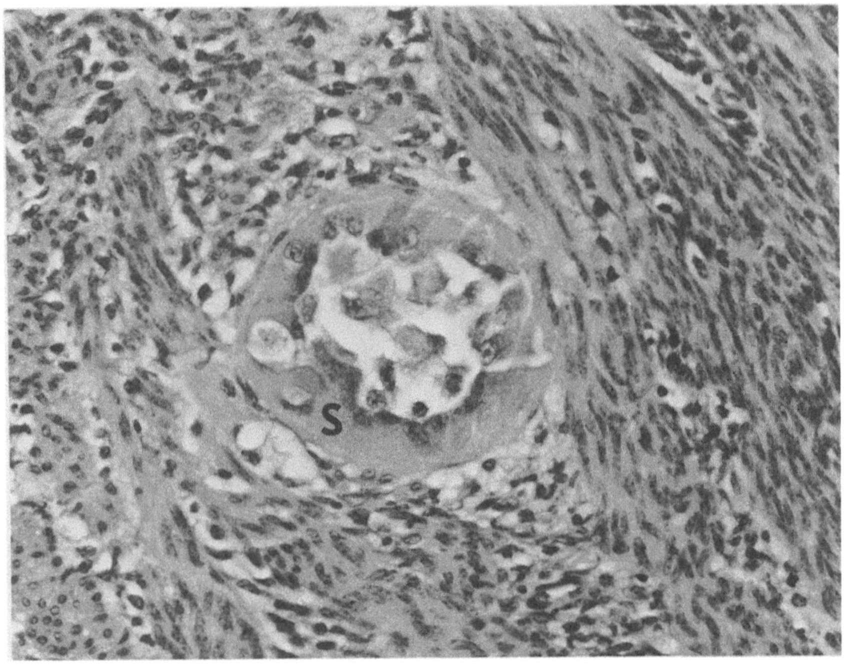

Fig. 9. Endovascular deposits deep in the myometrium. These deposits contain areas (*S*) where individual cells appear to have fused, generating multinucleated cell masses suggestive of syncytiotrophoblast. X 330. Reproduced from (70), by permission.

frequently forming endovascular tumor deposits in the uterine veins (Figs. 8 and 9).

In one case in which a pregnancy ended in abortion, both conceptus and placenta were recovered and subjected to necropsy. Tumor tissue identical to that in the uterine stroma and in pulmonary metastases was identified within the placenta. This observation, together with the morphology of the cells, the striking resemblance of the clinical features of the disease to human choriocarcinoma (including the absence of an exophytic tumor mass within the uterus and the tendency of the neoplasm to kill by hemorrhage, frequently from metastatic tumor deposits) have led us to the conclusion that this neoplasm constitutes gestational choriocarcinoma in the patas monkey. The histologic features of the tumor exclude a mesenchymal origin, and are consistent with choriocarcinoma in humans. The presence of intracytoplasmic glycogen within the tumor cells is a prominent histochemical feature of human choriocarcinomas (71), and is especially prominent in the patas neoplasms. Endovascular tumor tissue in our animals morphologically resembles normal endovascular trophoblast identified in the uterine spiral arteries of pregnant baboons, macaques, and patas monkeys and described by Panigel and his associates (72, 73).

Preliminary attempts to detect a chorionic gonadotropin in the urine or sera of either normally pregnant or tumor-bearing patas monkeys by immunoassays empirically developed for use with other primate species (74) have thus far been unsuccessful. Utilization of this parameter to confirm our histologic interpretations must possibly await development of an assay specific for the putative patas hormone. Chorionic gonadotropin is readily measured in other nonhuman primate species, such as the rhesus, but only during the first weeks of pregnancy, a pattern strikingly different from the persistence of this hormone throughout pregnancy in the great apes and in humans (75). It is possible that a similarly limited duration of chorionic gonadotropin production during early pregnancy will be found characteristic of the patas, perhaps to a more extreme degree. Tumors of trophoblastic origin in this species accordingly may not continue to produce chorionic gonadotropin and this characteristic feature of human choriocarcinoma may not be duplicated in the nonhuman primates, especially since the tumors tend to consist largely of cytotrophoblast-like tumor cells, with syncytium formation a relatively rare event.

With the exception of these recent findings in patas monkeys, gestational choriocarcinoma is almost uniquely a neoplastic disease of man. No reproducible animal model has been proposed, despite occasional identification of single cases in species such as the armadillo (76) and the rhesus monkey (77). Attempts to induce choriocarcinoma in the rat by direct implantation of carcinogenic hydrocarbons into placental sites within the gravid uterus (77, 78) are at best remotely related to the possible etiology of human disease, and moreover tend to yield a much higher incidence of neoplasms other than choriocarcinoma, especially sarcomas. Choriocarcinoma has not been seen, or at least not reported, in rodents given ENU or any other carcinogen during pregnancy in transplacental experiments. Very possibly the extremely short period between implantation and parturition in rodents does not afford adequate opportunity for potentially neoplastic trophoblastic elements to become established outside the placenta during normal pregnancy in these species. Trophoblast of patas monkeys appears highly susceptible to the carcinogenic effects of ENU and perhaps other carcinogens, and thus provides a useful animal model for gestational choriocarcinoma.

EXPERIMENTAL APPROACHES TO THE ETIOLOGY OF HUMAN GESTATIONAL CHORIOCARCINOMA

All animal models of human disease have limits to their

validity and invariably differ in some respects from the corresponding condition in humans. The patas monkey model differs most from human gestational choriocarcinoma in its apparent lack of immunochemically demonstrable chorionic gonadotropin, and to a lesser extent in some of its histologic and biologic features, such as the relative paucity of syncytiotrophoblast-like elements in tumor deposits and in its patterns of metastases, especially the apparent absence of dissemination to the brain. These aspects and others require additional study. It may be that a chorionic gonadotropin is secreted by these tumors and can be detected by biologic means, if not by currently available immunochemical reagents, and cytogenetic methods may be useful in confirming the apparent trophoblastic origin of the tumor cells. Both these approaches are currently being investigated. The major use of the inducible patas disease is as an etiologic rather than a pathophysiologic model, however, and if one is willing to accept the model even provisionally as truly a trophoblastic neoplasm, it presents major opportunities for investigating the premise that at least some human gestational choriocarcinoma is caused by exposure to genotoxic chemical carcinogens.

Another way in which the patas disease differs from that of man is the marked association of human gestational choriocarcinoma with molar pregnancies. We have never observed a hydatidiform mole in our monkeys, whether exposed to carcinogens or not, and have not found any reference to such an occurrence in the literature. As some chemical carcinogens, especially direct acting agents, are embryotoxic and teratogenic (42), one can envision a hypothetical mechanism for induction of hydatidiform mole by the toxic effect of a carcinogen on a normally pregnant female. Differential susceptibility to the toxic effects of the carcinogen might kill the fetus of the inner cell mass of a blastocyst, but leave damaged but viable extraembryonic trophoblast or placenta in a condition to generate a mole or a choriocarcinoma. However, cytogenetic studies have revealed the androgenetic origin of human complete moles (79-81), suggesting that attempts to prove the hypothetical mechanism outlined above would fail or, if successful, would be irrelevant to human disease. Further, cytogenetic studies on a limited number of human choriocarcinomas in women with a previous history of hydatidiform moles provided no evidence for a cellular lineage common to both complete moles and subsequent choriocarcinoma (82). The association between molar pregnancy and risk of choriocarcinoma may prove to be complex, and in any event cannot be studied with the patas model. All choriocarcinomas seen to date in patas monkeys have followed full term pregnancies (two) or abortions in which a dead fetus was recovered (five).

Our working hypothesis concerning the origin of patas gestational choriocarcinoma in females given carcinogen during early pregnancy and its relationship to transplacental carcinogenesis in their offspring is illustrated in Fig. 10. The mechanism requires direct action of a (presumably blood-borne) carcinogen on cells of the fetus for transplacental carcinogenesis, and on the trophoblast of the placenta for the induction of choriocarcinoma. Although to date we have seen choriocarcinoma only in gravid females given the direct acting carcinogen, ENU, there is every reason to expect that at least some metabolism-dependent agents could produce the same effect. Several categories of chemical carcinogen immediately suggest themselves as candidates for further study in patas monkeys and as possible causative agents of human gestational choriocarcinoma.

While many chemical carcinogens are substances created by man that do not occur in nature (1)(Table 1), nonetheless there are important classes of carcinogens that either form readily under naturally occurring conditions, or are natural products of higher plant or fungal origin. The N-nitroso compounds (47) readily occur during the cooking of food or in the gastric contents when inorganic nitrite and secondary, tertiary, or quaternary amines or amides are ingested together. In animal experiments, it is easy to demonstrate this endogenous synthesis of N-nitrosodialkylamines and N-nitrosoalkylureas in quantities sufficient for direct and for transplacental carcinogenesis (18, 19), and the nitroso compounds, of which ENU is representative, must be considered among the candidate agents. The carcinogenic natural products formed in higher plants occur in temperate, subtropical, and tropical areas of the world in plants that are or have been used for human and animal food. These include cycasin, from nuts of the cycad, consumed in the Pacific islands,

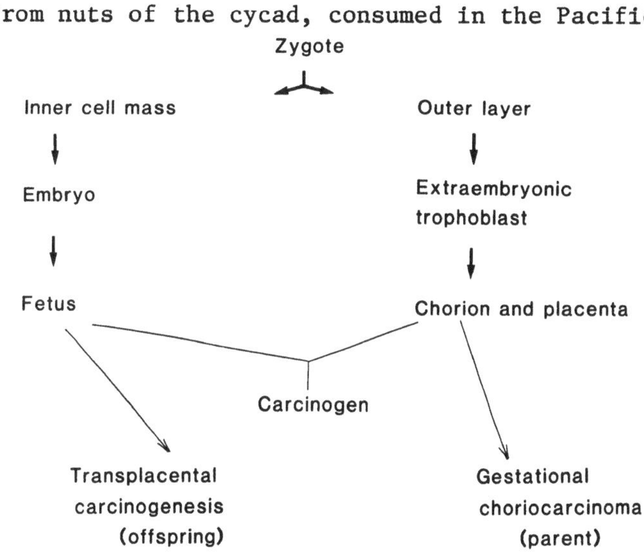

Fig. 10. Relation of choriocarcinoma induction to transplacental carcinogenesis. Presumptive origins of neoplastic disease originating from cells of the conceptus in patas monkeys given ENU during pregnancy and in their offspring.

especially Guam (47, 50); a potent carcinogen in croziers of the bracken fern, consumed by ruminants world-wide and eaten by humans in some areas, especially Japan (83); and substances in essential oils used as spices and flavorings (50). Some of these, especially the toxic principles in cycad nuts and bracken fern, have long been recognized as toxic by populations where these plants are eaten, and means of detoxifying the vegetables by soaking or by cooking are well known. It is nonetheless of some interest that these carcinogens occur in human foods in areas of the world, especially the Pacific basin, where gestational choriocarcinoma is said to be much more common than in Europe and North America.

Also especially prevalent in the same tropical and subtropical geographic regions are an entirely different category of carcinogenic toxic agents produced by fungi (50). Mycotoxins, produced by fungi that grow on human foods, include the aflatoxins, products of *Aspergillus flavus*, that are among the most potent chemical carcinogens known. Major epidemics of toxic hepatitis, the major effect of aflatoxicosis, are reported from time to time in human populations in Africa and Asia. The outbreaks in western India in 1974 (84) and in the Machakos district of Kenya, east of Nairobi, in 1981 (85) are representative. The principal agent most likely responsible for these epidemics is aflatoxin B_1, a genotoxic metabolism dependent carcinogen known to react with DNA *in vivo* (86)(Fig. 11). This agent strongly suggests itself as a candidate for study in the patas model system, and investigations of the capacity of aflatoxin B_1 to induce gestational choriocarcinoma in pregnant patas monkeys are in progress.

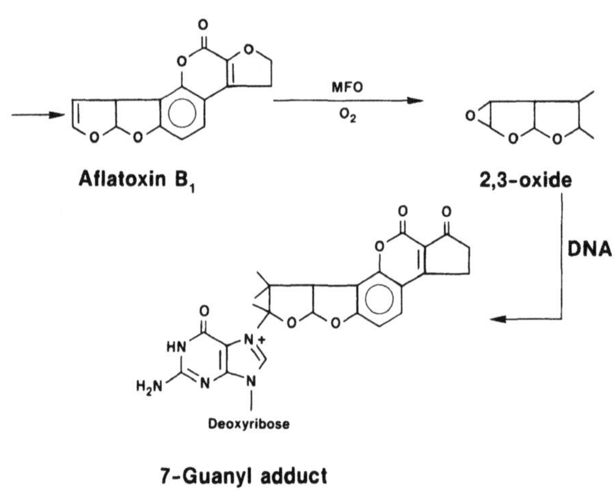

Fig. 11. Metabolism of aflatoxin B_1. Metabolism is oxidative and MFO-dependent, and generates a reactive 2,3-oxide intermediate that reacts with guanine residues in DNA to form a 7-guanyl adduct.

REFERENCES

1. International Agency for Research on Cancer, "IARC Monographs on the Evaluation of the Carcinogenic Risk of Chemicals to Humans," Supplement 4, IARC, Lyon, France (1982).
2. Druckrey, H., Kruse, H., Preussmann, R., Ivankovic, S., and Landschütz, C., Cancerogene alkylierende Substanzen. III. Alkyl-halogenide, -sulfate, -sulfonate, and ringspannte Heterocyclen, Z. Krebsforsch. 74:241 (1970).
3. Kleihues, P., Mende, C., and Reucher, W., Tumors of the peripheral and central nervous system induced in BD rats by prenatal application of methyl methane sulfonate, Eur. J. Cancer 8:641 (1972).
4. Druckrey, H., Kruse, H., Preussmann, R., Ivankovic, S., Landschütz, C., and Gimmy, J., Cancerogene alkylierende Substanzen. IV. 1,3-Propansulton and 1,4-Butansulton, Z. Krebsforsch. 75:69 (1970).
5. Jänisch, W., Schreiber, D., Warzok, R., and Schneider, J., Die transplacentare Induction von Geschwulsten des Nervensystems. Vergleichende Untersuchung der Wirksamheit von Methyl und Äthylnitrosoharnstoff, Arch. Geschwulstforsch. 39: 99 (1972).
6. Druckrey, H., Ivankovic, S., and Preussmann, R., Teratogenic and carcinogenic effects in the offspring after single injection of ethylnitrosourea to pregnant rats, Nature 210: 1378 (1966).
7. Ivankovic, S. and Druckrey, H., Transplacentare Erzeugung maligner Tumoren des Nervensystems. I. Äthylnitrosoharnstoff (ÄNH) an BD IX-Ratten, Z. Krebsforsch. 71:320 (1968).
8. Druckrey, H. and Landschütz, C., Transplacentare and neonatale Krebserzeugung durch Äthylnitrosobiuret (ÄNBU) an BD-IX Ratten, Z. Krebsforsch. 76:45 (1971).
9. Koestner, A., Swenberg, J. A., and Wechsler, W., Transplacental production with ethylnitrosourea of neoplasms of the nervous system in Sprague-Dawley rats, Amer. J. Pathol. 63:37 (1971).
10. Swenberg, J. A., Koestner, A., Wechsler, W., and Denlinger, R. H., Quantitative aspects of transplacental tumor induction with ethylnitrosourea in rats, Cancer Res. 32:2656 (1972).
11. Diwan, B. A. and Meier, H., Strain- and age-dependent transplacental carcinogenesis by 1-ethyl-1-nitrosourea in inbred strains of mice, Cancer Res. 34:764 (1974).
12. Rice, J. M., Transplacental carcinogenesis in mice by 1-ethyl-1-nitrosourea, Ann. New York Acad. Sci. 163:813 (1969).
13. Vesselinovitch, S. D., Koka, M., Rao, K. V. N., Mihailovich, N., and Rice, J. M., Prenatal carcinogenesis by ethylnitrosourea in mice, Cancer Res. 37:1822 (1977).
14. Fox, R. R., Diwan, B. A., and Meier, H., Transplacental induction of primary renal tumors in rabbits treated with 1-ethyl-1-nitrosourea, J. Natl. Cancer Inst. 54:1439 (1975).

15. Stavrou, D. and Hanichen, T., Oncogene Wirkung von Äthylnitrosoharnstoff beim Kaninchen während der pranatalen Periode, Z. Krebsforsch. 84:207 (1975).
16. Stavrou, D., Dahme, E., and Schroder, B., Transplacentare neuroonkogene Wirkung von Äthylnitrosoharnstoff beim Kaninchen während der fruhen Graviditätsphase, Z. Krebsforsch. 89:331 (1977).
17. Rice, J. M., Palmer, A. E., London, W. T., Sly, D. L., and Williams, G. M., Transplacental effects of ethylnitrosourea in the patas monkey, in: "Tumors of Early Life in Man and Animals," L. Severi, ed., Perugia Quadrennial International Conferences on Cancer, Perugia (1978), p. 893.
18. Osske, G., Warzok, R., and Schneider, J., Diaplazentare Tumorinduktion durch endogen gebildeten N-Äthyl-N-nitrosoharnstoff bei Ratten, Arch. Geschwulstforsch. 40:244 (1972).
19. Fox, R. R., Diwan, B. A., and Meier, H., Transplacental carcinogenic effects of combined treatment of ethylurea and sodium nitrite in rabbits, J. Natl. Cancer Inst. 59:427 (1977).
20. Alexandrov, B. A., Blastomogenic effect of dimethylnitrosamine on pregnant rats and their offspring, Nature 218:280 (1968).
21. Pielsticker, K., Wieser, O., Mohr, U., and Wrba, H., Diaplazentar induzierte Nierentumoren bei der Ratte, Z. Krebsforsch. 69:345 (1969).
22. Diwan, B. A. and Meier, H., Transplacental carcinogenic effects of diethylnitrosamine in mice, Naturwissenschaften 63:487 (1976).
23. Mohr, U., Althoff, J., and Authaler, A., Diaplacental effect of the carcinogen diethylnitrosamine in the golden hamster, Cancer Res. 26:2349 (1966).
24. Mohr, U., Reznik-Schuller, H., Reznik, G., and Hilfrich, J., Transplacental effects of diethylnitrosamine in Syrian hamsters as related to different days of administration during pregnancy, J. Natl. Cancer Inst. 55:681 (1975).
25. Bulay, O. M. and Wattenberg, L. W., Carcinogenic effects of subcutaneous administration of benzo[*a*]pyrene during pregnancy on the progeny, Proc. Soc. Exptl. Biol. Med. 135:84 (1970).
26. Bulay, O. M. and Wattenberg, L. W., Carcinogenic effects of polycyclic hydrocarbon carcinogen administration to mice during pregnancy on the progeny, J. Natl. Cancer Inst. 46:397 (1971).
27. Tomatis, L., Turusov, V., Guibbert, D., Duperray, B., Malaveille, C., and Pacheco, H., Transplacental carcinogenic effect of 3-methylcholanthrene in mice and its quantitation in fetal tissues, J. Natl. Cancer Inst. 47:645 (1971).
28. Goerttler, K. and Lohrke, H., Diaplacental carcinogenesis: initiation with the carcinogens dimethylbenzanthracene (DMBA) and urethane during fetal life and postnatal promotion with the phorbol ester TPA in a modified 2-stage Berenblum/Mottram experiment, Virch. Arch. [Path. Anat.] 372:29 (1976).

29. Goerttler, K. and Lohrke, H., Diaplacental carcinogenesis: tumor localization and tumor incidence in NMRI mice after diaplacental initiation with DMBA and urethane and postnatal promotion with the phorbol ester TPA in a modified 2-stage Berenblum/Mottram experiment, Virch. Arch. [Pathol. Anat.] 376:117 (1977).
30. Napalkov, N. P. and Alexandrov, V. A., Neurotropic effects of 7,12-dimethylbenz[*a*]anthracene in transplacental carcinogenesis, J. Natl. Cancer Inst. 52:1365 (1974).
31. Rice, J. M., Joshi, S. R., Shenefelt, R. E., and Wenk, M., Transplacental carcinogenic activity of 7,12-dimethylbenz[*a*]-anthracene, in: "Carcinogenesis, Vol. 3, Polynuclear Aromatic Hydrocarbons," P. W. Jones and R. I. Freudenthal, eds., Raven Press, New York (1978), p. 413.
32. Grice, H. C., Moodie, C. A., and Smith C. D., The carcinogenic potential of aflatoxin or its metabolites in rats from dams fed aflatoxin pre- and postpartum, Cancer Res. 33:262 (1973).
33. Spatz, M. and Laqueur, G. L., Transplacental induction of tumors in Sprague-Dawley rats with crude cycad material, J. Natl. Cancer Inst. 38:233 (1967).
34. Vesselinovitch, S. D., Rao, K. V. N., and Mihailovich, N., Transplacental and lactational carcinogenesis by safrole, Cancer Res. 39:4378 (1979).
35. Larsen, C. D., Pulmonary tumor induction by transplacental exposure to urethane, J. Natl. Cancer Inst. 8:63 (1947).
36. Ivankovic, S., Erzeugung von Malignomen bei Ratten nach transplacentarer Einwirkung von N-Isopropyl-α-2(methylhydrazino)-*p*-toluamid HCl, Arzneim. Forsch. 22:905 (1972).
37. Maltoni, C., Predictive value of carcinogenesis bioassays, Ann. New York Acad. Sci. 271:431 (1976).
38. Kleihues, P., Developmental carcinogenicity, in: "Developmental Toxicology," K. Snell, ed., Praeger, New York (1981), p. 211.
39. Rice, J. M., Effects of prenatal exposure to chemical carcinogens and methods for their detection, in: "Developmental Toxicology," C. A. Kimmel and J. Buelke-Sam, eds., Raven Press, New York (1981), p. 191.
40. Rice, J. M., ed., "Perinatal Carcinogenesis," NCI Monograph 51, United States Government Printing Office, Washington, D.C. (1979).
41. Severi, L., ed., "Tumors of Early Life in Man and Animals," Perugia Quadrennial International Conferences on Cancer, Perugia, Italy (1978).
42. Tomatis, L. and Mohr, U., eds., "Transplacental Carcinogenesis," International Agency for Research on Cancer, Lyon, France (1973).
43. Miller, E. C. and Miller, J. A., The metabolism of chemical carcinogens to reactive electrophiles and their possible mechanisms of action in carcinogenesis, in: "Chemical Carcinogens, ACS Monograph 173," C. E. Searle, ed., American Chemical Society, Washington, D. C. (1976), p. 737.

44. Sims, P., Grover, P. L., Swaisland, A., Pal, K., and Hewer, A., Metabolic activation of benzo[*a*]pyrene proceeds by a diol-epoxide, Nature 252:326 (1974).
45. Langenbach, R., Newnow, S., and Rice, J. M., eds., "Organ and Species Specificity in Chemical Carcinogenesis," Plenum Press, New York (1983).
46. Mochizuki, M., Anjo, T., Takeda, K., Suzuki, E., Sekiguchi, N., Huang, G. F., and Okada, M., Chemistry and mutagenicity of α-hydroxy nitrosamines, in: "N-Nitroso Compounds: Occurrence and Biological Effects," H. Bartsch, M. Castegnaro, J. K. Oneill, and M. Okada, eds., IARC Scientific Publications No. 41, International Agency for Research on Cancer, Lyon, France (1982), p. 553..
47. Magee, P. N., Montesano, R., and Preussmann, R., N-Nitroso compounds and related carcinogens, in: "Chemical Carcinogens, ACS Monograph 173," C. E. Searle, ed., American Chemical Society, Washington, D. C. (1976), p. 737.
48. Salmon, A. G., Cytochrome P-450 and the metabolism of vinyl chloride, Cancer Lett. 2:109 (1976).
49. Zajdela, F., Croisy, A., Barbin, A., Malaveille, C., Tomatis, L., and Bartsch, H., Carcinogenicity of chloroethylene oxide, an ultimate reactive metabolite of vinyl chloride, and bis (chloromethyl)ether after subcutaneous administration and in initiation-promotion experiments in mice, Cancer Res. 40: 352 (1980).
50. Schoental, R., Carcinogens in plants and microorganisms, in: "Chemical Carcinogens, ACS Monograph 173," C. E. Searle, ed., American Chemical Society, Washington, D. C. (1976), p. 626.
51. Levitt, R. C., Pelkonen, O., Okey, A. B., and Nebert, D. W., Genetic differences in metabolism of polycyclic aromatic carcinogens and aromatic amines by mouse liver microsomes. Detection by DNA binding of metabolites and by mutagenicity in histidine-dependent *Salmonella typhimurium in vitro*, J. Natl. Cancer Inst. 62:947 (1979).
52. Wattenberg, L. W. and Leong, J. L., Inhibition of the carcinogenic action of benzo[*a*]pyrene by flavones, Cancer Res. 30:1922 (1970).
53. Yuspa, S. H., Hennings, H., Lichti, U., and Kulesz-Martin, M., Organ specificity and tumor promotion, in: "Organ and Species Specificity in Chemical Carcinogenesis," R. Langenbach, S. Nesnow, and J. M. Rice, eds., Plenum Press, New York (1983), p. 157.
54. Peraino, C., Fry, R. J. M., and Staffeldt, E., Reduction and enhancement by phenobarbital of hepatocarcinogenesis induced in the rat by 2-acetylaminofluorene, Cancer Res. 31:1506(1971).
55. Stevens, F. J. and Peraino, C., Liver as a model system for analyzing mechanisms of tumor initiation and promotion, in: "Organ and Species Specificity in Chemical Carcinogenesis," R. Langenbach, S. Nesnow, and J. M. Rice, eds., Plenum Press, New York (1983), p. 231.

56. Cohen, S. M., Promotion of urinary bladder carcinogenesis, in: "Organ and Species Specificity in Chemical Carcinogenesis," R. Langenbach, S. Nesnow, and J. M. Rice, eds., Plenum Press, New York (1983), p. 253.
57. Reiners, J., Jr., Davidson, K., Nelson, K., Mamrack, M., and Slaga, T., Skin tumor promotion: a comparative study of several stocks and strains of mice, in: "Organ and Species Specificity in Chemical Carcinogenesis," R. Langenbach, S. Nesnow, and J. M. Rice, eds., Plenum Press, New York (1983), p. 173.
58. Boutwell, R. K., Some biological aspects of skin carcinogenesis, Progr. Exptl. Tumor Res. 4:207 (1964).
59. Rice, J. M., Palmer, A. E., Ward, J. M., and Cicmanec, J. L., Hepatocellular neoplasia in nonhuman primates after transplacental diethylnitrosamine and postnatal phenobarbital, Fed. Proc. 42:1022 (1983).
60. Williams, G. M., Epigenetic effects of liver tumor promoters and implications for health effects, Environmental Health Persp. 50:177 (1983).
61. Ivankovic, S., Erzeugung von Genitalkrebs bei trächtigen Ratten, Arzneimitted Forsch. 19:1040 (1969).
62. Jurgelski, W., Jr., Hudson, P., and Falk, H. L., Tissue differentiation and susceptibility to embryonal tumor induction by ethylnitrosourea in the opossum, Natl. Cancer Inst. Monogr. 51:123 (1979).
63. Klinger, W., Muller, D., Kleeberg, U., and Barth, A., Peri- and postnatal development of phase I reactions, in: "Developmental Pharmacology," C. A. Kimmel and J. Buelke-Sam, eds, Raven Press, New York (1981), p. 83.
64. Herbst, A. L., Scully, R. E., and Robboy, S. J., Prenatal diethylstilbestrol exposure and human genital tract abnormalities, Natl. Cancer Inst. Monogr. 51:25 (1979).
65. Metzler, M. and McLachlan, J. H., Peroxidase-mediated oxidation, a possible pathway for metabolic activation of diethylstilbestrol, Biochem. Biophys. Res. Commun. 85:874 (1978).
66. Rice, J. M., London, W. T., Palmer, A. E., Sly, D. L., and Williams, G. M., Direct and transplacental carcinogenesis by ethylnitrosourea in the patas monkey (*Erythrocebus patas*), Proc. Amer. Assoc. Cancer Res. 18:53 (1977).
67. Rice, J. M., London, W. T., and Sly, D. L., Transplacental carcinogenesis by ethylnitrosourea in the rhesus monkey (*Macaca mulatta*), Proc. Amer. Assoc. Cancer Res. 22:74 (1981).
68. Jänisch, W., Schreiber, D., Warzok, R., and Scholtze, P., Versuche mit den Kanzerogenen Methyl- und Äthylnitrosoharnstoff bei Macaca mulatta, Arch. Geschwulstforsch. 47:123 (1979).
69. Rice, J. M., Palmer, A. E., London, W. T., Sly, D. L., and Williams, G. M., Induction of gestational choriocarcinoma in patas monkeys by ethylnitrosourea given during pregnancy, Proc. Amer. Assoc. Cancer Res. 21:84 (1980).

70. Rice, J. M., Williams, G. M., Palmer, A. E., London, W. T., and Sly, D. L., Pathology of gestational choriocarcinoma induced in patas monkeys by ethylnitrosourea given during pregnancy, Placenta (Suppl. 3):223 (1981).
71. Bur, G. I., Hertig, A. T., McKay, D. C., and Adams, E. C., Histochemical aspects of hydatidiform mole and choriocarcinoma, Obstet. Gynecol. 19:156 (1962).
72. Panigel, M., Structure et ultrastructure comparées de la membrane placentaire chez certains primates non humains, Bulletin de l'Association des Anatomistes 145:319 (1969).
73. Legrand, C. and Panigel, M., L'ultrastructure des cellules intravasculaires dan les artères spiralées utéroplacentaires au debut de la gestation chez le Babouin, *Papio cynocephalus*, Comptes Rendus de l'Academie des Sciences de Paris, Série D 272:429 (1971).
74. Hodgen, G. D., Tullner, W. W., Vaitukaitis, J. L., Ward, D. N., and Ross, G. T., Specific radioimmunoassay of chorionic gonadotropin during implantation in rhesus monkeys, J. Clin. Endocrinol. Metab. 39:457 (1974).
75. Hodgen, G. D., Niemann, W. H., and Tullner, W. W., Duration of chorionic gonadotropin production by the placenta of the rhesus monkey, Endocrinology 96:789 (1975).
76. Marin-Padilla, M. and Benirschke, K., Thalidomide-induced alterations in the blastocyst and placenta of the armadillo, *Dasypus novemcinctus mexicanus*, including a choriocarcinoma, Amer. J. Pathol. 43:999 (1963).
77. Stein-Werblowsky, R., Induction of chorionepitheliomatous tumors in the rat, Nature 186:980 (1960).
78. Shintani, S., Glass, L. E., and Page, E. W., Studies of induced malignant tumours of placental and uterine origin in the rat. II. Induced tumors and their pathogenesis with special references to choriocarcinoma, Amer. J. Obstet. Gynecol. 95: 550 (1966).
79. Kajii, T., and Ohama, K., Androgenetic origin of hydatidiform mole, Nature 268:633 (1977).
80. Wake, N., Takagi, N., and Sasaki, M., Androgenesis as a cause of hydatidiform mole, J. Natl. Cancer Inst. 60:51 (1978).
81. Lawler, S. D., Genetic studies on hydatidiform moles, in: R. A. Pattillo and R. O. Hussa, eds., "Human Trophoblast Neoplasms," Plenum Press, New York (1984), p. 147.
82. Wake, N., Tanaka, K., Chapman, V., Matsui, S., and Sandberg, A. A., Chromosomes and cellular origin of choriocarcinoma, Cancer Res. 41:3137 (1981).
83. Evans, I. A., The bracken carcinogen, in: "Chemical Carcinogens, ACS Monograph 173," C. E. Searle, ed., American Chemical Society, Washington, D. C. (1976), p. 690.
84. Krishnamachari, K. A. V. R., Bhat, R. V., Nagarajan, V., and Tilak, T. B. G., Hepatitis due to aflatoxicosis. An outbreak in western India, Lancet i:1061 (1975).

85. Ngindu, A., Kenya, P. R., Ocheng, D. M., Omondi, T. N., Ngare, W., Gatei, D., Johnson, B. K., Ngira, J. A., Nandwa, H., Jansen, A. J., Kaviti, J. N., and arap Siongok, T., Outbreak of acute hepatitis caused by aflatoxin poisoning in Kenya, Lancet i:1346 (1982).
86. Croy, R. G., Essigmann, J. M., and Wogan, G. N., Aflatoxin B_1: correlations of patterns of metabolism and DNA modification with biological effects, in: "Organ and Species Specificity in Chemical Carcinogenesis," R. Langenbach, S. Nesnow, and J. M. Rice, eds., Plenum Press, New York (1983), p. 49.

IMMUNOLOGY, GESTATION, AND NEOPLASIA

It has been demonstrated that malignant cells from murine trophoblastic cells and malignant cells from teratocarcinomas produce a compound of low molecular weight that inhibits macrophage migration and prevents the inflammatory response normally associated with invasion by this tumor. In this regard, the relationship between the properties of the malignant cells and the physiologic function of trophoblast cells follow parallel patterns. These results indicate that malignant cells from teratocarcinoma and trophoblastic cells, as well as other tumors, bypass the host immunologic surveillance system and thus avoid immunologic rejection. Since malignancy and pregnancy both represent tolerance of foreign tissue by the host immune system, this parallel is not unexpected. A large body of evidence suggests that blocking factors are present in normal pregnancy and in tumors. In tumor immunology there is a paradox, however, in that there appears to be a discordance between humoral and cell-mediated immune responses. A considerable amount of information demonstrates that antibodies may protect tumors against otherwise effectively sensitized lymphocytes. The presence of such blocking or enhancing antibodies may result from the early development of humoral immunity preceding the appearance of cellular immunity, with the resulting occurrence of noncytotoxic antibodies. Such blocking factors may be antibody, antigen, or antigen-antibody complex. The following chapters will present information bearing upon immunology of gestation and neoplasia, with particular consideration given to blocking factors.

It has been demonstrated that two prominent curves of biological interest intersect at a point where decreasing immunological competence associated with advancing age criss-crosses a curve of increasing incidence of neoplasia in the same aging population. These observations suggest that diminished host resistance permits the unregulated growth of neoplastic cells incapable of being destroyed and eliminated by the host. The chapter by Parmley describes a possible placental "aging pigment", lipofuchsin, consisting of a chemically heterogeneous group of compounds that accumulate in all fixed post-mitotic cells in proportion to the chronologic age of the placenta. Since these pigments are believed to result from the peroxidation of intracellular lipids by oxygen free radicals, a by-product of cellular respiration, it is noted to be of interest that one of the theories of neoplasia induction is the presence of increased free radical formation.

Choriocarcinoma following a full-term gestation does not permit chronologic placental study, since the diagnosis is not made until the placenta is discharged. It is, nonetheless, of interest to explore whether the hormonal profiles associated with aging events predispose to free radical formation, increased lipofuchsin pigment deposition, and a greater susceptibility to neoplastic transformation. At the other end of the spectrum, *i.e.*, gestational trophoblastic neoplasm of the hydatidiform mole category, which occurs at the inception of trophoblast or placental proliferation, it would be of equal interest to determine if lipofuchsin pigment were likewise found in increased quantities even without a prolonged period of time for the "aging" process. Such a hormonal abnormality as increased production of melanocyte-stimulating hormone could conceivably accompany the neoplastic transformation early or as a characteristic of hydatidiform mole formation as well as post full-term gestational choriocarcinoma. These events would be internal to trophoblast function and the host immune response mechanisms might be obtunded for maternal recognition and immunobiological response.

At this time, a very preliminary impression of host immune responses and possible hormonal changes, such as melanocyte-stimulating hormone activity and gonadotropin activity, are possible factors in generation of trophoblast neoplasms. The role of hCG in host immune response has been extensively studied, and although a role for circulating hCG on suppression of immune competence has not been proven definitively, it has been suggested that this hormone may act at the cellular level by decreasing the capacity of the host for cytotoxic expression. It remains for further investigation to uncover any significant link between placental aging, lipofuchsin pigment, melanocyte-stimulating hormone, hCG, and neoplasia generation, and it can only be said at this point that such investigation may open some new insights into the field of gestational trophoblastic neoplasms.

GENETIC ORIGIN, IMMUNOBIOLOGY, AND GONADOTROPIN EXPRESSION IN TROPHOBLAST AND NONTROPHOBLAST NEOPLASMS

Roland A. Pattillo

Department of Gynecology and Obstetrics
Medical College of Wisconsin
8700 W. Wisconsin Avenue
Milwaukee, WI 53226, USA

ETIOLOGY OF A HUMAN TROPHOBLAST NEOPLASM

Development from an External Gene Donor, the Spermatozoa

A sequence of chronologic steps leading to the identification of exclusively paternal chromosomes in most hydatidiform moles has been developed. It had long been recognized that most moles were chromatin-positive at the nuclear margin. This was confusing, however, since one would ordinarily expect a 50:50 ratio of chromatin-positive to chromatin-negative moles. The initial large study by Baggish and Woodruff (1) on moles treated in Singapore revealed that all 90 moles studied showed well-defined heterochromatin bodies.

A small portion of moles, however (< 13%)(83) are not XX, but rather XY. These cannot arise by reduplication of a single paternal haploid set. A single case of a complete mole with a 46, XY karyotype has been reported by Surti and associates (2). However, in that study it could not be determined whether two separate sperm, one bearing an X and one bearing a Y chromosome, were involved. The polymorphic chromosomal and enzyme markers of the paternal and molar chromosomes derived from both paternal haploid sets totally, without a maternal contribution. The study was carried out on a hydatidiform mole which progressed to metastatic trophoblastic disease with pulmonary metastasis. The molar tissue was cultured and quinacrine dihydrochloride markers for the polymorphic fluorescent patterns were studied. In addition, polymorphic enzyme systems were done using standard electrophoretic technique. Studies of the unique marker chromosome bonds demonstrated that those patterns in the mole were referable solely to those present in the father's karyotype.

Both sets of molar chromosomes derived from the father, or none of the patterns of maternal homologues could be identified. Enzyme analysis likewise confirmed the paternal origin of the chromosomes wherein the mother was shown to be glucose-6-phosphate dehydrogenase type B, whereas the mole and the father's were type A. Esterase in the mother was B, type I, while the mole and the father were type 2. This mole is the only literature report derived from the total paternal genome instead of representing a reduplicated haploid X carrying set. By contrast, partial or incomplete moles have been shown to be associated with an ascertainable fetus and a triploid karyotype. Many of the villi of this placenta are not hydropic, and many functioning vascular villi are present. Diploidy, trisomies, double trisomies and tetraploidy, along with multiple congenital anomalies in the fetus have also been found in other incomplete or partial moles.

It is conceivable that the previously mentioned finding of an increased number of translocation carrier women in the molar patients interferes with female meiosis and results in non-development of the female pronucleus while the 23,X male pronucleus duplicates, forming the molar tumor. The analogous situation in the ovary may result in duplication of the 23,X ovum with production of the commonly observed dermoid cyst of the ovary. Duplication of the 23,XY pronucleus is not viable and has not been reported.

Choriocarcinoma of Gestational Origin

Choriocarcinoma of gestational origin is a neoplasm of the placental trophoblast. In order to determine the chromosomal origin of choriocarcinoma following a molar versus normal conceptus, polymorphic chromosomal and enzyme markers were analyzed in the choriocarcinoma patients, together with those of the respective patient and her husband. When the choriocarcinoma was preceded by an antecedent mole, the Y chromosome was absent and the markers were homozygous at all loci. When the choriocarcinoma followed a full-term delivery of a male child, the tumor showed a Y chromosome and was heterozygous at some of the observed loci. This indicated that the choriocarcinoma following a full-term gestation had both maternal and paternal chromosomes, suggesting inability to effect a complete immune response. In contrast, the choriocarcinoma following a complete mole was found to have only paternal chromosomes, comprising a complete allograft. This choriocarcinoma portended a good prognosis, the patients now being complete cures up to five years in follow-up. In future investigation, the results of chromosomal constitution and HL-A studies may have important predictive ability with regard to the patient's host resistance mechanisms as well as chemotherapy response. Since gestational trophoblastic tumors of the complete molar type may be complete allografts, and therefore antigenically foreign, the overall good prognosis of benign and malignant moles with appropriate treatment seems to reflect a favorable scene for development of strong host immunological rejection mechanisms. Lawler (3) and Shaw (4) have shown that pregnancy with a hydatidiform mole is more immunogenic to HLA stimuli than in normal pregnancy. While choriocarcinoma can occur following birth of an HLA-incompatible infant, patients with choriocarcinoma as a group have more compatible offspring, and high-risk patients are more compatible with their husbands (5). This suggests that lesser antigenic stimuli are operative in high-risk choriocarcinoma patients than in the complete allograft associated with complete moles. It is conceivable that mechanisms, such as enhancement, possibly operating in normal pregnancy to prevent the maternal host from rejecting her fetus, may also be operative in trophoblastic tumors. Tolerance of patients with choriocarcinoma to skin grafts from their husbands has previously been demonstrated by Robinson (6) and by Bagshawe (7).

Mogensen and Kissmeyer-Nielsen (8) proposed that survival of placental choriocarcinoma in the maternal host presupposes a high degree of histocompatibility between the fetus and mother as regards major transplantation antigens. This concept theorized that choriocarcinoma, an allograft of fetal tissue in the maternal host, develops in an environment of homogeneity of maternal and fetal antigens. Accordingly, such tumors should receive one of the father's chromosomes carrying his histocompatibility antigens. Failure of tumor rejection may result if that chromosome fails to contain an antigenic determinant that can be recognized as foreign by the mother. Haplotype studies, obtained by serotyping the children of pregnancies in which choriocarcinoma developed, showed that the children in five of these six families possessed no antigens not also present in their mother's cells (9). This finding provided the basis for their concept that the paternal chromosome inherited by these children and the associated choriocarcinoma contained no serologically detectable strong transplantation antigen not already present in the maternal genetic composition. However, evidence against this concept was presented by Rudolph and Thomas (10), from histocompatibility studies in three patients with trophoblastic tumors and 14 of their children. Using one-way mixed leukocyte cultures (MLC), cells from all 14 of the children stimulated the mother's lymphocytes, indicating the presence of antigenic differences. Significantly, leukocyte serotyping detected antigenic differences in only six children. It could be surmised, therefore, in contrast to Mogensen and Kissmeyer-Nielsen's original findings, which employed only leukocyte serotyping with antisera, that all antigenic differences are not detectable by antisera alone and that the question of a maternal contribution to choriocarcinoma was unresolved.

Theory of Trophoblast Oncogenesis

The Nobel laureate, Temin (11) has presented a new genetic hypothesis for cancer which proposed that the germ line, in its chromosomes, contains only "the potential for genetic evolution by the somatic cells that may lead to the de novo formation of the information for cancer." This concept portrays vertical transmission of the information for cancer, even though the germ line does not contain this information in its chromosomes as proviruses or oncogenes, or as full virions. Temin believes that the mechanisms of RNA to DNA information transfer may play a role in normal cellular differentiation by providing a mechanism for variability in the genome of somatic cells without disturbing the stability of the germ line. Since only DNA-to-DNA, DNA-to-RNA, and RNA-to-protein modes of information transfer occur in the germ line, variability of DNA is permitted only by mutations and random selections. The protovirus hypothesis allows, therefore, that variability may occur without mutation through formation of new sequences of DNA from RNA-to-DNA information transfers. This is accomplished using the normal cellular RNA-dependent DNA polymerase enzyme system in somatic cells. The findings of the reverse transcriptase in normal cells have given strong support to this hypothesis.

Temin does point out, however, that RNA-to-DNA information transfer could occur in the germ line without affecting the progeny, if integration did not occur. On the other hand, in extreme cases, it was speculated that a DNA product of protovirus evolution could become integrated in the germ line, thereby providing a mechanism for genetic transmission of characteristics evolved from environmental influences. In considering the physiologic function of protovirus evolution to be that of normal differentiation, Temin appears to be postulating the origin of information which determines colonization of cells, functionally and organotypically. This may have genetic control relationship to "organizer substance" elaboration during normal organogenesis, a process requiring stable differentiation which might be achieved in DNA from RNA-to-DNA information transfer. Temin proposed that predetermined regions for RNA-to-DNA information transfer in the cell's genome would be specified through polymerase and integration systems, selecting these regions on the basis of base sequences. For adaptation, variability, or evolutionary development, this system may be equally suitable. Temin postulates that cancer may represent a variation in normal physiologic evolution of protovirus DNA which can occur either by mutation of base sequences, by integration in incorrect places, or by both mechanisms. He notes that this information for cancer, brought about by the action of chemicals or irradiation on DNA, RNA, or protein, would not necessarily require the formation of an RNA tumor virus. However, he proposes that protovirus evolution could give rise to a virus which could enter the organism from the outside, insert the information for cancer, and thereby supersede the "usual process" of protovirus evolution. The neoplastic phenotype would persist since no further information transfer would be required in the cell in which the information for cancer had already been transferred from RNA to DNA.

Temin's protovirus hypothesis is based on his previous provirus (12) hypothesis which stated that permanent establishment of RNA tunor virus genetic information required information transfer from viral RNA to DNA. That RNA tumor virus replication is associated with a DNA intermediate was firmly established by demonstration of complementarity between Rous virus RNA and Rous cell DNA in molecular hybridization experiments. The RNA-dependent DNA polymerase (reverse transcriptase) enzyme responsible for this conversion was subsequently documented by Temin and Mizutani and by Baltimore. The protovirus hypothesis is distinct from the former proposal, however, in that no DNA provirus is present; rather, the potential for genetic evolution of the information for cancer is transmitted in the DNA (protovirus DNA). This hypothesis envisions the information for cancer to be present in the genome normally and to be evolved in somatic cells as either normal differentiation or cancer. The process, Temin believes, occurs in a series of cumulative steps: segments of the cell's genome, designated as "protovirus" region (contains normal DNA controlling various cell functions), synthesize RNA which is transferred from cell A to cell B. Using the reverse transcriptase enzyme, the original DNA from cell A is transcribed in cell B and, by appropriate integration systems involving ligases and endonucleases, is inserted into the host DNA sequence. Depending upon the site and specificities of information inserted, a proximate series of function directions deriving from the "protovirus" regions (*i.e.*, regions specifying polymerase control for cell replication, surface properties, and so forth), could assemble in a contiguous region of the chromosome appropriate information for cancer or for an enveloped virion or for a normal physiologic adaptation through this differentiation process.

Only in extreme cases, Temin notes, could one envision a product of protovirus evolution infecting the germ line, becoming integrated there, and thus affecting progeny organisms. This process might, however, provide a mechanism for inheritance of desirable adaptations to environmental influences. Inclusive in Temin's hypothesis are the possibilities that cancer may occur as a result of normal physiologic evolution of the protovirus DNA but with integration in incorrect places or by mutation of base sequences. Since DNA, RNA, and proteins are involved in the sequence of DNA-to-RNA-to-DNA information transfer, the formation of variants leading to malignancy may result from the disruptive effects of radiation or chemicals. Tumor formation in animals and plants apparently related only to the genetic constitution of the organism, exclusive of external stimuli, have also been reported.

A major thrust of the protovirus hypothesis is its projected role in normal differentiation. In considering the requirement of cells to group functionally and organotypically, Temin cites the stability of RNA-to-DNA information transfer as the most plausible means of accomplishing this objective. The presumption is made that the "cell's particular differentiated state could be partially specified by the types of new protovirus derived DNA it contained. RNA transcribed from this new protovirus derived DNA could be transferred to other cells and thus induce an orderly conversion of adjacent cells into the same, or a related differentiated state." Examples of this process include embryonic induction and secondary antibody response.

In considering the origin of the trophoblast, it is significant that teleologically, trophoblastic tissue can be said to derive from "protoderm," the totipotential stage of development prior to differentiation into epithelial and mesenchymal elements. In the framework of the Temin hypothesis, because the normal role of protoviruses from the germ line and from somatic cells appears to be to differentiate these genomes physiologically, there may be some advantage in separating these two stages as "protogerm DNA" and "protosome DNA" as distinct from the protovirus which would contain information for cancer. The link between human cancer and a cancer virus has been identified in "T" cell leukemia reported by Gallo of the National Cancer Institute. The virus causes a type of malignancy called T-cell leukemia, cancer of specific white blood cells. These white cells, the T-lymphocytes, are produced by the body to fight infection. When infected by the virus, they lose control and multiply rapidly. T-cell leukemia is rare in the United States but common in Japan and parts of the Caribbean. Many animal cancer viruses are known, but the T-cell leukemia virus is the first human cancer virus to have been discovered. Diseases like T-cell leukemia seem to occur in clusters of people, suggesting that they are passed from one person to another as an infectious disease.

ECTOPIC hCG IN NONTROPHOBLAST CANCERS

Ectopic gonadotropin production in organs not normally engaged in the synthesis of this glycoprotein hormone - which may represent retrogenic reexpression of trophoblast genes in somatic and germ cells - is being reported with increasing frequency. A review of the literature by Civantos and Rywlin (13) reported 54 cases of choriocarcinomas in cancers of nongenital organs and cited another 11 cases reported by Regan and Cremin (14). One hundred cases of ovarian choriocarcinomas were also reviewed (13), including three cases of mucinous and papillary cystadenocarcinomas with trophoblast differentiation. Chorionic gonadotropin activity was identified by various methods, including tissue localization by specific immunofluorescence with rhodamine-labeled anti-hCG, and by bioassay and immunoassay.

Cancers of various organs which have been shown to have trophoblastic or choriocarcinomatous differentiation and gonadotropin activity include stomach (14), lung (15), esophagus (16), kidney

(17), bladder (18), pineal, pituitary gland (19), mediastinum (20), retroperitoneal space, and thymus (21). Gonadotropin secretion in carcinomas of breast, adrenal gland, and malignant melanoma was described, although histologic descriptions were not included (22). Gonadotropin production of chorionic and pituitary-like characteristics was reported in hepatoblastomas, although trophoblastic differentiation was not described histologically. Choriocarcinomas in ovary and testis (23) are well known. Increasing numbers of lung carcinomas with gonadotropin activity have been reported and discussed by Rosen and associates (15). Generally, the patients have been men with histologic patterns of undifferentiated carcinoma; however, squamous, mixed adeno and squamous, oat cell, and bronchio-alveolar carcinomas have also been reported. Other hormones, in addition to hCG, have been found also in trophoblastic tumors. A recent report by Hershman and co-workers summarized the findings of human chorionic thyrotropin in benign trophoblastic tumors (24).

Gonadal trophoblastic cancers of ovary and testis have generally been felt to be of germ cell origin. In the ovary, tumors of probable germ cell origin including adult cystic teratomas, embryonal carcinomas, and dysgerminomas with and without trophoblastic differentiation comprise some 33 to 76 percent of ovarian tumors encountered in the child (25).

Although testicular neoplasms comprise somewhat less than one percent of all cancers occurring in males - because they occur predominantly in young men and because more than 90 percent prove to be malignant - the significance of this form of cancer becomes apparent. Testicular tumors constitute the leading form of lethal cancer in men from 25 to 34 years of age (23).

Histogenic classification of ovarian and testicular tumors is exceedingly difficult because of the range of pluripotentiality in these germ cell cancers. It is estimated that more than 97 percent of the tumors are of germinal origin (25). In the male the germinal tumors include predominantly seminomas (approximately 40 percent), embryonal carcinomas (15 to 20 percent), teratocarcinomas (15 to 20 percent), combined tumors (15 to 20 percent), and choriocarcinomas (1 percent). In the female child, dysgerminomas account for approximately 25 percent, malignant teratomas 25 percent, embryonal carcinomas 14 percent, adenocarcinomas 14 percent, granulosa cell and arrhenoblastomas 5 percent, and approximately 3 percent of these show trophoblastic differentiation (25).

It is believed that embryonal carcinomas represent primitive and undifferentiated neoplasms composed of pluripotential germ cells which have the potentiality and the manifest capacity for differentiation along either trophoblastic lines, giving rise to the lethal choriocarcinomas, or along somatic lines, giving rise to varying degrees of teratomas with assorted types of tissue or organoid formations. Recent investigations of genetic control of experimental teratogenesis have suggested that the appearance of these embryonic tumors is influenced by the action of a single gene (26).

TROPHOBLAST ANTIGENICITY AND CARCINOGENESIS

The fetal and placental unit, from the standpoint of transplantation biology, represents a tolerated intrauterine graft of genetically alien tissue. In spite of the vast amount of new knowledge in this field, the immunologic enigma of mammalian pregnancy, a most provocative exception to the fundamental laws of allograft rejection, remains largely unresolved. The basic mechanism yet unsolved is the process which permits survival of the heterozygous trophoblast and embryo in intimate association with genetically dissimilar maternal tissues. The immunobiology of pregnancy is therefore of major interest to oncologists for reasons related to possible common denominators in the tolerant state of the two processes. It may be anticipated that basic processes of normal growth, metabolism, and immunologic factors which permit survival of the allograft of trophoblast and embryo are also likely to be operative in the maintenance of malignancy.

The various theses which have been called upon to explain tolerance of the pregnancy allograft include (27) contentions that (a) the fetus is antigenically immature, (b) the uterus is an immunologically privileged site, (c) the immunologic reactivity of the maternal host is suppressed during gestation because of placental and maternal steroids, and (d) the trophoblast, in direct contact with the maternal host tissues by virtue of a "fibrinoid coat," is antigenically unexpressed.

The mechanism believed most likely to be operative in this unique biologic milieu is that of trophoblast mediation. Trophoblastic nonreactivity, when the mother had been specifically immunized against paternal antigens, has been demonstrated by Simmons and co-workers (28). Using mouse ectoplacental cones comprised of essentially pure trophoblastic elements at 6½ to 7½ days of gestation, transplants were placed beneath the kidney capsule of presensitized adult CBA mice which had previously rejected paternal strain grafts. Survival, growth, and proliferation of the trophoblast were observed without appreciable lymphocytic reaction, whereas grafts of the embryonic tissue were regularly rejected. Midgestational placenta, because it is a composite anatomic structure containing vessels, connective tissue, and leukocytes from the fetus, in addition to trophoblastic tissue, was rejected by recipients of the maternal strain. The natural conclusion drawn from these experiments is that immunologic protection of the fetus is an important function of the trophoblast. From this failure of the allograft rejection it is suggested that transplantation or histocompatibility antigens on the trophoblast are either not present or are protected from expression, possibly by cell surface masking.

Currie and Bagshawe (29), using an in vitro histocompatibility test based on allogeneic inhibition phenomenon, reported that the addition of maternal lymphocytes to human trophoblast monolayer cultures resulted in marked cytotoxicity, maximal on the fourth day of incubation. They suggested that a sialomucin coating on the trophoblast may mask underlying histocompatibility antigens, thus preventing detection by immunologically competent cells of the maternal host. Since enzymatic dispersion with trypsin had been used for preparation of these trophoblast monolayers, the intactness of the in vivo trophoblast cell surface components could not be assured in these experiments.

In considering the concept of retrogenic trophoblast and embryonic redifferentiation in multiple forms of malignancy, it must be emphasized that a gene may directly influence the immune reaction by specific control, or surface antigen synthesis (*i.e.*, induction by viral transformation), or indirectly by enzymatically modifying availability of these antigens through control of a "fibrinoid" surface masking coat. Topographically, the trophoblast cells are physically interposed between fetus and mother. These cells have been observed to have an electron-dense fibrinoid coat (30, 31) containing sialomucin and staining positively with PAS and colloidal iron. Treatment of placental tissue with neuraminidase, the enzyme capable of removing terminal sialic acid groups from cell membrane sialomucin, has been reported to unmask transplantation antigens of early mouse trophoblast (32). For whatever cause, though not finally resolved and not withstanding the reports (33) that blood group substances have been observed on the trophoblast, present evidence would suggest trophoblastic nonantigenicity (34). In addition to the inertness of mouse placental trophoblast (28), somewhat similar experiments with rabbits (35) resulted in successful pregnancy after fertilized ova of a breeding pair were placed in the uterus of a different female sensitized to tissues of the original paternal strain. From the foregoing it is apparent that a comprehensive summation of the immunobiologic properties of trophoblast as a tolerated "graft" will be closely mirrored in malignancy. It is pertinent, therefore, to consider the results of homograft and histocompatibility experience in normal and cancer patients.

HISTOCOMPATIBILITY ANTIGENS IN TROPHOBLAST NEOPLASMS

Although tumor-associated antigens can be detected on

trophoblast tumor cells from choriocarcinoma patients, HLA antigens no doubt play an important role in the development of a host immune response to this tumor. The genetic makeup of an individual may determine the capacity of the individual to successfully combat cancer and other disease states, *e.g.*, abnormal pregnancies, abortions, infertility, and preeclampsia. These factors appear to be based upon the individual's immunogenetics, as histocompatibility-restricted T-cell cytotoxicity may be deficient in the observed instances of increased histocompatibility between husband and wife found in trophoblast tumor patients and in other instances of abnormal pregnancies.

Isoantibodies against paternal antigens on fetal cells are formed during pregnancy as a maternal response to foreign fetal antigens. Identification of the biological role of these immunoactive molecules constitutes a major objective of the developing field of reproductive immunology.

Clinical application of the HLA system developed in the early 1950's with the recognition that multiple blood transfusions, even though compatible by cross-matching, immunized a patient to the white blood cells of the transfused blood. On further investigation, the alloantigens responsible for this immunization were found to be located on the white blood cells that were present on closely-linked genes in the A region of chromosome 6. Accordingly, the term HLA is derived from human leukocyte antigen of the A region, and is synonymous with transplantation or histocompatibility locus antigens.

In the mid-60's, panels of leukocyte-typing sera and several allelic systems were defined. It has now been found that the HLA antigens present on all nucleated human cells are coded for by at least four separate genes on autosomal chromosome 6. Each individual locus is designated by the letter A, B, C, or D. The specificities of the HLA types are defined by antisera, identified in turn by serologic definition, that is, the A, B, and C subloci. The D locus is defined only by mixed lymphocyte cultures. Since these loci are separated by less than 0.5 recombinant units, the alleles do not separate on segregation. Thus, at fertilization an individual receives chromosomal contributions from the paternal and maternal chromosomes, giving rise to his haplotype.

A second basis for the present interest in histocompatibility is that recent discoveries have accentuated the importance of HLA type in tumor immunology. Gerald Edelman's laboratory at the Rockefeller Institute has identified the amino acid sequence of beta$_2$-microglobulin and identified it as similar to portions of the IgG molecule. Edelman's group has thus suggested that the immune response genes controlling immunological tumor phenomena (as well as other immune reactions to foreign antigens, such as those expressed during repeated abortions or in severe preeclampsia) and the histocompatibility genes are controlled on the same gene loci. In an even broader sense, Edelman and J. A. Gally at Meharry Medical College have suggested that the immune system, with its specialized functions, has probably evolved from a system of histocompatibility antigens. While the selection of donor-recipient pairs for organ transplantation remains the primary use of histocompatibility testing, human leukocyte antigen typing in pregnancy and disease is rapidly gaining acceptance.

Biochemistry of HLA

The histocompatibility antigens are glycoproteins and consist of two components. The larger component carries the antigenic specificity; its molecular weight is about 45,000. The smaller component appears to be common to histocompatibility antigens of all specificities; it has a molecular weight of about 11,000 to 12,000 (36).

The smaller component of the HLA antigen is a unique protein present on the surface of all mammalian cells, including B and T lymphocytes. This small component is the $beta_2$-microglobulin. The $beta_2$-microglobulin is in fact a component of the HLA antigen found on the surface of all nucleated cells. It consists of 100 amino acids and is similar in amino acid composition to a segment of the constant region of the heavy chain of IgG. The remaining portions of IgG (the two identical light chains, each of molecular weight 20,000 and containing the variable regions that confer specificity as they contain the sites that combine with the corresponding antigens, as well as the additional segments of the two identical heavy chains, of molecular weight 50,000) are all totally distinct from the $beta_2$-microglobulins.

Genetic Control of HLA

Histocompatibility antigens are genetically controlled structures on the cell surface, which differ from individual to individual. In principle, they are defined by the fact that grafts exchanged between individuals whose HLA antigens differ are rejected by the immune mechanisms of the recipient, except during normal pregnancy when the allograft of pregnancy is sustained through the period of gestation. The importance of these differences for reproductive biology is quickly becoming apparent in the fields of habitual abortion, infertility, preeclampsia, and trophoblastic tumors. Much evidence from different points of view indicates the great biological significance of these cell surface structures. Possible biological functions for these gene products, such as control of the immune response and susceptibility to certain viruses, have been suggested (37-43).

Histocompatibility antigen systems are, by definition, polymorphic. Polymorphism is most simply defined operationally as the existence in the same population of two or more alleles at a given genetic locus, each of which has an appreciable frequency.

Changes in gene frequencies in a population with time is evolution. Its basic driving forces are mutation, which produces the genetic variation that is the basis for evolution, and natural selection, which adaptively molds gene frequency changes to fit the prevailing environment. This is the basis on which it has been postulated that the immune response genes and their functions are derived from a system of histocompatibility antigens that controlled the host's capacity to reject offending invaders and thus to survive and proliferate.

Pregnancy Immunology and the HLA System

It has been suggested that placental weight in the human is related to histocompatibility antigen-dependent reactivity between maternal and fetal cells (44). Some reports indicated that histocompatibility does influence placental weight and that increased histocompatibility differences are associated with larger placentas. In view of the known relationship between placental weight and birth weight, and between placental weight and perinatal mortality, it has been suggested that the outcome of pregnancy could be predicted to some extent by a knowledge of the parental genetic relationship. Animal experiments have already indicated the greater histocompatibility differences between mother and conceptus may be associated with larger placentas and selective prenatal survival advantage (45). The fetus in human pregnancy is correctly viewed as an allograft, and thus histocompatibility differences between it and the maternal host would be expected to influence graft survival. The mixed lymphocyte cultures between cells from the mother and her neonate were used as a dynamic model of cell-mediated immunity in the experiments referred to above. It was shown that larger placentas were associated with those pairs that had significantly higher mixed lymphocyte cell reactions. The implication of increased perinatal survival potential is clear from prior animal experiments.

The expression of HLA on normal trophoblast has been controversial because of the conflicting reports on this matter. Faulk and Temple (46) failed to identify HLA or associated beta$_2$-microglobulin in full term placental trophoblast using immunofluorescence and peroxidase staining in association with electron microscopy. Mesenchymal stroma easily showed positive staining, although enzymatic attempts to uncover masked antigens on the trophoblast were simultaneously unsuccessful. Johnson and Faulk (47) found no beta$_2$-microglobulin in first trimester trophoblast, although it was readily identified in endothelial cells. Using purified placental plasma membranes, Goodfellow (48) quantitated the concentration of

HLA-A and -B locus antigens and $beta_2$-microglobulin, and only found levels consistent with contamination by blood vessel endothelium and mesenchymal stroma. In contrast, using the BeWo choriocarcinoma cell line, Trowsdale and co-workers (49) recently identified HLA-A, -B, -C, and $beta_2$-microglobulin in the trophoblast in culture. This is consistent with the earlier demonstration by Loke (50) of HLA in tissue culture of normal trophoblast using multi-specific anti-HLA antisera in a complement-dependent cytotoxicity reaction.

That the trophoblast is antigenic can be inferred by the presence of HLA antibody in 20 to 30 percent of postpartum patients. This may be an incomplete reflection of antibody activity, however, since the allogeneic placenta appears to function as a paternal strain immunoabsorbent (51), and HLA antibodies are easily eluted from the placenta (52). In this way, the placenta could serve as a barrier between the maternal immune response and the semiallogeneic fetus. In the experiments referred to above (52), eluted placenta gamma-globulin demonstrated specific antibody against HLA antibodies of the HLA-A, -B, and -C allotype. However, most antibodies were directed against HLA-D-related determinants. It is of interest that clinical trials are currently underway in a large program using these eluted alloantibodies for passive immunologic enhancement of renal transplants. The immunoglobulins are prepared by acid elution from large pools of placenta. These eluted placental gamma-globulins have already been shown to possess antibody activity against the entire spectrum of histocompatibility antigens.

Cell-Mediated and Humoral Immunity in Gestation

As Barnstable and Bodmer have pointed out (53), the late development of the fetal lymphoid system excludes it as a primary force in preventing rejection of the fetal allograft. Rather, avoidance of rejection is more likely produced by a lack of a cell-mediated, rather than antibody-mediated, immune response. Humoral antibodies against HLA antigens are made in 20 to 30 percent of pregnant women (53). The production of these antibodies in the mother indicates that the maternal humoral immune system has not "turned off." However, it must be noted that, since not all pregnant patients demonstrate the antibodies, their presence cannot represent a general mechanism of enhancement.

The mechanisms surrounding acceptance of the fetal allograft bear strongly on the depressed immunogenicity of the trophoblast and fetus. A very depressed expression of HLA on the trophoblastic tissue in contact with the maternal circulation may prevent cell-mediated immune attack on the fetus.

It has been shown in the mouse that cell-mediated killing is restricted by the major histocompatibility (H_2) system in that species. Recognition of either H2K or D determinants, complexed to a foreign determinant in order to give rise to an "altered self," was found to be necessary before generation of cytotoxic T cells was possible. Bach has suggested a similar HLA-restricted T cell-mediated cytotoxicity in man. This is in keeping with Bach's earlier suggestion that, under certain circumstances, T cells recognize foreign antigens in association with self-determinants. For instance, T cell-mediated cytotoxic reactions can occur only when target and effector cells carry some common histocompatibility antigens. This phenomenon was observed with virus-infected cells when cytotoxic T cells from an animal immune to a specific virus could specifically lyse infected target cells only if the target cells shared the same histocompatibility antigens as the cytotoxic T cells. Therefore, the lack of significant quantities of HLA-A, -B, and -C antigens on trophoblast could act either to prevent the generation of cytotoxic T lymphocytes, as suggested by Barnstable and Bodmer, or to prevent the action of such cells when directed against any fetal or polymorphic antigens for which there is feto-maternal incompatibility. Barnstable and Bodmer thus concluded that suppressed trophoblast immunogenicity for HLA with respect to cellular immunity, rather than depression of maternal immunocompetence, was more probably the major force inducing acceptance of the allograft of pregnancy. Similarities with tumor immunology were also suggested.

Normal Pregnancy and Trophoblast Tumor Immune Parallels

Parallels between immunological mechanisms in normal pregnancy and in tumor immunology have recently been delineated by the new concept of leukocyte migration enhancement as proposed by Gleicher and colleagues (54-56). These authors propose that the phenomenon of leukocyte migration enhancement in vitro is representative of graft enhancement in vivo, and is associated with plasma antibody excess. On the other hand, a relative excess of antigen is associated with leukocyte migration inhibition. Interesting correlations with amniotic fluid and pregnancy plasma in this regard have been shown, to the effect that an immunoglobulin of the IgG class may be the immunoactive substance. The suggestion was made that common embryonic antigens in pregnancy and malignancy may result in the induction of specific IgG fractions, heralding specific lymphocyte subpopulations, and producing suppressor effects that prevent leukocyte migration inhibition. This is seen in the phases of tumor growth associated with antigen excess.

Trophoblast Rejection in Abortions

It has been shown that a high degree of wife-husband antigen compatibility at the HLA-A locus is associated with recurrent abnormal pregnancies, including spontaneous abortion (57). As noted previously, experimental work supporting the concept that strong selective pressures contribute to superior reproductive outcome of heterozygotes derives mainly from studies conducted in animals (58, 59). Placental size and weight of allogeneic conceptuses in mice is significantly increased by dissimilarity in major histocompatibility antigens between mother and fetus. In addition to the fact that spontaneous abortion occurs with greater frequency in couples who have a higher degree of husband-wife compatibility, women in these couples are significantly less reactive against paternal stimulating cells in one-way mixed lymphocyte reactions. A significantly increased frequency of HLA-A9 was found in women with recurrent abnormal pregnancies of unknown etiology (60).

The different distribution of one or more common antigen specificities, as well as the different associations of common HLA antigen specificities in couples with repeated abortions as compared to controls, led Komlos and Halbrecht (61) to propose the following hypothesis to explain maternal cytotoxic responses toward the fetus in fetomaternal HLA antigen-restricted allogeneic reactions. They proposed that "the induction of cytotoxic cell mediated responses in the mother, toward the immunizing fetus, is influenced by gene dose effects for certain HLA antigens carried by the fetus." Thus, the immunizing effect of the fetal cells, probably influenced by certain haplotype combinations, seemed to depend on the number of homozygous HLA antigens (locus A and B) shared by the mother and the fetus. It was hypothesized that fetuses homozygotic for one single HLA antigen (locus A and B) shared with the mother tend to induce maternal cytotoxic responses, as compared to fetuses homozygotic for two or more HLA antigen specificities shared with the mother.

These researchers observed an increased incidence of two or three common HLA antigens shared by couples in the control group and not in the group of repeated abortions. This finding led them to postulate that immune response genes, closely linked to genes controlling histocompatibility antigens, may have a regulatory effect on genes (locus A and B) controlling histocompatibility antigen-restricted cytotoxic reactions. Thus, it was suggested that, when two or three homozygous HLA antigen specificities are shared by fetus and mother, larger doses of identical genes controlling histocompatibility antigens (locus A and B), as well as immune response genes, are involved in the fetomaternal interaction.

Observations of histocompatibility antigen-restricted cytotoxic reactions to viruses in the mouse, chemically modified (43) and allogeneic cells suggested that the compatibility requirements for immune response genes between effector and target cells are irrélevant in cytotoxic reactions. The requirement for compatibility in the immune region was observed in suppression reactions between T cells producing suppressive factors and the target cells. Thus, it was postulated that a large number of immune response genes shared by mother and fetus in specific haplotype combinations may have a depressing effect on genes controlling histocompatibility antigen-restricted (locus A and B) cytotoxic reactions (61). The regulatory effect of immune response genes linked to genes controlling histocompatibility antigen-restricted cytotoxic reactions was proposed as a possible explanation for the increased incidence of two or three common HLA antigens (locus A and B) shared by fertile couples, as compared to couples with repeated abortions. The regulatory effect of immune response genes controlling HLA antigen-restricted cytotoxic reactions is not always beneficial, which may also depend on a preferential antigenicity for certain histocompatibility antigens, or antigen associations, on the induction of cytotoxic reaction.

Cell-mediated histocompatibility antigen-restricted cytotoxic reactions were interpreted as being mediated mainly by T cells. However, it was noted that any possible explanation for the complex biological function of the HLA system had to take into account the tissue distribution of the major histocompatibility antigens, as well as cell-to-cell interactions according to this distribution. Since optimal cooperative interactions between T and B cells, as well as between T cells and macrophages, require identity among certain genes of the major histocompatibility antigens, it was presumed that the genetic control of the fetomaternal immune response must be a multicellular event.

Immunogenicity of HLA Antigens in Trophoblast Tumors

Because gestational trophoblastic tumors may be complete allografts, and therefore antigenically foreign, they reflect a favorable situation for the development of strong HLA immunologic rejection mechanisms. While choriocarcinoma can occur following the birth of an HLA-incompatible infant, patients with choriocarcinoma as a group usually have more compatible offspring, and high-risk patients are more compatible with their husbands (62). This suggests that weaker antigenic stimuli are operative in high-risk choriocarcinoma patients than in the complete allograft situation of a complete mole. It is conceivable that mechanisms such as enhancement, possibly operating in normal pregnancy to prevent the maternal host from rejecting her fetus, may also be operative in trophoblastic tumors. The tolerance of patients with choriocarcinoma to skin grafts from their husbands has previously been demonstrated by Robinson (63) and Bagshawe (64).

The hypothesis that the survival and dissemination of postgestational choriocarcinoma are dependent on a high degree of histocompatibility between the malignant graft deriving from the child's placenta and the maternal host has not been proven. Mixed lymphocyte culture experiments from maternal and paternal pairs by Lewis and associates show that histocompatibility differences could be readily demonstrated by a responsive state between the paternal and maternal lymphocytes in patients with trophoblastic tumors.

The above observations bear on Bach's findings (65). He has differentiated these findings in the human HLA and mouse H-2 systems by defining two regions of the respective chromosome's serologically-defined loci, and lymphocyte-defined loci. The latter can be defined only by lymphocyte interaction in mixed lymphocyte culture. These regions are the major histocompatibility loci; their alleles control the respective tissue type antigens. Genetic mapping of the H-2 locus in the mouse (65) has shown it to be composed of a serologically defined region beginning proximally to the centromere, comprised of H-2K and H-2D loci. On the other hand, it contains the immune response (Ir) locus and another locus controlling serum protein levels. In the mouse, the Ir-1 gene product seems to be expressed in T lymphocytes, and it has been suggested that it may control a T cell receptor site (39). Bach and associates have suggested that, if the lymphocyte-defined locus and the immune response locus are found to be the same, then the receptors noted above could act as both recognition molecules on responding cells and foreign molecules on stimulating cells. Thus, any cell with one or more immune response receptors that a second cell does not have might stimulate the second cell in mixed lymphocyte culture. If the lymphocyte-defined locus product is different from the immune response locus product, the latter might be recognized by T cells, but may be incapable of stimulating B cells. An alternate possibility is that T lymphocytes may recognize differences in the spatial arrangement of antigens, which may be controlled by the lymphocyte-defined locus.

At this point, it can only be stated that the definition of immune response control mechanisms still poses a major challenge. Using information gained in the HLA typing of choriocarcinoma patients, their husbands, and their children, preliminary trials in immunotherapy for these resistant tumors have been initiated. To date no cures have been achieved; however, inhibitory (66) effects have been observed.

Biological Evolution of Trophoblast Tumors

The biological events in neoplastic transformation of the trophoblast of human conception results in the formation of grossly swollen, hydropic avascular villi in the absence of a fetus, cord, or amniotic membrane and with varying degrees of hyperplasia and anaplasia in the trophoblastic elements. The classical hydatidiform mole may progress to invasive malignant trophoblastic sequelae and require cytotoxic chemotherapy in approximately 20 percent of cases as indicated in the studies of Hammond, Parker and Curry *et al.* (67, 68). In over 80 percent of cases, regression of the human chorionic gonadotropin titer to negative occurs within 60 days of evacuation of the tumor (Table 1). Elimination of the residual trophoblastic tumor cells by autologous cytotoxic destruction is a function of the "host" response system. The inherent malignant potential of the

Table 1. Chorionic Gonadotropin After Delivery of Hydatidiform Mole

Days	Titer	
	Positive	Negative
At evacuation	100%	0%
10	57%	43%
20	40%	60%
30	28%	72%
40	24%	76%
50	22%	78%
60	20%	80%

trophoblastic tumor on the one hand and the host response on the other hand determines the clinical course of a trophoblastic neoplasm. Host response capability is an expression of both genetic and immunologic characteristics. Recent human and animal studies have shown that an individual's capacity to respond immunologically depends on tissue type (38, 39, 40), major histocompatibility complex, and human leucocyte antigen - HLA. This system appears to control the individual's "T" cell cytotoxicity (thymus dependent or cell-mediated immunity). Residual trophoblastic tumor cells, whether at the molar implantation site, within the myometrium or embolized to a distant metastatic site, must be cytotoxically destroyed if persistent tumor is to be rejected. As previously stated, under the histocompatibility restriction of "T" cell-mediated cytoxicity, T cells recognize foreign antigens only in association with self determinants, that is, destruction of foreign antigen can occur only when the target cells and effector cells carry a common histocompatibility antigen.

Host Reactions to Trophoblast Tumor Challenge

The biological basis of host resistance to neoplastic trophoblast cells can be deduced by critical analysis of a number of observations in nature. It is well recognized that skin grafts derived from genetically distinct individuals are rapidly rejected, principally by lymphoid reactions. These grafts come from foreign donors and, as their genetically distinct antigens are absorbed into the host's lymphatic system, a prompt cellular reaction is generated and subsequent rejection occurs. Malignant tumors, on the other hand, arise within the host and although circulating tumor cells with their tumor-specific antigens are present in the blood stream, adequate immunity and rejection do not occur. In pertinent experiments, Fisher and Fisher (72) have recently shown that the blood stream is a highly ineffective means of producing tumor sensitization. In contrast, tumor rejection can be produced only when the lymph nodes are intact. When the inguinal and popliteal lymph nodes were surgically excised and C_3H mouse tumors were inoculated subcutaneously in the hind leg, no immunity developed. From these two important observations, it appears reasonable to assume that immune stimulation of peripheral lymph nodes from their afferent arms could provide a means for increasing host reaction to neoplastic trophoblast. Tumor-specific antigens, as well as nonspecific immunostimulants, such as *Bacillus calmette-guerin* (BCG) could also accomplish this objective. However, before such immunostimulation could be considered, it would be necessary to evaluate the immunologic status of the patients to be treated. Note must be taken of the fact that previous literature reports have indicated that patients with advanced malignancy have suppressed immune systems, both by laboratory tests using T- and B-cell stimulating agents and by clinical skin testing of responses to commonly encountered antigens (73-79).

T and B Lymphocyte Reactions to Trophoblast Neoplasms

Lymphocytes comprise the major cell type of the immune reaction. The lymphocyte is characterized by its unique surface receptors or recognition sites which allows it to pick out particular three-dimensional molecular configurations known as antigenic determinants. A single lymphocyte is believed to be programed for only one or two antigenic determinants. The contact of a quiescent lymphocyte with its corresponding antigenic determinant activates its cell membrane. This event triggers metabolic activation which is followed by blast transformation and DNA synthesis. The cell enlarges and divides, giving rise to daughter cells with the same recognition site as the parent cell. This expansion continues until a whole colony of lymphocytes with the same recognition sites is produced (Fig. 1).

T lymphocytes are thymic dependent. They mature under the influence of the thymus, through the action of single peptide hormones of thymic origin. These cells are programed to recognize particular antigenic determinants.

T cells derive originally from epithelial cells in the third and fourth pharyngeal pouches and are concentrated in the fetal thymus, where they synthesize the thymic hormone, thymosin. Lymphocytes developing in the thymus are dependent upon thymosin for the development of characteristic T cell functions. Included in these functions are (a) immunosurveillance, a major aspect of cancer immunity; (b) delayed hypersensitivity reactivity; (c) transplantation immunity, as in graft rejection; and (d) cell-mediated host defenses against certain viruses, fungi, and intracellular facultative bacteria. In addition, the activity of these T cells is stimulated by persistent antigens, or indirectly by antigen which has been processed by macrophages (80). Three subsets of T-lymphocyte

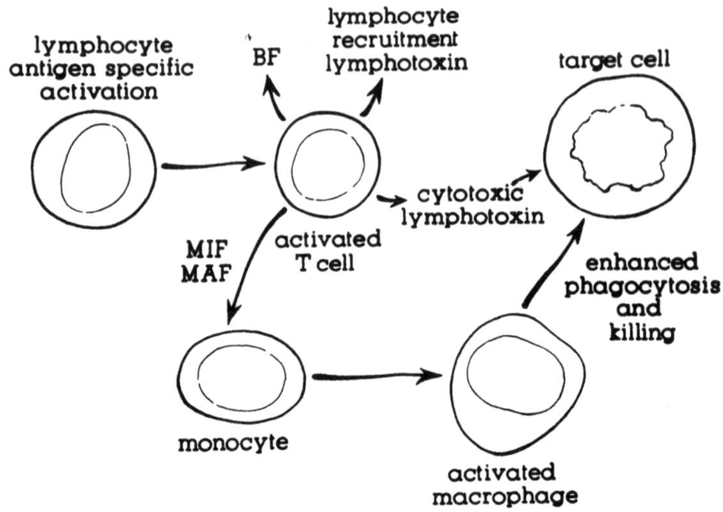

Fig. 1. Development of immune rejection of trophoblast tumor cells requires recognition of the foreign antigen by stem cells which proliferate and ultimately attack the target cell, producing lysis.

expression may occur: (a) After being stimulated by its antigenic determinant, effector T cells are generated. The effector T lymphocytes, upon encountering their antigenic determinant on the surface of the cell, produce a response that is cytotoxic to the cell. This cell-mediated lymphocyte toxicity produces the typical delayed hypersensitivity skin reaction as is observed in the PPD reaction. (b) Helper T cells develop. The helper T cells have the ability to cooperate with B lymphocytes in promoting antibody synthesis. (c) Generation of suppressor T cell proliferation. The suppressor T cells suppress or impede synthesis of immunoglobulin by B cells.

B lymphocytes are derived directly from the bone marrow, and in birds their maturation is dependent upon the bursa of Fabricius, a rudimentary blind pouch in the gut. The precise location of the B cell maturing factors is not clearly understood in the case of the human, and accordingly B cells are said to be under the control of "bursal equivalents" in the mammalian species. B cell encounter with antigen, for which the B cell has a receptor, stimulates the proliferative response. The end product of this proliferative response, however, is the production of immunoglobulin by cells that have been stimulated to undergo proliferation and morphologic change into plasma cells with characteristic marginal chromatin in the nucleus and highly basophilic cytoplasm. Five classes of immunoglobulins are secreted by these cells, including IgG, IgM, IgA, IgD, and IgE. These antibodies all combine with the antigenic determinant and constitute the major portion of the antibody-mediated immunity system, which requires complement for activation. B cells make up 15 to 30 percent of circulating lymphocytes, have abundant surface immunoglobulin, and bind both complement and the Fc fragmant of gamma globulin. By contrast, T cells, which make up the remaining 70 to 85 percent of circulating lymphocytes, have little surface immunoglobulin, but form rosettes when incubated with sheep red blood cells and proliferate when stimulated with PHA and Con A.

After stimulation by specific antigens, T lymphocytes release a series of substances called lymphokines, which are involved in the amplification of the antigen-specific immune process. These soluble antigens affect surrounding cells. They are released from activated lymphocytes and encompass a number of substances, including (a) blastogenic factor; (b) migration inhibitory factor; and (c) macrophage aggregation factor. In addition, antibody-mediated cytolysis requires activation by complement. This involves a series of cascading enzymes, ultimately permitting antibody combination with antigen on the target cell surface. This process produces defects in the cell membrane and ultimate lysis.

Monitoring of T and B Cells in Trophoblast Tumor Patients

T Cells. In vivo T cell reactions can be monitored by delayed hypersensitivity skin tests. By use of *Candida albicans*, a common fungal antigen; mumps, a viral antigen; and PPD and SKSD, bacterial antigens; it can be expected that 85 percent of a normal population will have at least one positive response to one of these antigens. With the addition of dinitrochlorobenzene sensitization, over 95 percent of a normal population may be expected to react to a 100 mg sensitizing dose of dinitrochlorobenzene. In vitro T cell responses may be assessed by use of plant lectins or mitogens which stimulate lymphocytes to undergo blast transformation, synthesize DNA, and undergo mitosis. Commonly, PHA and Con A are clinically significant T cell mitogens.

Histocompatibility antigens. Histocompatibility antigens are studied in mixed lymphocyte cultures, wherein the lymphocytes of two different individuals are incubated in culture after one of the individual's lymphocytes have previously been treated (stimulator population) with an agent such as mitomycin C to prevent DNA synthesis in these cells, while permitting blast transformation cells in the other individual's lymphocytes (responder population). By virtue of antigenic differences on lymphocyte-definable loci, blast transformation occurs in the responder population, and thymidine incorporation into DNA can be measured and expressed as counts per minute in the mixed lymphocyte culture reaction. Likewise, the T cell rosette test represents a nonspecific in vitro agglutination of sheep red blood cells in a rosette pattern by a subpopulation of peripheral lymphocytes which have T cell characteristics.

Macrophage Inhibitory Factor (MIF). Macrophage inhibitory factor, as measured by the indirect method of David (81), is an in vitro T cell monitoring test wherein guinea pig peritoneal macrophages packed in capillary tubes and immersed in tissue culture medium are incubated with products of lymphocytes that have been stimulated by the antigen being tested. Under these circumstances, the antigen-stimulated lymphocytes will produce a factor, macrophage inhibitory factor, which will inhibit the migration of the guinea pig peritoneal macrophages from the capillary tube. This macrophage inhibitory factor can be quantitated when compared to established standards. In a direct leukocyte migration inhibition assay, the leukocytes are packed into capillary tubes and incubated with the test antigen. Inhibition observed in this incubation directly inhibits migration (82).

B Cell Testing. B cells in the peripheral blood may be monitored by quantitative immunoglobulins after immunoelectrophoresis of peripheral serum samples. Lymphoid cells separated from the peripheral cell population can be tested by B cell rosettes in which sensitized sheep red blood cells are incubated with peripheral blood lymphocytes, forming B cell rosettes. These B cells contain surface immunoglobulins which can be detected by fluorescein-conjugated anti-globulin preparations or by the previously-mentioned sensitized or antibody-coated sheep red blood cells. In addition, they contain specific receptors for certain complement components. Likewise, quantitative isohemagglutinins can be determined in all patients except those of the blood group AB. Patients can also be immunized with *Salmonella* H and O antigens, to which the normal host responds by making antibody. Diptheria and tetanus antigens are administered as vaccines and are followed by skin test reactivity as observed in the Schnick test in an immunologically competent host.

Immunologic Monitoring of Trophoblast Tumor Patients

Using the principles of immunobiology outlined in this chapter, it has been possible in the author's laboratory to utilize cytotoxicity assays to longitudinally monitor trophoblast tumor patients. The test system utilized has been a modification of the Hellstrom assay. Terminal thymidine labeling of target cells incubated with the patient's lymphocytes in the absence and the presence of the patient's serum has permitted the identification of host lymphocyte cytotoxicity or blocking of cytotoxicity against cancer antigen on malignant trophoblast cells. The target cell systems have been maintained in continuous culture (BeWo and JAr lines). The presence of blocking of cytotoxicity has been determined to be present when the patient's serum is seen to block cytotoxicity. This is negative in the absence of tumor and reappears in the presence of active tumor growth. Using this assay, a direct correlation has been observed between tumor regression by the cytotoxicity assay and regression of the chorionic gonadotropin titer by the hCG radioimmunoassay. It is anticipated that extensive use of these assays will provide important new knowledge in the delineation of the origin and in the treatment of trophoblast neoplasms.

REFERENCES

1. Baggish, M. S., Woodruff, J. D., Tow, S. H., and Jones, N., Sex chromatin pattern in hydatidiform mole, Amer. J. Obstet. Gynecol. 102:362 (1968).
2. Surti, U. and Szulman, A., Complete hydatidiform mole with 46 XY karyotype, Human Genetics 51:153 (1979).
3. Lawler, S., HLA and trophoblastic tumours, Brit. Med. Bull. 34: 305 (1978).
4. Shaw, A. R. E., Dasgupta, M. K., Kovithavongs, T., Johny, K. V., LeRiche, J. C., Dossetor, J. B., and McPhearson, T. A., Humoral and cellular immunity to paternal antigens in trophoblastic neoplasia, Int. J. Cancer 24:586 (1979).
5. Tomoda, Y., Fuma, M., Saiki, N., Ishivuka, Z., and Akaza, T., Immunologic studies in patients with trophoblastic neoplasia, Amer. J. Obstet. Gynecol. 126:661 (1976).
6. Robinson, E., Ben-Hur, N., Zuckerman, H., and Neuman, Z., Further immunologic studies in patients with choriocarcinoma and hydatidiform mole, Cancer Res. 27:1202 (1967).
7. Bagshawe, K., Choriocarcinoma: the clinical biology of the trophoblast and its tumors, London, Arnold (1969), p. 292.
8. Mogensen, B. and Kissmeyer-Nielson, F., Histocompatibility antigens on the HLA locus in generalized gestational choriocarcinoma, Lancet 1:721 (1968).
9. Mogensen, B., Kissmeyer-Nielsen, F., and Hauge, M., Histocompatibility antigens on the HLA locus in gestational choriocarcinoma, Transplant. Proc. 1:76 (1969).
10. Rudolph, R. and Thomas, E., Histocompatibility studies in patients with trophoblastic tumors, Amer. J. Obstet. Gynecol. 108:1126 (1970).
11. Temin, H. M., The protovirus hypothesis: speculations on the significance of RNA directed DNA synthesis for normal development and for carcinogenesis, J. Natl. Cancer Inst. 46:III (1971)(Guest editorial).
12. Temin, H. M., Nature of the provirus of Rous sarcoma, Natl. Cancer Inst. Monogr. 17:557 (1964).
13. Civantos, F. and Rywlin, A. M., Carcinomas with trophoblastic differentiation and secretion of chorionic gonadotrophins, Cancer 29:789 (1972).
14. Regan, J. F. and Cremin, J. H., Chorioniepthelioma of the stomach, Amer. J. Surg. 100:224 (1967).
15. Rosen, S. W., Becker, C. E., Schlaff, S., Easton, J., and Gluck, M. C., Ectopic gonadotropin production before clinical

recognition of bronchogenic carcinoma, New Engl. J. Med. 279: 640 (1968).
16. McKechnie, J. C. and Fechner, R., Choriocarcinoma and adenocarcinoma of the esophagus with gonadotropin secretion, Cancer 27:694 (1971).
17. Castleman, B., Scully, R. E., and McNeely, B. U., Case records of the Massachusetts General Hospital, New Engl. J. Med. 286: 713 (1972).
18. Ainsworth, R. W. and Gresham, G. A., Primary chorioncarcinoma of the urinary bladder in a male, J. Pathol. Bacteriol. 79: 185 (1960).
19. Edmonds, L. C. and Cerrera, G. M., Extragenital choriocarcinoma, J. Pediatr. 67:94 (1965).
20. Bennington, J. L., Haber, S. L., and Schweid, A., Primary mediastinal choriocarcinoma, Dis. Chest 46:623 (1964).
21. Jernstrom, P. and McLaughlin, H., Choriocarcinoma of the thymus, J. Amer. Med. Assoc. 182:147 (1962).
22. McArthur, J. W., Para-endocrine phenomena in obstetrics and gynecology, Progr. Gynecol. 4:146 (1963).
23. Rubin, P., Cancer of the urogenital tract: testicular tumors, J. Amer. Med. Assoc. 213:89 (1970).
24. Hershman, J. M., Starnes, W. R., Kenimer, J. G., and Pattillo, R. A., Human chorionic thyrotropin, Proc. 4th Intl. Congr. Hormonal Steroids, Amsterdam, Excerpta Medica.
25. Breen, J. L., Ovarian malignancy in children, with special reference to the germ-cell tumors, Ann. N. Y. Acad. Sci. 12: 658 (1967).
26. Stevens, L. C., Genetic control of experimental teratocarcinogenesis in mice, Anat. Rec. 151:420 (1965)).
27. Billingham, R. E., Transplantation immunity and the maternal-fetal relation, New Engl. J. Med. 270:667 (1964).
28. Simmons, R. L. and Russell, P. S., The antigenicity of mouse trophoblast, Ann. N. Y. Acad. Sci. 99:717 (1962).
29. Moller, G., Beckman, V., and Lundgren, G., In vitro destruction of human fibroblasts by non-immune lymphoid cells, Nature 212:1203 (1966).
30. Kirby, D. R., Bradbury, W. D., and Goldstein, D. J., Antigen barrier in the mouse placenta, Nature 204:548 (1964).
31. Bradbury, S., Billington, W. D., and Kirby, D. R., A histochemical and electron microscopical study of fibrinoid of the mouse placenta, J. Roy. Microsc. Soc. 84:199 (1965).
32. Currie, G. A., Doornick, A., and Bagshawe, K. D., Effect of neuraminidase on the immunogenicity of early mouse trophoblast, Nature 219:191 (1968).
33. Haskova, V., Transplantation non-antigenicity of the fetal placenta, Nature 193:278 (1962).
34. Douglas, G. W., The immunological role of the placenta, Obstet. Gynecol. Survey 20:442 (1965).
35. Lanman, J. T., Herod, L., and Fikrig, S., Homograft immunity in pregnancy survival rates in rabbits born of ova transplan-

ted into sensitized mothers, J. Exptl. Med. 119:781 (1964).
36. Tanigaki, N., Nakamuro, K., Natori, T., et al., Common antigenic structures of HLA antigens, Transplantation 18:74 (1974).
37. Doherty, P., Blanden, R., and Zinkernagel, R., Specificity of virus T cells for H-2K and H-2D compatible interaction: implication diversity, Transplant. Proc. 29:89 (1976).
38. Bevan, M., The major histocompatibility complex determines susceptibility to cytotoxic T cells directed against minor histocompatibility antigens, J. Exptl. Med. 142:1349 (1975).
39. Benacerraf, M. and McDevitt, H., The histocompatibility linked immune response genes, Science 175:273 (1972).
40. McDevitt, H. and Bodmer, W., HL-A immune-response genes and disease, Lancet 1:1269 (1974).
41. Blanden, R., Doherty, P., Dunlop, M., et al., Genes required for cytotoxicity against virus infected target cells in K and D regions of H_2 complex, Nature 254:269 (1975).
42. Shearer, G., Rehn, T., and Garbarino, C., Cell-mediated lympholysis of trinitrophenyl-modified autologous lymphocytes. Effector cell specificity to modified cell surface components controlled by the H-2K and H-2D serological regions of the murine major histocompatibility complex, J. Exptl. Med. 141:1348 (1975).
43. Shearer, G., Cell-mediated cytotoxicity to trinitrophenyl-modified syngeneic lymphocytes, Eur. J. Immunol. 4:527 (1974).
44. Jensen, D. and Good, S., Mixed lymphocyte reaction and placentation, Nature New Biol. 240:211 (1972).
45. Billington, W., Influence of immunological dissimilarity of mother and fetus on size of placenta in mice, Nature 202:317 (1964).
46. Faulk, W. and Temple, A., Distribution of $beta_2$microglobulin and HLA in chorionic villi in human placentae, Nature 262: 799 (1976).
47. Johnson, D. and Faulk, W., Immunological studies of human placentae: identification and distribution of proteins in immature chorionic villi, Immunology 34:1027 (1975).
48. Goodfellow, P., Barnstable, C., Bodmer, W., et al., Expression of HLA antigen systems on placenta, Transplantation 22:595 (1976).
49. Trowsdale, J., Bodmer, W., Pattillo, R., and Travers, P., Expression of HLA-ABC and $beta_2$microglobulin in human choriocarcinoma cell lines, J. Exptl. Med. 152 (1980) In press.
50. Loke, Y., Joysey, V., and Borland, R., HL-A antigens on human trophoblast cells, Nature 232:403 (1971).
51. Wegmann, T., Singh, B., and Carlson, G., Allogeneic placenta is a paternal strain antigen immunoabsorbent, J. Immunol. 122:270 (1979).
52. Brochier, J., Bonneau, M., Robert, M., et al., Anti-HLA-R alloantibodies eluted from human placental tissue, Transplant.

Proc. 9:779 (1979).
53. Barnstable, C. and Bodmer, W., Immunology and the fetus, Lancet 1:326 (1978).
54. Gleicher, N., Beers, P., Cohen, C. J., Kerenyi, T., and Gusberg, S. B., Leukocyte migration enhancement as an indicator of immunologic enhancement. I. Pregnancy, Amer. J. Obstet. Gynecol. 136:1 (1980).
55. Gleicher, N., Beers, P., Cohen, C. J., Kerenyi, T., and Gusberg, S. B., Leukocyte migration enhancement as an indicator of immunologic enhancement. II. Malignancy, Amer. J. Obstet. Gynecol. 136:126 (1980).
56. Gleicher, N., Deppe, G., and Cohen, C. J., Common aspects of immunologic tolerance in pregnancy and malignancy, Obstet. Gynecol. 54:335 (1979).
57. Gerencer, M., Kastelan, A., Drazancic, A., et al., The HLA antigens in women with recurrent abnormal pregnancies of unknown etiology, Tissue Antigens 12:223 (1978).
58. Billingham, R., Transplantation immunity and the maternal-fetal relation, New Engl. J. Med. 270:667 (1964).
59. Anderson, J., Transplantation - nature's success, Lancet 2: 1077 (1971).
60. Gerencer, M., Drazancic, A., and Kuvacic, I., HLA studies in women with recurrent gestational disorders, Fertil. Steril. 31:401 (1979).
61. Komlos, L. and Halbrecht, I., Repeated abortions and histocompatibility antigens. Can HLA antigen restricted gene dose effects influence the feto-maternal relationship, Med. Hypotheses, 5:901 (1979).
62. Tomoda, U., Fuma, M., Saiki, N., et al., Immunologic studies in patients with trophoblastic neoplasia, Amer. J. Obstet. Gynecol. 126:661 (1976).
63. Robinson, E., Ben-Hur, N., Zuckerman, H., et al., Further immunologic studies in patients with choriocarcinoma and hydatidiform mole, Cancer Res. 27:1202 (1967).
64. Bagshawe, K., Choriocarcinoma: The clinical biology of trophoblast and its tumors, London: Arnold (1969).
65. Bach, F., Bach, M., and Klein, J., Genetic and immunological complexity of major histocompatibility regions, Science 176: 1024 (1972).
66. Pattillo, R. A., HLA haplotypes in choriocarcinoma, in: "Transcripts of 7th Rochester Trophoblast Conference," H. Thiede, ed., p. 110 (1977).
67. Hammond, C. and Parker, R. T., Diagnosis and treatment of trophoblastic disease: a report from the Southeastern Regional Center, Obstet. Gynecol. 35:132 (1970).
68. Curry, S., Hammond, C. B., Tyrey, L., Creasman, W. T., et al., Hydatidiform mole: diagnosis, management and long-term follow up, Obstet. Gynecol. 45:1 (1975).
69. Doherty, P. C., Blanden, R. V., Zinkernagel, R. M., Specificity of virus-immune effector T-cells for H-2K and H-2D compatible

interaction: implications for H-antigen diversity, Transplant. Rev. 29:89 (1976).
70. Gordon, R. D., Simpson, E., and Samelson, L. C., In vitro cell-mediated immune responses to the male specific (H-Y) antigen in mice, J. Exptl. Med. 142:1108 (1975).
71. Shearer, G., Cell-mediated cytotoxicity to trinitrophenyl-modified syngeneic lymphocytes, Eur. J. Immunol. 4:527 (1974).
72. Fisher, B. and Fisher, E. T., Studies concerning the regional lymph node in cancer, Cancer 27:1001 (1971).
73. Khoo, S. K. and Mackay, E. R., Immunologic reactivity of female patients with genital cancer: status in preinvasive, locally invasive, and disseminated disease, Amer. J. Obstet. Gynecol. 119:1018 (1974).
74. Nalick, R. H., DiSaia, P. J., Rea, T. H., and Morrow, C. P., Immunocompetence and prognosis in patients with gynecologic cancer, Gynecol. Oncol. 2:81 (1974).
75. Chen, S. S., Koffler, D., and Cohen, C. J., Cellular hypersensitivity in patients with squamous-cell carcinoma of the cervix, Amer. J. Obstet. Gynecol. 121:91 (1975).
76. Chen, S. Y., Koffler, D., and Cohen, C. J., Cell-mediated immunity in patients with ovarian carcinoma, Amer. J. Obstet. Gynecol. 115:467 (1973).
77. DiSaia, P. J., Sinkovics, J. G., Rutledge, R. N., and Smith, J. P., Cell-mediated immunity to human malignant cells, Amer. J. Obstet. Gynecol. 114:979 (1972).
78. Nalick, R. H., DiSaia, P. J., Rea, T. H., and Morrow, M. H., Immunologic response in gynecologic malignancy as demonstrated by the delayed hypersensitivity reaction: clinical correlations, Amer. J. Obstet. Gynecol. 118:398 (1974).
79. Khoo, S. K. and Mackay, E. V., Relation of vell-mediated immunity in women with genital tract cancer to origin, hisoloty, clinical stage and subsequent behavious of neoplasm, Obstet. Gynaecol. Brit. Commonw. 81:229 (1974).
80. Feldman, M., Williams, R. C., et al., Cell collaboration between T and B lymphocytes and macrophages in antibody production in vivo, in: "Lymphocytes and Their Interactions: Recent Observations," New York, RAven Press (1975).
81. David, J. R., Macrophage migration, Fed. Proc. 27:6 (1968).
82. McCoy, J. L., Jerome, L. F., Dean, J. H., et al., Inhibition of leukocyte migration by tumor-associated antigens in soluble extracts of human breast carcinoma, J. Natl. Cancer Inst. 53:11 (1974).
83. Pattillo, R. A., Sasaki, S., Katayama, K. P., Roesler, M., and Mattingly, R. F., Genesis of 46,XY hydatidiform mole, Amer. J. Obstet. Gynecol. 141:104 (1981).

IMMUNOLOGY IN GENESIS OF PARTIAL AND TOTAL HYDATIDIFORM MOLE

Shoshichi Takeuchi

Department of Obstetrics and Gynecology
School of Medicine
Niigata University
Niigata, Japan

INTRODUCTION

In early pregnancy, a variety of pathology of trophoblastic cells is observed in trophoblastic disease and in spontaneous abortion. Trophoblastic disease includes hydatidiform mole, metastatic and/or invasive mole, and choriocarcinoma. Therefore, for better understanding of trophoblastic disease and spontaneous abortion, an exact knowledge of the morbid anatomy of trophoblasts is required. Especially needed is profound insight into regulatory mechanisms of *in vivo* trophoblastic growth which may undergo either damage or proliferation and survival. But the regulatory mechanisms are not clear because of their complexity, involving cellular factors such as benign or malignant neoplastic cellular changes, and/or environmental factors such as nutritional, endocrinological, and immunological factors.

Since the advent of chemotherapy, research on trophoblastic disease has been dominated by the idea that hydatidiform mole, invasive mole, and choriocarcinoma are not individual disease entities, but rather constitute a single entity, that of trophoblastic neoplasm. The results of many experimental and clinical studies have been interpreted, for clinical convenience alone, that trophoblastic disease occurs as a result of neoplastic changes of normal trophoblasts. In other words, molar trophoblasts have become more active than normal trophoblasts, through cellular change. The modified molar trophoblast changes into sort of a benign neoplasm, and progresses further through cellular change to semimalignant invasive mole, which in turn further advances to malignant choriocarcinoma (1-3). This concept is clearly based on the idea that the cellular factors may be more dominant than the environmental factors in genesis of trophoblastic disease. We must, however, admit that clear evidence for neoplastic changes in hydatidiform mole has never been reported, with the exception of its propensity for remote metastases and myometrial invasion. Just as molar trophoblasts undergo myometrial invasion and/or remote metastases (deportation), so do normal trophoblasts. Therefore, it may be difficult to find any reason, at least for hydatidiform mole, to be categorized into neoplasm, though the term, neoplasm, is very complex conceptually and is difficult to define precisely.

On the other hand, cytogenetic studies on trophoblastic disease and spontaneous abortion have been made. The recent consensus is that total hydatidiform moles come mainly from zygotes of androgenetic origin (4-11), partial moles often come from triploid conceptuses (12-15), and spontaneous abortions, in about 60% of cases, come from conceptuses with chromosomal anomalies such as trisomies, monosomies, etc. (16-18). Furthermore, it has been recognized that trophoblasts must play a pivotal role in an immunologically hostile mother in order for successful maintenance of pregnancy (19-23), and that the correlation between trophoblastic cell growth and immunologic factors may be close (22-25). Needless to say, the consensus holds that immunology is strictly dependent upon genetics. Therefore, to elucidate the genesis or nature of hydatidiform mole and spontaneous abortion, studies are clearly required from both immunologic and cytogenetic aspects. Unfortunately, however, immunologic studies on hydatidiform mole as well as spontaneous abortion are scant.

In this context, extensive immunologic studies on hydatidiform mole and spontaneous abortion have been made in our laboratory for more than a decade, and have led us to the view that an immune selection mechanism regulated by blocking (or enhancing) antibodies may play an important role in determining the destiny of the conceptuses, be they normal pregnancy, spontaneous abortion, partial mole or total hydatidiform mole (26-28). Immune dependency of trophoblastic cell growth was also strongly suggested in our studies, which led us to an alternative concept on the nature of hydatidiform mole, including invasive mole. Both invasive mole and hydatidiform mole are types of abortion with a variety of trophoblastic hyperplasia resulting from continuing production of blocking antibodies after early demise of embryo proper (or inner cell mass) due to lethal abnormality and higher MHC antigenicity of androgenetic fertilized ova. Therefore, the whole story of genesis of hydatidiform mole, we believe, may be described without the presumption of neoplastic change of molar trophoblast.

TROPHOBLASTIC CELL GROWTH IN EARLY NORMAL AND ABNORMAL PREGNANCY

Hydatidiform mole as well as normal placenta in first trimester show a variety of trophoblastic hyperplasia. By contrast, spontaneous abortion shows mostly trophoblastic damage and degeneration. In these situations of early pregnancy, the phenotype has been found to relate to the genotype of the chromosomes. In particular, trophoblastic cell growth and size or grade of villous swelling are closely correlated with kinds of chromosomal anomalies.

Correlation Between Trophoblastic Cell Growth and Genotypes in Conceptuses

Spontaneous abortion. Spontaneous abortions are usually subdivided into subclinical (occult) and clinical forms. The former, usually not diagnosed by the clinician, occur the ovular phase of development before the sixth week of gestation. The latter, usually easily diagnosed clinically, is further subgrouped into early abortion and late abortion. Early abortion occurs during embryonal development, between the sixth and tenth weeks of gestational age; late abortion occurs during the fetal phase of development, between 11 and 28 weeks of gestational age. About 60% of early spontaneous abortions have been demonstrated to reveal chromosomal aberrations. The aberrations, in descending order of frequency, include trisomies, triploidies, monosomies, tetraploidies, and structural anomalies (16, 17).

Those aberrations with lethal chromosomal anomalies may result in primary demise of the embryo proper, followed by secondary trophoblastic cell damage, thus giving rise to spontaneous abortions. Clinical early spontaneous abortions are considered to occur 3 to 5 weeks after embryonal demise (16). During this period, the trophoblastic cells may undergo damage. In spontaneous abortions there is, needless to say, another type in which primary trophoblastic cell damage occurs and is followed by secondary embryonal death. The latter is usually observed in an unexplained habitual abortion occurring during the embryonal phase of development.

Habitual abortion is defined as three or more consecutive spontaneous abortions within 24 weeks of gestation and not resulting in a live birth. Habitual abortions constitute 0.1% to 0.5% of all women becoming pregnant for the third time (63). Possible causes of habitual abortion are maternal anatomical defects, infections, hormonal disturbances, chronic renal failure, coagulation defects, pollutants, and chromosomal aberrations which are often of the translocation type. In unexplained habitual abortions, the frequency of chromosomal anomalies is notably far less than in incidental single early spontaneous abortions. Trophoblastic cell damage is usually observed in unexplained habitual abortions.

Thus, we may conclude that almost all spontaneous abortions in early pregnancy reveal more or less trophoblastic damage.

Total (complete) hydatidiform mole. Complete moles reveal a variety of hyperplasia of the surviving trophoblastic cells, and were proved to arise from zygotes of androgenetic origin. In 96% of cases, the complete moles have a 46,XX karyotype and in 4%, a 46,XY karyotype (29). Androgenesis is the development of an ovum under the influence of a spermatozoan nucleus, the egg nucleus being either absent or inactivated. This process would account for the predominance of 46,XX mole, because the YY counterparts are probably lost during the early cleavage stage. Although complete moles appear to have a normal karyotype, they have a serious chromosomal anomaly, that is, androgenesis in which the zygote inherits two haploid sets from the father but none from the mother. Androgenesis of the zygote may arise from duplication of the chromosomes fertilized by a haploid sperm, resulting in a 46,XX karyotype of which all is homozygous. This process has been proved to be the main mechanism of genesis of hydatidiform moles, as shown in Fig. 1. The complete mole may also arise from an ovum fertilized by two spermatozoa (dispermy), giving a 46,XX or 46,XY karyotype which is heterozygous (6-8). Genesis from an ovum fertilized by diploid sperm such as 46,XX or 46,XY coming from nondisjunction of the first meiosis during spermatogenesis can be considered theoretically, but has not been proved (9-11).

Total, or complete, hydatidiform moles are usually not accompanied by an embryo. Androgenesis may be a serious anomaly

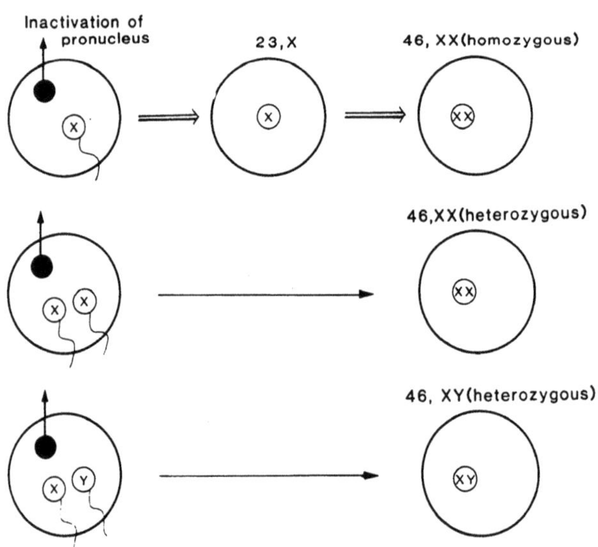

Fig. 1. Probable mechanism of androgenetic fertilization.

Table 1. Close Correlation Between Kinds of Chromosomal Anomalies and Trophoblastic Cell Growth

Pathology in early pregnancy	Kinds of chromosomal anomalies	Trophoblastic cell growth
Spontaneous abortion	Trisomy, monosomy, maternally derived triploidy	Degenerated and damaged
Partial hydatidiform mole	Mostly paternally derived triploidy	Survived and slight hyperplastic
Total (complete) hydatidiform mole	Mostly androgenesis	Survived and variously hyperplastic

for the embryo, so its demise would occur earlier during ovular (inner cell mass) development. It is likely that the more serious the chromosomal anomalies, the earlier the demise of the embryo.

Partial hydatidiform mole. Partial moles usually reveal only slight hyperplasia of the trophoblasts on the surface of the swollen villi, but not so rarely show a variety of focal hyperplasia.

Chromosomal anomalies of partial moles consist mainly of triploidy and, rarely, trisomies 2, 13, 16, and 18, in addition to double trisomies and tetraploidy (12, 15). Jacobs and associates (12) reported, from cytogenetic study of 106 triploidies, that all 51 paternally derived triploidies (diandry) in which a pathologic diagnosis could be made were partial moles, whereas only 3 of 15 maternally derived triploidies (digyny) in which a diagnosis could be made were partial moles. In other words, partial moles arising from triploidies come mainly from paternally derived triploidies. Furthermore, these workers demonstrated that the mean gestational age of the paternally derived triploidies was 122 days, while that of the maternally derived triploidies was only 74 days (12). Thus, in the case of triploidy, it is likely to be derived paternally through fertilization of dispermy, thereby constituting diploid from the father and haploid from the mother.

Partial hydatidiform moles are usually accompanied by the embryo. In most of them, demise of the embryo may be considered to occur during the embryonal phase, after the ovular phase of development has occurred. As summarized in Table 1, the correlation between kinds of chromosomal anomalies and trophoblastic cell growth

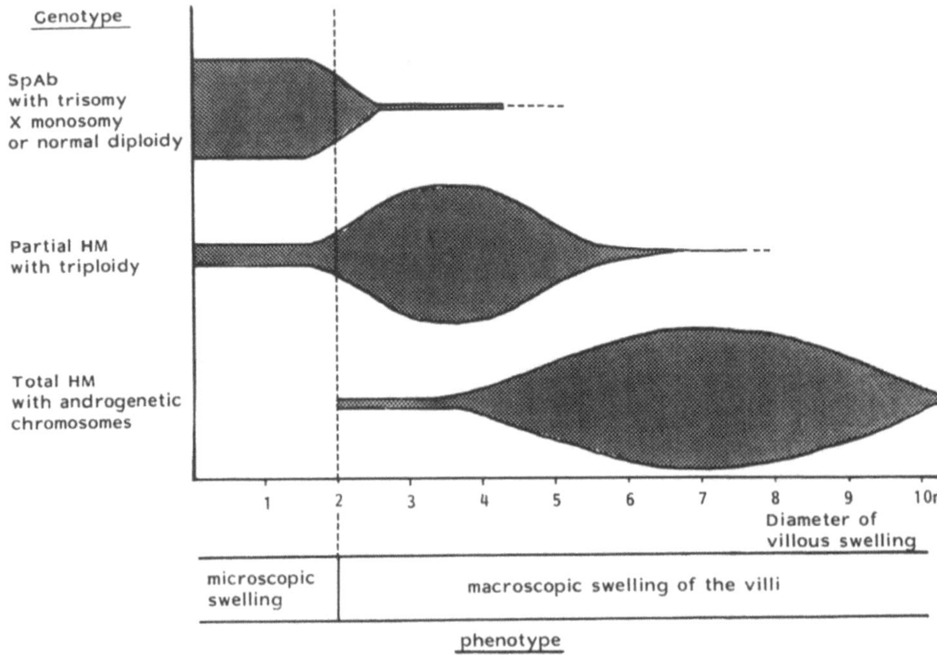

Fig. 2. Relative frequency of size of villous hydropic swelling (phenotype) related to chromosomal anomalies (genotype). Hydropic swellings more than 2 cm in diameter are easily recognized grossly by most observers.
Abbreviations: SpAb, spontaneous abortion; HM, hydatidiform mole.

may therefore be very close.

Correlation Between Size of Villous Hydropic Swelling and Genotypes in Conceptuses

Spontaneous abortion. Microscopic hydatidiform change recognized only by microscope is observed in about two-thirds of spontaneous abortions with chromosomal anomalies such as trisomies, X-monosomies, or triploidies, while it is found in only 10% of therapeutically induced abortions in early pregnancy.

Partial hydatidiform mole. Hydatidiform change ranging from microscopic to macroscopic villous hydrops is observed in some villi. Chromosomal anomalies of partial mole were previously described.

Total (complete) hydatidiform mole. Macroscopic swelling involving all the villi is observed in complete mole in which embryo, cord, or amniotic membrane are usually absent. Typical central cistern formation is observed in many villi, but mazy cistern formation or edematous change are also found in some villi. When preserved, the stroma of the villi have the appearance of immature mesenchyme, and occasionally fetal capillaries are seen. Nucleated blood cells are never observed.

Thus, correlation between size of villous hydrops and genotype may be very close, as illustrated in Fig. 2.

Nature's Experimental System for Elucidation of Immune Dependency of Trophoblastic Cell Growth

It is now very clear that more consideration must be given to the work of Hertig and Edmonds (30) on the genesis of total hydatidiform mole and to that of Hertig (31), in which the morphological progressive changes from early microscopic mole in spontaneous abortions with chromosomal anomalies, through transitional mole to total hydatidiform mole, were faced.

Important but neglected facts in their investigations are that the destiny of conceptuses after early demise of embryo proper due to pathologic ovum may be either the spontaneous abortion with trophoblastic damage or the partial or total mole with a variety of trophoblastic hyperplasia (32). Blighted or pathologic ova, as Hertig and associates termed them, have now been clarified by cytogenetic study as having various chromosomal anomalies. Blighted ova with frequent chromosomal anomalies such as trisomy or monosomy may be lost as spontaneous abortions after demise of the embryo, but the remaining blighted ova, when derived by paternal triploidy, may develop to partial mole and, with androgenesis, eventually develop to total hydatidiform moles, as depicted in Fig. 3.

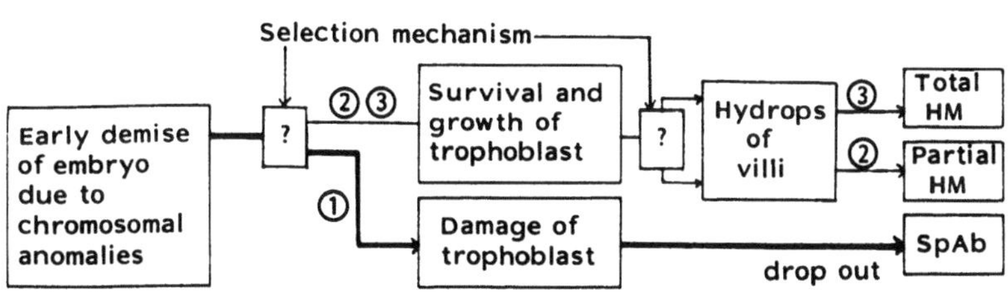

Fig. 3. Nature's experimental system in early pregnancy. The destiny of the conceptus after early demise of the embryo due to chromosomal anomalies is either spontaneous abortion or hydatidiform mole. The selection mechanism must be closely related to kinds of chromosomal anomalies. *Circled numbers: 1*, trisomy, monosomy, triploidy, etc.; *2*, paternally derived triploidy; *3*, androgenesis. Abbreviations: SpAb, spontaneous abortion; HM, hydatidiform mole.

Therefore, it is now very likely that there may be a close correlation between phenotype and genotype found in spontaneous abortion, partial hydatidiform mole, and total (complete) hydatidiform mole. The published studies, however, do not solve the problem of correlating morphological and cytogenetic aspects of these diseases. In this context, it may be very important to clarify the following two mechanisms according to kinds of chromosomal anomalies, by introduction of the immunologic aspect. The first mechanism is the immunologic regulatory mechanism involved in trophoblastic cell growth; the second concerns problems in formation of villous hydrops, especially related to duration of the existence of villous circulation, depending on the timing when demise of the embryo occurs, and trophoblastic cell activity.

Thus the immunological study on spontaneous abortion, partial mole and total mole in relation to normal first trimester pregnancy would clearly constitute a natural experimental system for elucidation of these problems. To the best of our knowledge, however, immunologic studies on this system have been neglected and thus, heretofore never studied. In our laboratory, comparative studies on the immunology of this system have been made intensively for more than a decade. Consequently, we would like to place more emphasis on the importance and usefulness of study on this system in order to better understand the nature of these diseases and further the advancement of reproductive immunology by associating immunology with cytogenetics in spontaneous abortion and hydatidiform mole.

IMMUNOLOGICAL STUDY ON NATURE'S EXPERIMENTAL SYSTEM IN EARLY PREGNANCY

Antithetic Difference Between Spontaneous Abortion and Partial or Total Hydatidiform Mole in Production of Blocking Antibodies by Patients

Comparative study on the immunology of this system has been made intensively in our laboratory to determine how the immunological mechanism selects a destiny for the conceptus after the early demise of the embryo (23-25). We have found that the antigens of the conceptus are immunogenic to the mother. As a consequence, the mother produces both humoral and cell-mediated immunity against the conceptus in abnormal pregnancy, such as spontaneous abortion and hydatidiform mole, in addition to normal first trimester pregnancy. A distinct antithetic difference between spontaneous abortion and hydatidiform mole was found in the amount of blocking antibodies produced by the mother, and blocking antibody-related phenomena.

Amount of blocking antibodies produced by the patients. The amount of blocking antibodies in sera of patients was estimated by their blocking effect on one-way mixed leucocyte reaction (MLR) performed between spouses:

$$\% \text{ Blocking effect} = (1 - \frac{\text{MLR in autologous serum}}{\text{MLR in control serum}}) \times 100\%$$

It is clear that the higher the blocking effect, the more blocking antibodies are present. Therefore, the amount of blocking antibodies would be represented by the blocking of the patient's serum.

The blocking effect of sera from patients with spontaneous abortion was 7% ± 13%, whereas that from patients with complete mole was 34% ± 20%, showing a statistically significant difference between the two diseases, as summarized in Fig. 4. Furthermore, the blocking effect of sera from patients with partial mole was 22% ± 10%, indicating a significant increase relative to that of spontaneous abortion. A noteworthy result in spontaneous abortion was that production of blocking antibodies, as evidenced by blocking effect, showed some decrease in the threatened stage (blocking effect = 20% ± 5%), and then declined rapidly in the inevitable abortion stage (blocking effect = 7% ± 13%)(Fig. 4).

In habitual aborters, the blocking antibodies produced were found to be sparse or absent, as pointed out by Rocklin and associates (45, 46) and as shown in Fig. 5.

Blocking antibody-related immunological phenomena (trophoblast-bound antibodies and placenta-bound IgG). Trophoblast-bound antibodies were studied by the indirect immunofluorescence technique. Positive findings in hydatidiform mole as well as in normal first trimester pregnancy included the observation of IgG in a granular pattern on the trophoblast cells. By contrast, in spontaneous abortion mainly IgM was observed, arranged in a linear pattern on the trophoblasts (33).

Placenta-bound IgG was prepared from each placenta obtained from hydatidiform mole and normal term pregnancy, thus providing us with enough IgG for our mixed leucocyte reaction blocking assays. Our impression was that IgG might bind to molar trophoblasts in greater amounts than to normal placenta (34). On the other hand, it was difficult to obtain sufficient IgG when the source was pooled aborted trophoblasts from 10 patients. This suggested that the amount of placenta-bound IgG in spontaneous abortions was scanty (35). No notable differences were observed in the IgG prepared from placenta and sera (34).

Capability of trophoblastic cells to bind with autologous antibodies. Immune adherence tests were performed on the trophoblasts after pretreatment with autologous serum. Positive results were found in 23.5% of spontaneous abortions, in 0% of hydatidiform

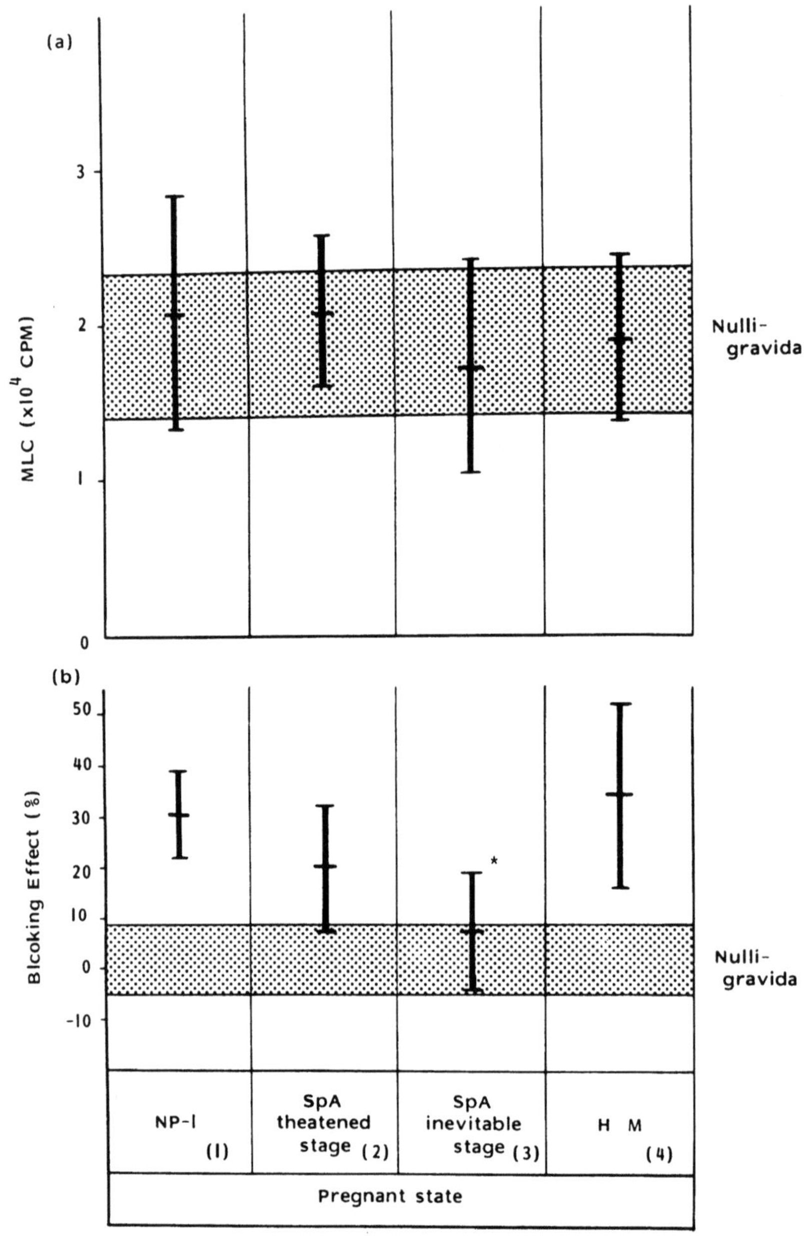

*: Statistically significant ($p < 0.05$)
(3) : [(1),(2) or (4)]

Fig. 4. One-way MLC in couples in the pregnant state, and the blocking effect of maternal sera on MLC.
Abbreviations: NP-1, normal first trimester pregnancy; SpAb, spontaneous abortion; HM, hydatidiform mole.

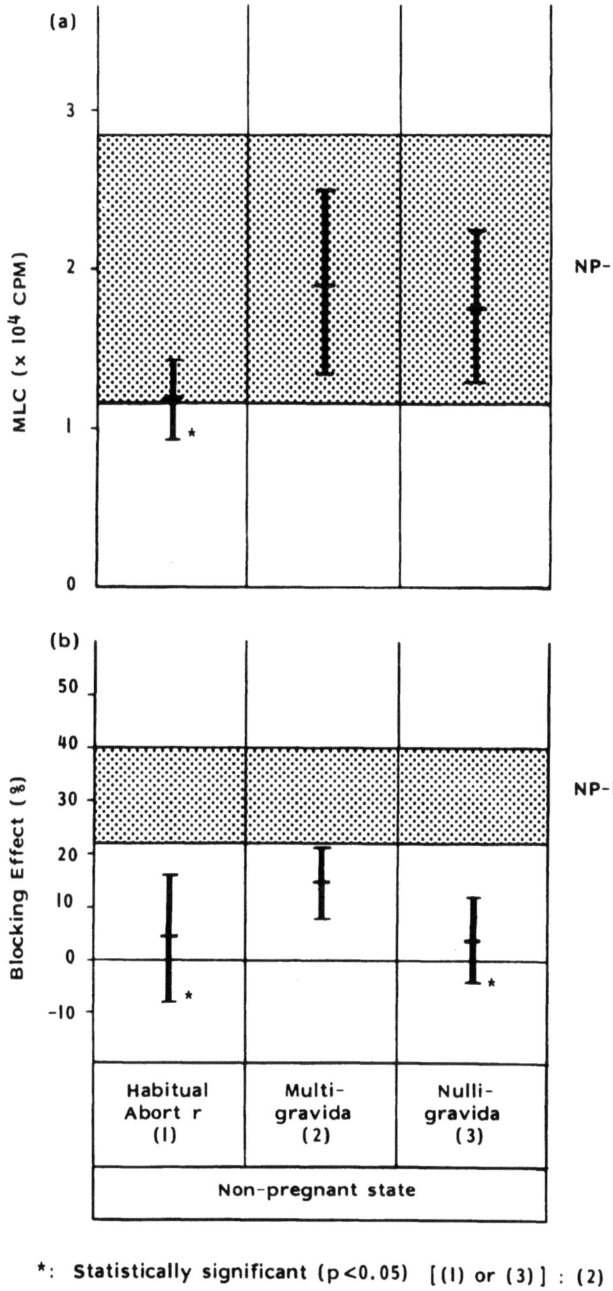

Fig. 5. One-way mixed leucocyte reaction (MLC) in couples in the nonpregnant state, and the blocking effect of maternal serum on the MLC. Abbreviation: NP-1, normal first trimester pregnancy (range indicated by *shaded area*).

moles, and in 9.4% of normal first trimester pregnancies (23). This result may suggest that capability of trophoblastic cells to bind with autologous antibodies in spontaneous abortion was greater than that of hydatidiform mole and normal first trimester pregnancy, and thus antigenic expression on the trophoblastic cells was greater in spontaneous abortion than that in hydatidiform mole and normal pregnancy.

MHC antigenicity of conceptuses. Anti-HLA A or B antibody was found in 26% of hydatidiform moles (para 1.2 average) and in 7.1% of normal first trimester pregnancies (para 1.0 average), suggesting that molar conceptuses are more immunogenic to the mother than the conceptuses of normal first trimester pregnancy (23).

The higher antigenicity of molar trophoblast, as determined by production of anti-HLA A or anti-HLA B was reported earlier by Lawler (36). It must be considered from these results that MHC antigen is expressed on trophoblastic cells responsible for production of anti-MHC antibodies, because antigenic embryo proper is absent in hydatidiform moles.

Considerations in MHC Antigenicity of Trophoblastic Cells

Studies on mature human placentas have virtually failed to reveal class 1 MHC (HLA A, B, or C) antigens, β_2-microglobulin, or class 2 MHC (HLA D/DR) antigens on the plasma membranes of syncytiotrophoblast (37). That a thick sialomucin glycocalyx associated with the trophoblast plays an antigenic quarantining role was the once-popular belief, but has failed to withstand later critical investigations (38). In this context, some reports have shown the class 1 MHC antigens on experimentally dissociated trophoblastic cells (38-42) and on nonvillous trophoblastic cells in histological specimens (43, 44).

It has been unanimously recognized that class 2 MHC antigens on syncytiotrophoblast in direct contact with maternal blood are absent. The presence or absence of class 1 MHC antigens, however, has not come to universal agreement. Although most reports deny the presence of MHC antigens on syncytiotrophoblast, some reports reveal *in situ* expression of paternal class 1 MHC antigens on the sinusoidal face of human syncytiotrophoblast and murine labyrinthine trophoblastic cells exposed to maternal circulation (45, 46). Weak immunogenicity of trophoblast cells was suggested to be responsible for the absence of class 2 antigens, despite the presence of class 1 MHC antigens (45, 46). The next problem is the presence or absence of MHC antigens on cytotrophoblast not in direct contact with maternal tissue or blood, and some reports have suggested their presence (47). As described above, the high levels of anti-HLA A or B antibodies found in the blood of women with total hydatidiform moles in which antigenic embryo proper is absent may be responsible for class 1 MHC antigens expressed on subpopulations of trophoblastic cells (23, 36).

Thus, the expression of MHC antigens on trophoblasts is strongly suggested to be changing dynamically by a mechanism such as antigenic modulation, depending on the presence or absence of anti-MHC antibodies. We should not neglect the significance of the trophoblast as a potential source of alloantigens responsible for stimulating the feto-maternal unit. Our results showing sharp antithetic immunological difference between spontaneous abortion and hydatidiform mole may be reasonably understood only on these considerations.

Characterization of Blocking Antibodies

A number of investigators have recognized the presence of blocking antibodies in the serum of multigravid women, which block the mixed leucocyte reaction or macrophage migration inhibition test performed between spouses (48-59).

Blocking effect was markedly decreased in absorbed serum from which IgG had been removed by anti-IgG affinity chromatography, and was regained by the addition of IgG extracted from multigravid women to the absorbed serum. Thus, the main component of blocking antibodies is IgG antibody (23, 48-51).

The blocking antibodies are not removed by exhaustive absorption with pooled human platelets, but are removed by absorption with corresponding B lymphocytes. Thus, the main IgG was indicated to be antibodies to HLA D locus determinants, which have Ia-like antigens (34, 59).

As shown in Fig. 6, individual specificity of blocking antibodies was uncertain. Sera from normal first trimester pregnancy and from hydatidiform mole demonstrated the presence of blocking antibodies, not only to the respective autologous mixed leucocyte reaction, but also to the unrelated mixed leucocyte reaction in spontaneous abortion. Furthermore, sera from spontaneous abortion patients revealed the absence of, or only sparce, blocking antibodies on both autologous and unrelated mixed leucocyte reactions performed between spouses in spontaneous abortion and even in normal first trimester pregnancy and hydatidiform mole. Considering that blocking antibodies are antibodies against HLA D/DR of the conceptus inherited from the husband, this result may not be understandable (59).

We found, however, that individual specificity of blocking antibodies was great when mixed leucocyte reaction between mother and baby was performed with B lymphocytes as stimulator, as shown in Fig. 7. By contrast, the mixed leucocyte reaction was not great when performed with whole lymphocytes (59). Furthermore, we found

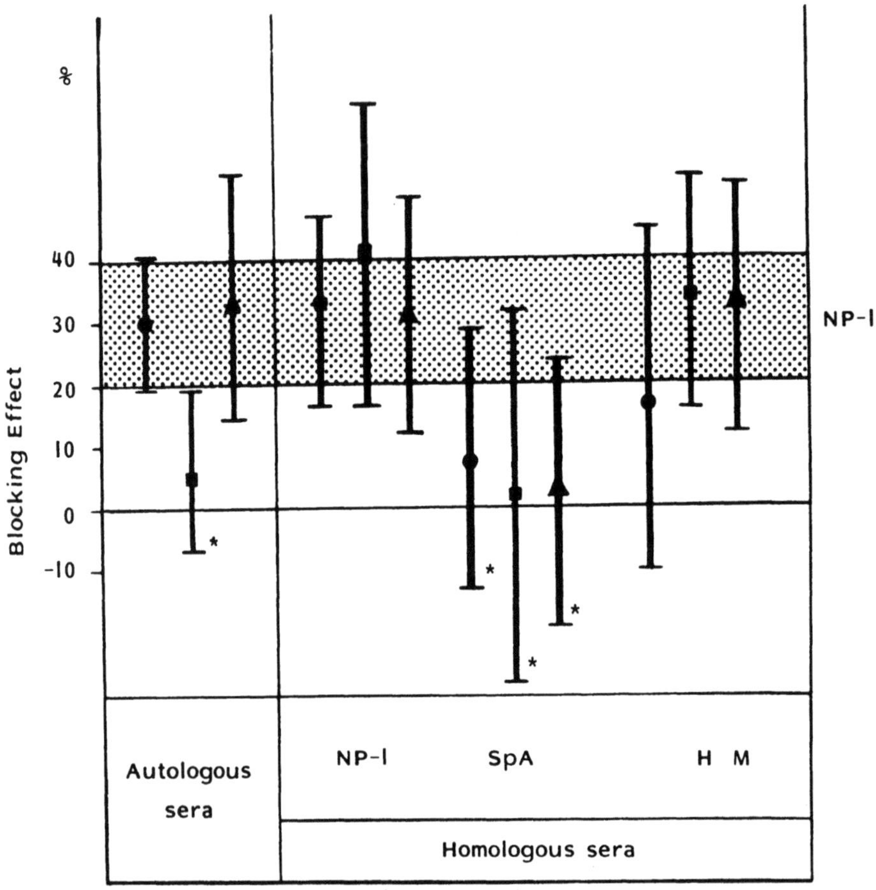

MLC in couples of NP-I (●), SpA (■), HM (▲)
*: Statistically significant (P<0.05)

NP-I: normal pregnancy in the first trimester,
SpA: spontaneous abortion,
H M: hydatidiform mole.

Fig. 6. Blocking effect of autologous and homologous sera on the mixed leucocyte reaction performed in couples of normal first trimester pregnancy, spontaneous abortion, and hydatidiform mole, showing its less individual specificity.

that IgGs prepared from placenta showed greater individual specificity than those from sera, even when mixed leucocyte reaction was performed with whole lymphocytes (34, 56). These results may indicate the presence of antibodies that are not individually specific in blocking antibodies, in addition to individually specific anti-HLA D antibodies. The antibodies must clearly be related to pregnancy, so that stage-specific onco-developmental antigens

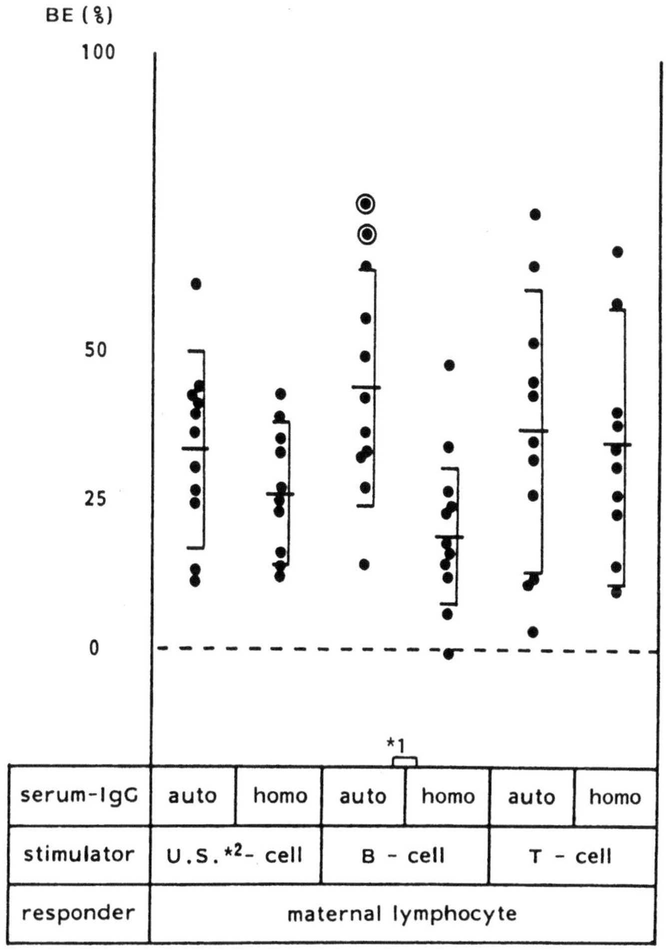

Fig. 7. Blocking effect of IgG from autologous and homologous sera on mixed leucocyte reaction performed between mother and baby. Individual specificity was observed when B cells were used as stimulator in the mixed leucocyte reactin. *BE*, blocking effect; *solid dots within circles*, positive cytotoxicity for B cell; **1*, P<0.01; **2*, unseparated; *auto*, autologous; *homo*, homologous.

appearing during development of the conceptus may be the most probable candidate, and their presence has never been clearly characterized so far. Thus, characterization of blocking factors, including blocking antibodies appearing in pregnancy, may be summarized at the present time as shown in Table 2.

Table 2. Blocking Factors Found in Pregnancy

I. Non-antibody factors

- A. Placental protein hormones: hCG, hPL
- B. Placental steroids: estrogens, progesterone
- C. Adrenal steroids: corticosteroids
- D. Proteins proper to placenta
  - 1. β_1-Glycoprotein: SP_1, PSBG, PAPP-C
  - 2. Placental proteins: PP_5, PAPP-A, PAPP-B
  - 3. Placenta-associated protein
    - a. Placenta-associated glycoprotein: α_2PAG, SP_3, PPZ
    - b. Placental protein: PP-1, PP-2, PP-3, PP-4, PP-6, PP-7, transcortin, transferrin
- E. Proteins proper to embryo
  - 1. Early pregnancy factors (EPF)
  - 2. α-Fetoprotein (AFP)

II. Antibody factors (blocking antibodies)

- A. Anti-MHC antibodies (individually specific)
  - 1. Anti-class 1 MHC antibodies
    Class 1 MHC: HLA A, HLA B, HLA C
  - 2. Anti-class 2 MHC antibodies
    Class 2 MHC: HLA D/DR
- B. Anti-ODP antibodies (not individually specific, but pregnancy related)

ODP: Onco-developmental proteins (stage/phase-specific embryonic/fetal proteins)

Correlation Between Amount of Blocking Antibodies Produced by the Mothers and Strength in MHC Antigenicity of the Conceptuses

Close correlation between blocking antibodies and MHC antigenicity. It was found in our laboratory that the amount of blocking antibodies produced by the mother was 7% ± 13%, 22% ± 10%, and 34% ± 20%, in terms of blocking effect in spontaneous abortion, partial mole, and total (complete) mole, respectively.

Here we need to note the varieties of chromosomal anomalies of these pathologic forms of early pregnancy. Spontaneous abortions are mainly trisomy or monosomy, partial moles are mainly paternally derived triploidy due to diandry, and total moles are androgenesis. We may interpret these chromosomal aberrations in terms of paternal

Table 3. Grouping of Conceptuses by Karyotype and MHC Antigenicity

Group	Karyotype	Paternal chromosomal contribution	MHC antigenicity to the mother
A1	Triploidy of digyny	33%	Lower
A2	Normal, trisomy, X-monosomy	50%	Average
B	Triploidy of diandry	67%	Higher
C	Androgenesis	100%	Highest

contribution of chromosomes as 50% in trisomy or monosomy, 67% in triploidy due to diandry, and 100% in androgenesis. It is very likely that the higher the percentage of paternal contribution, the stronger the MHC antigenicity of the conceptuses, and thus the greater the amount of blocking antibodies that are produced by the mothers.

From this consideration we may reasonably conclude that varieties of genotypes of the conceptuses should be understood in terms of strength in MHC antigenicity from the percentage of paternal chromosomal contribution, as shown in Table 3. Thus, there must be a close correlation between amount of blocking antibodies produced by the mother and strength in MHC antigenicity of the conceptuses.

Decrease in amount of produced blocking antibodies related to decrease in MHC antigenicity of the conceptuses after demise of the embryo proper. We found that the amount of blocking antibodies produced by the patients rapidly decreased from the threatened stage to the imminent stage of spontaneous abortions, as already described. The amount of produced blocking antibodies in habitual aborters was found to be sparse or absent despite repeated pregnancies (Fig. 8). Furthermore, similarity, especially in class 2 MHC antigens, between spouses with habitual abortion has been reported (60-67).

These results strongly suggest that a decrease in amount of blocking antibodies in spontaneous abortion may be responsible for decrease in MHC antigenicity of the conceptuses after demise of the embryo proper.

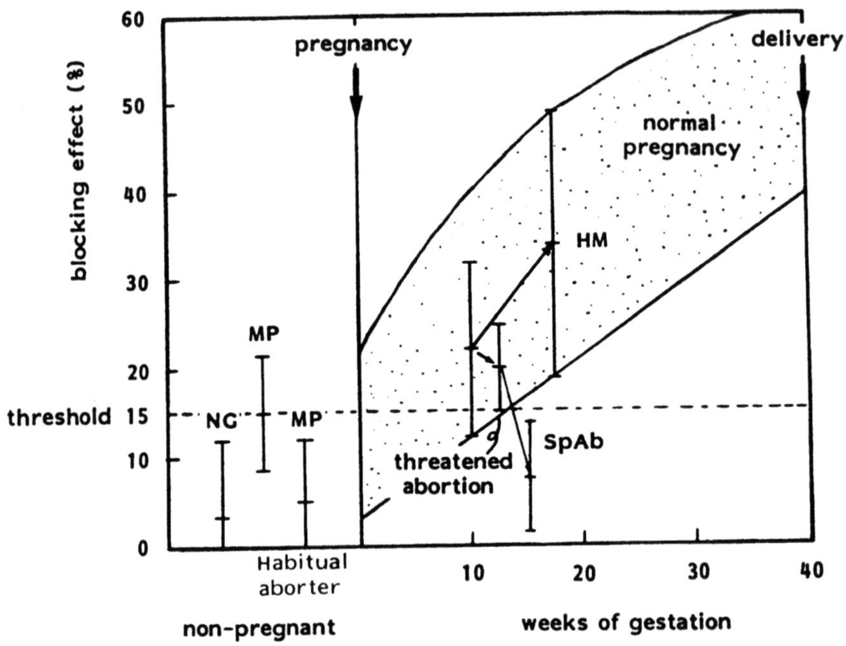

Fig. 8. Dynamic change in amount of blocking antibodies produced relative to the threshold. Abbreviations: NG, nulligravida; MP, multipara; SpAb, spontaneous abortion; HM, hydatidiform mole.

Correlation Between Amount of Blocking Antibodies Produced and Pattern of Trophoblastic Cell Growth in the Mothers

As shown in Table 1, there may be no doubt about the close correlation among pathology in early pregnancy, kinds of chromosomal anomalies, and pattern of trophoblastic cell growth. Here, we would like to discuss a role for amount of blocking antibodies produced in relation to this close correlation.

Trophoblastic cell growth depends on the amount of blocking antibodies produced by the mother. As shown in Table 4, we observed that the amount of blocking antibodies produced was sparse or absent in spontaneous abortions with degenerated and damaged trophoblasts, slightly greater in partial moles with slight hyperplasia of surviving trophoblasts, and greatest in complete moles with marked trophoblastic hyperplasia. It was sparse or absent in unexplained habitual abortion.

It is tempting to conclude from these results that damage or growth and survival of trophoblastic cells may depend on the amount of blocking antibodies produced by the mothers. In this context,

Table 4. Close Correlation Between Trophoblastic Cell Growth and Amount of Blocking Antibodies Produced

Pathology	Trophoblastic cell growth	Amount of blocking antibodies produced (blocking effect)
Spontaneous abortion	Damaged	Sparse or absent (7% ± 13%)
Partial hydatidiform mole	Slight hyperplasia	Slightly higher (22% ± 10%)
Total hydatidiform mole	Various hyperplasia (slightly to marked)	Highest (34% ± 20%)

however, the problem is that expression of MHC antigens may be absent on the surface of the syncytiotrophoblast. This problem has not been completely solved, but we are considering the possibility that antigenic modulation may be responsible for lack of expression of MHC antigen on the syncytiotrophoblast. This phenomenon has been under study in our laboratory.

Presumption of the presence of a threshold in amount of blocking antibodies produced for determining either damage or growth and survival of trophoblastic cells *in vivo*. The damage of trophoblast cells in spontaneous abortion, and their variable hyperplasia in hydatidiform mole, provide a sharp contrast between the two diseases. This is an all or none phenomenon in terms of trophoblastic growth pattern. Therefore, if it is right that trophoblastic cell growth may depend mainly on the amount of blocking antibodies produced, there must be a threshold that separates total lack of effect from total effect.

In our study, a threshold for rejection or nonrejection of trophoblast was presumed to be at a blocking effect of approximately 15%, because it was 3% ± 8% in nulligravida, 7% ± 13% in spontaneous abortion, and 20% ± 5% in normal first trimester pregnancy of primigravida, as shown in Fig. 8.

GENESIS OF PARTIAL HYDATIDIFORM MOLE FROM ZYGOTES OF PATERNALLY DERIVED TRIPLOIDY AND GENESIS OF TOTAL HYDATIDIFORM MOLE FROM ZYGOTES OF ANDROGENESIS

As shown in Fig. 3, the destiny of the conceptuses in Nature's Experimental System in early pregnancy is clearly either spontaneous abortions or hydatidiform moles after early demise of the embryo proper due to chromosomal anomalies. However, the question of what mechanism destines the conceptuses to be either spontaneous abortion or hydatidiform mole has never been answered from both morphologic and cytogenetic studies.

Our comparative immunological study on spontaneous abortions and hydatidiform moles strongly suggested that the unknown selection mechanism shown in Fig. 3 should an immunological one which is closely related to the genotype of the conceptuses.

Immunological Selection Mechanisms of Conceptuses into Either Spontaneous Abortion or Hydatidiform Mole after Early Embryonic Death

Fig. 9 describes our hypothesis relating to the immune selection mechanism. This mechanism is also an immunological regulatory mechanism for trophoblastic cell growth.

Women produce blocking antibodies in early pregnancy, when conception occurs, against MHC antigens of the conceptuses. These blocking antibodies maintain a successful pregnancy, as shown in Fig. 8. When production of blocking antibodies by the mother is scant or absent, the pregnancy may result in spontaneous abortion. Women in this situation may be prone to habitual abortion.

When the conceptuses have lethal chromosomal anomalies, the embryo proper may give rise to early demise during ovular or embryonal development, but the remaining trophoblasts may continue to survive for some time. Antigenicity of the conceptuses may decrease after the embryonal death, and thus the amount of blocking antibodies produced may decrease beneath the threshold in due course after demise of the embryo.

The amount of blocking antibodies firstly determine, by their threshold, whether the trophoblasts are to undergo damage or survival, in an all or none principle. When the amount of blocking antibodies decrease below the threshold, trophoblastic cell damage occurs. Thus, conceptuses are secondly lost clinically as spontaneous abortions. When the amount of blocking antibodies does not decrease below the threshold, trophoblastic cells may continue to survive, showing a variety of trophoblastic hyperplasia depending on the amount of blocking antibodies produced over the threshold. When the amount of blocking antibodies is slightly greater than the

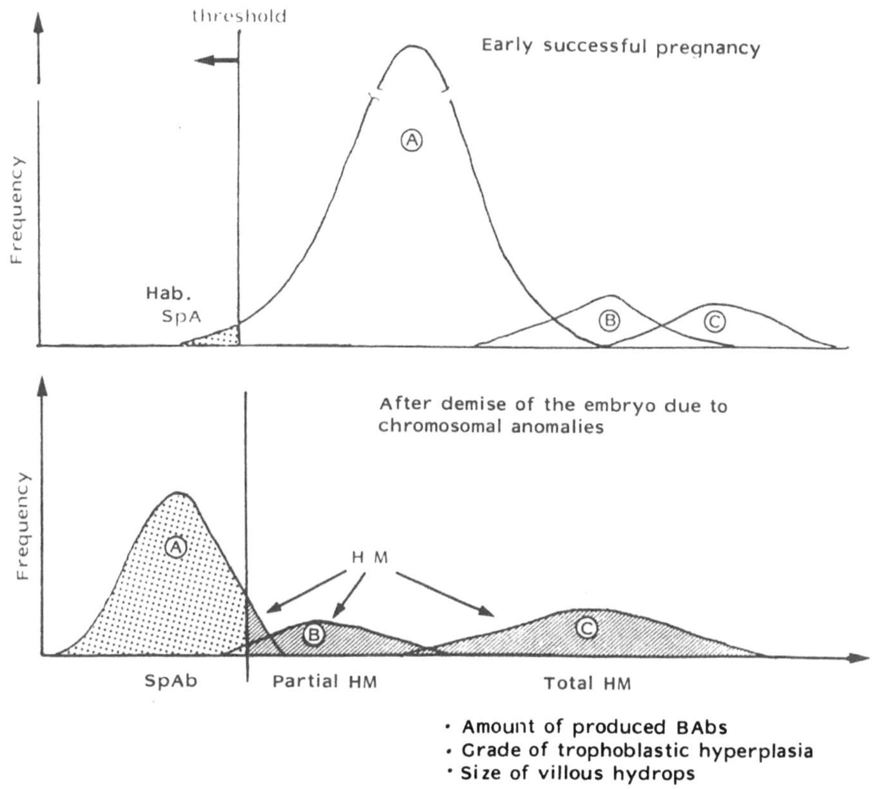

Fig. 9. Schematic drawing to explain the mechanism of immune selection of conceptuses to either spontaneous abortion, partial hydatidiform mole, or total hydatidiform mole, by the amount of blocking antibodies produced related to the threshold after early demise of the embryo. Letters *A*, *B*, and *C* refer to Table 3. Abbreviations: Hab, habitual abortion; SpAb, spontaneous abortion; HM, hydatidiform mole; BAbs, blocking antibodies.

threshold, as seen in partial hydatidiform moles, the trophoblasts may show marked hyperplasia.

Therefore, we now conclude that the immune selection mechanism, determined by the amount of blocking antibodies produced in relation to the threshold, may play a decisive role in determining the destiny of conceptuses into either spontaneous abortion or hydatidiform mole. The immune selection mechanism may be important in determining grade of trophoblastic hyperplasia, and thus a clinical picture of either partial or total mole. Of course, while selection of a destiny, whether spontaneous abortion or hydatidiform mole, is made on an all or none basis, selection of a hydatidiform mole into either partial or total may not be made on an all or none basis, but in a biologically wide variation. In fact, some overlap in amount of blocking antibodies produced was observed between partial and total hydatidiform moles. Therefore, the presence of some biological overlap between the two kinds of mole must be taken into account when considering the antigenicity of conceptuses and amount of blocking antibodies produced by the mothers, and also when considering grade of trophoblastic hyperplasia.

Mechanism of Hydropic Swelling of the Villi

Hertig (19) explained that hydatidiform change of the villi in hydatidiform mole may result from the progressive accumulation of fluid within the villi, by the functioning of the trophoblast in the absence of fetal circulation after early demise of the embryo. This explanation may also hold for the formation of villous hydrops. Thus, whenever input of fluid to the villous stroma from the mother by the functioning of the trophoblast exceeds output of fluid to the embryo by fetal circulation, the outcome may be hydropic swelling of the villi. Therefore, two factors, namely grade of the trophoblastic function and duration of absence of the villous circulation, may be related to the formation of villous hydrops and its size.

In the case of zygotes of androgenesis, embryonal demise may occur during the ovular phase of development within the fifth week of gestation due to its serious chromosomal anomaly. Thus the fate of the conceptus would be subclinical (occult) spontaneous abortion, unless the conceptus, because of high MHC antigenicity, induced production of sufficient blocking antibodies. In reality, marked hyperplasia of the trophoblasts due to marked production of blocking antibodies prevents them from dropping out as spontaneous abortion. In addition, a long duration of lack of fetal circulation may affect all the villi, thus resulting in total hydatidiform mole.

In the case of conceptuses with triploidy of diandry, demise of the embryo usually occurs later than in conceptuses with androgenesis during embryonal or fetal phases of development. Thus the conceptuses would result in clinical spontaneous abortion, unless they failed to induce the production of sufficient blocking antibodies to exceed the threshold because of their relatively higher MHC antigenicity. However, the slight hyperplasia of surviving trophoblasts due to production of blocking antibodies slightly over the threshold prevent them from being lost as spontaneous abortion. The lower functioning of the trophoblasts and short duration of lack of fetal circulation may affect only some of the villi, thus resulting in partial moles.

In the case of conceptuses with trisomy or monosomy, demise of the embryo usually occurs during embryonal development. After this time, the trophoblasts continue to survive for some time in the absence of fetal circulation, and eventually undergo damage due to decrease in amount of blocking antibodies produced, to below the threshold. Consequently, the conceptuses are lost as spontaneous abortions, with microscopic hydatidiform change of the villi in two thirds of them.

Therefore, formation of villous hydrops is likely to occur by the same mechamism in microscopic mole, partial mole, and total (complete) mole.

Difference Between Partial and Total Hydatidiform Mole

Some cytogeneticists have claimed that partial moles arising from triploidy, and total moles arising from androgenesis, are different diseases because of their clear difference in cytogenetic characteristics (68-70). It has also been suggested that partial moles lack the potential to progress to invasive mole or choriocarcinoma and consequently the patients are not at risk, whereas total moles give rise to invasive mole and choriocarcinoma and the patients are at risk (68-70). These workers further claimed that there is no transition from partial to total mole and that total moles undergo total hydatidiform changes early in pregnancy, while partial moles undergo slow hydatidiform changes, similar to total moles but affecting only some of the villi (69, 70). We can agree with these statements in a general sense only. We observed some total moles with triploidy and some partial moles with androgenesis, indicating the presence of some biologic overlap between the two diseases (discussed above). Furthermore, patients with partial moles are never without risk. Brewer and Bagshawe have pointed out that patients with partial moles are at risk (72). We also experienced some patients with partial moles who required treatment. We can only say now that partial moles may be at lower risk relative to the high risk of total moles.

In this context, it should be noted that there is some confusion in applying the established criteria for the clinical and morphologic diagnoses of partial or total mole. Such confusion may be responsible for poor recognition of the presence of the overlap between the two diseases, as mentioned above.

The Most Important Morphologic Features Characterized by Our Proposed Model for Genesis of Hydatidiform Mole

In early pregnancy the trophoblastic cells may be damaged, probably by the immunologic mechanism, when demise of the embryo proper occurs. Thus, the damaged embryo-trophoblast unit (conceptus) may be lost clinically as a spontaneous abortion. This notion is also supported by the experiment in which the remaining trophoblasts resulted in degeneration and damage after early embryectomy in Rhesus monkeys (71).

In this context, the most important characteristics of hydatidiform mole lie in the fact that trophoblastic cells continue to survive and grow, resulting in formation of gross villous hydrops in the absence of villous circulation after demise of the embryo. The viable functioning trophoblasts in the absence of fetal circulation may lead to the formation of hydropic swelling in the villi.

Thus the most important morphologic feature of hydatidiform mole is the villous hydropic swelling with viable trophoblasts and with no evidence of trophoblastic cell damage in absence of the embryo. When the trophoblastic growth and survival associated with hydropic swelling of some or all villi is evident, it would be categorized as hydatidiform mole. On the contrary, when trophoblastic damage is evident, it would be categorized as spontaneous abortion, irrespective of the presence or absence of the villous hydrops and the embryo, because determination of whether damage or survival of trophoblasts will occur after demise of the embryo is very likely to be an all or none phenomenon.

The second important morphologic feature is the grade of trophoblastic hyperplasia, usually considered to be the most important characteristic of hydatidiform mole. Methods of classifying moles on the basis of trophoblastic proliferation have been proposed, and attempts have been made to correlate them with prognosis, but no uniform agreement has been reached as to the prognostic value of considering the grade of trophoblastic hyperplasia. Consensus may hold that the trophoblastic growth pattern is not diagnostic for the prognosis of the individual patients and that one cannot predict the future occurrence of choriocarcinoma by morphologic criteria. In large series, however, some correlation may exist between morphology and the presence of invasive mole, such that the innocuous hydatidiform moles rarely have invasive mole and the percentage of invasive mole progressively rises with the degree of trophoblastic hyperplasia. This may be quite natural because invasive mole is a hydatidiform mole showing a variety of myometrial invasion, and there may be a discontinuity between benign invasive mole and malignant choriocarcinoma (26-28). In addition, there is a problem of sampling. When we examine the entire specimen of hydatidiform mole, we observe marked trophoblastic hyperplasia in some regions, a little hyperplasia in other regions, and no hyperplasia in the rest of the specimen (72). Therefore, the true morphologic characteristics of hydatidiform moles can be determined only by histologic examination of the entire mole and, if possible, of the uterus as well. In reality, however, the opportunity to examine an entire specimen usually does not exist. In this context, it is not absolute but only relative that partial moles arising from triploidy show only a slight hyperplasia of trophoblasts, whereas total moles arising from androgenetic fertilization show marked trophoblastic hyperplasia. We must therefore recognize that it is far more important to determine whether a product of conception specimen is spontaneous aboriton or hydatidiform mole than to determine whether the mole is a partial hydatidiform mole or a small total hydatidiform mole.

So, from the viewpoint of rational follow-up, we would like to emphasize the importance of morphologic criteria of hydatidiform mole in which conceptuses showing villous hydropic swelling with viable trophoblasts should be included in the category of hydatidiform mole, in situations of absent or pathologic embryo, even if the hydropic swelling is microscopic. Furthermore, those moles showing gross villous hydrops with viable trophoblasts should not be excluded from this category, even if there is no evidence of hyperplasia.

CONCLUSION

It may be clear by this presentation that it may now be possible to describe the whole story of genesis of partial and total hydatidiform moles from the aspects of morphology, cytogenetics, and immunology. To do so, however, requires further studies regarding the following problems:

a) details of regulatory mechanisms of trophoblastic cell growth by blocking antibodies;
b) details of differences in amount of produced blocking antibodies relative to maternally derived triploidy (digyny) or paternally derived triploidy (diandry);
c) mechanisms responsible for production of blocking antibodies against HLA D/DR antigens of feto-placental unit instead of generation of cytotoxic T cells found in immunological response to antigens of adult tissues;
d) epidemiologic study on incidence of hydatidiform mole to make causal genesis of androgenetic fertilization clear; and
e) experimental formation of hydatidiform mole in monkeys.

In any event, we may now reasonably conclude that hydatidiform moles are a pathological state of immunologic failure in intrauterine loss (i.e., selection) of the dead embryo as spontaneous abortion, which erroneously permits the remaining trophoblasts to proliferate. Furthermore, the difference between partial mole arising from triploidy, and total mole arising from androgenetic fertilization may not be absolute, but only relative as to degree of trophoblastic hyperplasia, size of villous hydrops, and risk of the patient, in spite of the clear difference of cytogenetic findings between the two.

The more the embryonal allograft differs in MHC from the mother, the more blocking antibodies that are likely to be produced by the mother and thus the more actively the trophoblasts proliferate. In this context, we can now understand that the stronger the difference in MHC between mother and conceptus, the better the mother's reproductive performance.

This general rule in normal pregnancy is likely to also be the case in early abnormal pregnancy. In the case of conceptus with chromosomal anomalies such as triploidy of diandry or androgenesis, the mother continues to produce blocking antibodies in amounts above the threshold for immune rejection of trophoblasts. This occurs because of the high antigenicity of the conceptus with chromosomal anomalies. As a consequence, the mother's immune system fails to recognize that the embryo has been lost, and trophoblasts continue to proliferate, leading to formation of hydatidiform mole.

REFERENCES

1. Hertz, R., "Choriocarcinoma and Related Gestational Trophoblastic Tumors in Women," Raven Press (1978).
2. Park, W. W., "Choriocarcinoma. A Study of Its Pathology," F. A. Davis, Philadelphia (1971).
3. Goldstein, D. P. and Berkowicz, R. S., "Gestational Trophoblastic Neoplasms - Clinical Principles of Diagnosis and Management," W. B. Saunders Co., New York (1982).
4. Kajii, T. and Ohama, K., Androgenetic origin of hydatidiform mole, Nature 268:633 (1977).
5. Wake, N., Takagi, N., and Sasaki, M., Androgenesis as a cause of hydatidiform mole, J. Natl. Cancer Inst. 60:51 (1978).
6. Jacobs, P. A., Angel, R. R., Buchananan, I. M., Hassold, T. J., Matsuyama, A. M., and Mannuel, B., Chromosome constitution of gestational trophoblastic disease, Lancet ii:49 (1978).
7. Lawler, S. D., Pickthall, V. J., Fisher, R., Povey, S., Evens, M. W., and Szulman, A. E., Genetic studies of complete and partial hydatidiform mole, Lancet 11:580 (1979).
8. Yamashita, K., Wake, N., Araki, T., et al, Human lymphocyte antigen expression in hydatidiform mole: androgenesis following fertilization by a haploid sperm, Amer. J. Obstet. Gynecol. 135:597 (1979).
9. Ohama, K., Kajii, T., Okamoto, E., et al., Dispermic origin of XY hydatidiform mole, Nature 292:551 (1981).
10. Surti, U., Szulman, A. E., and O-Brien, S., Complete (classic) hydatidiform mole with 46,XY karyotype of paternal origin, Human Genet. 51:153 (1979).
11. Pattillo, R., Sasaki, S., Katayama, K., Roesler, M., and Mattingly, R., Genesis of 46,XY hydatidiform mole, Amer. J. Obstet. Gynecol. 141:104 (1981).
12. Jacobs, P. A., Szulman, A. E., Funkhouser, J., Matsuura, J. S., and Wilson, C. C., Human triploidy: relationship between parental origin of the additional haploid complement and development of partial hydatidiform mole, Ann. Hum. Genet. 46: 223 (1982).

13. Lawler, S. D., Pickthall, V. J., Povey, S., and Evens, M. W., Genetic studies on hydatidiform moles. 1. The origin of partial moles, Cancer Genetics and Cytogenetics (1982).
14. Szulman, A. E., Philipp, E., Boue, J. G., and Boue, A., Human triploidy: association with partial hydatidiform moles and non-molar conceptuses, Human Pathology 12:1016 (1981).
15. Szulman, A. E. and Surti, U., The clinico-pathological profile of the partial hydatidiform mole, Obstet. Gynecol. (1982).
16. Boue, J., Boue, A., and Lazal, P., Retrospective and prospective epidemiological studies of 15,000 karyotyped spontaneous human abortions, Teratology 12:11 (1975).
17. Car, D. H., Chromosomes and abortion, in: "Advances in Human Genetics," H. Harris and K. Hirshhorn, eds., Plenum Press, New York (1971), p. 201.
18. Kajii, T. and Ferrier, A., Cytogenetics of aborters and abortuses, Amer. J. Obstet. Gynecol. 131:33 (1978).
19. Beer, A. E. and Billingham, R. E., "The Immunobiology of Mammalian Reproduction," Prentice-Hall, Englewood Cliffs, N. J. (1976).
20. Beer, A. E. and Billingham, R. E., Mechanisms of nonrejection of feto-placental allografts, Folia Biologica (1980).
21. Loke, Y. W., "Immunology and Immunopathology of the Human Foetal Maternal Interaction," Elsevier-North Holland, Amsterdam (1978).
22. Voisin, G. A., Role of antibody class in the regulatory facilitation reaction, Immunol. Rev. 49:3 (1980).
23. Takeuchi, S., Immunology of spontaneous abortion and hydatidiform mole, Amer. J. Reprod. Immunol. 1:23 (1980).
24. Takeuchi, S., An immune dependency of trophoblastic growth implied by the antithetic difference in immunology between spontaneous abortion and hydatidiform mole, in: "Reproductive Immunology," N. Gleicher, ed., Alan R. Liss, Inc., New York (1981), p. 245.
25. Takeuchi, S., Immunology of growth and demise of embryo-trophoblast unit indicated by comparative study between abortion and hydatidiform mole - A nature's experiment system, in: "Immunobiology of Transplantation, Cancer and Pregnancy," P. K. Ray, ed., Pergamon Press, New York (1983).
26. Takeuchi, S., Definition and classification of trophoblastic disease based on its nature, in: "Human Reproduction," K. Semm and L. Mettler, eds., Excerpta Medica, Amsterdam-Oxford-Princeton (1981).
27. Takeuchi, S., Nature of invasive mole and its rational management, Seminars in Oncology 9:181 (1982).
28. Kato, M., Tanaka, K., and Takeuchi, S., The nature of trophoblastic disease initiated by transplantation into the immunosuppressed animals, Amer. J. Obstet. Gynecol. 142:497 (1982).
29. Kajii, T., Personal communication.

30. Hertig, A. T. and Edmond, H. W., Genesis of hydatidiform mole, Arch. Pathol. 30:260 (1940).
31. Hertig, A. T., Hydatidiform mole and chorionepithelioma, in: "Progress in Gynecology," J. V. Meigs and S. H. Sturgis, eds., Vol. 2 (1950), p. 372.
32. Takeuchi, S., Hando, T., Honda, T., Ohno, T., and Kanazawa, The nature of "trophoblastic tumours": immunological and pathological approach, J. Asian Fed. Obstet. Gynecol. 2: 218 (1971).
33. Tokunaga, A., Studies of humoral immunological response on the aborted trophoblasts (in Japanese), J. Japan Assoc. Obstet. Gynecol. 33:2125 (1981).
34. Hanoka, J. and Takeuchi, S., Individual specificity of blocking antibodies in molar and normal term placenta-bound IgGs, Amer. J. Reprod. Immunol., in press (1983).
35. Unpublished data.
36. Lawler, S. D., HLA and trophoblastic tumors, Brit. Med. Bull. 34:30- (1978).
37. Faulk, W. P. and Temple, A., Distribution of β_2 microglobulin and HLA in chorionic villi of human placentae, Nature 262: 799 (1976).
38. Billingham, R. B. and Head, J. R., Current trends in reproductive immunology: an overview, J. Rep. Immunol. 3:253 (1981).
39. Loke, Y. W., Joysey, V. C., and Borland, HL-A antigens on human trophoblast cell, Nature 232:403 (1971).
40. Chatterjee-Hasrouni, S. and Lala, P., Localization of H-2 antigens on mouse trophoblast cell, J. Exptl. Med. 149:1238 (1979).
41. Sellens, M. H., Jenkinson, E. J., and Bellington, W. D., Major histocompatibility complex and non-major histocompatibility complex antigens on mouse ectoplacental cone and placental trophoblastic cells, Transplantation 25:173 (1978).
42. Wegman, T. S., The presence of class 1 MHC antigens at the maternal-fetal interface and hypotheses concerning the survival of the murine fetal allograft, J. Reprod. Immunol. 3:267 (1981).
43. Sunderland, C. A., Redman, C. W. G., Stirrat, G. M., HLA A, B, C antigens are expressed on nonvillous trophoblast of the early human placenta, J. Immunol. 127:2614 (1981).
44. Sunderland, C. A., Naiem, M., Mason, D. Y., Redman, C. W. G., and Stirrat, G. M., The expression of major histocompatibility antigens by human chorionic villi, J. Reprod. Immunol. 3: 323 (1981).
45. Chatterjee-Hasrouni, S. and Lala, P. K., In situ localization of paternal H-2 K antigens on murine trophoblast cells, Amer. J. Reprod. Immunol. 2:170 (1982).
46. Montgomery, B. and Lala, P. K., Major histocompatibility antigens on human trophoblast cells, Amer. J. Reprod. Immunol. 2:171 (1982).

47. Brami, C. J., Sanyal, M. D., Johnson, C. C., Kohorn, E. I., Dwyer, J. M., and Naftolin, F., HLA-DR antigens on cultured human trophoblast cells, Amer. J. Reprod. Immunol. 2:109 (1982).
48. Rocklin, R. E., Kitzmiller, J. L., Carpenter, C. B., Bravoy, M. R., and David, J. R., Maternal-fetal relation: absence of an immunologic blocking factor from the serum of women with chronic abortions, New Engl. J. Med. 295:1209 (1976).
49. Stimson, W. H., Strachan, A. F., and Shepherd, A., Studies on the maternal immune response to placental antigens: absence of a blocking factor from the blood of abortion-prone women, Brit. J. Obstet. Gynecol. 86:41 (1979).
50. Hellstrom, K. E., Hellstrom, I., and Brawn, J., Abrogation of cellular immunity to antigenically foreign mouse embryonic cells by a serum factor, Nature 224:914 (1969).
51. Hellstrom, K. E. and Hellstrom, I., The role of serum factors ("blocking antibodies") as mediators of immunological nonreactivity to cellular antigens, in: "Ontogeny of Acquired Immunity," Ciba Foundation Symposium, Elsevier, New York (1972), p. 133.
52. Hirschberg, H., Albrechtsen, D., Solheim, B. G., and Thorsby, E., Inhibition of human mixed leucocyte culture stimulation by anti-HLA-D-associated antisera studies with primed responding cells, Eur. J. Immunol. 7:26 (1977).
53. Revillard, J. P., Robert, M., Dupont, E., et al., Inhibition of mixed lymphocyte culture by alloantibodies in renal transplantation and in pregnancy, Transplant. Proc. 5:331 (1975).
54. Pence, H., Petty, W. H., and Rocklin, R. E., Suppression of maternal responsiveness to paternal antigen by maternal responsiveness to paternal antigen by maternal plasma, J. Immunol. 114: 525 (1975).
55. Riggio, R. R., Saal, S. D., Steuzel, K. H., and Rubin, A. L., Retroplacental factors and passive enhancement, Transplant. Proc. 8:281 (1976).
56. Revillard, J. P., Brocier, J., Robert M., et al., Immunologic properties of placental eluates, Transplant. Proc. 8:275 (1976).
57. Voisin, G. A. and Chaouat, G., Demonstration, nature, and properties of antibodies fixed on placenta and directed against paternal antigens, J. Reprod. Fertil. 21 (Suppl.): 89 (1974).
58. Moe, T., David, C. S., Rijinbeek, A. M., Nabholz, M., Miggiano, V. C., et al., Inhibition of mouse MLR by anti-Ia sera, Transplant. Proc. 7 (Suppl.):127 (1975).
59. Kajino, T., Kanazawa, K., and Takeuchi, S., Blocking effects of maternal serum-IgG and placental eluate-IgG on materno-fetal MLR and their individual specificity, Amer. J. Reprod. Immunol., in press (1983).

60. Komlos, L., Zamis, R., Johnson, H., and Halbrecht, I., Common HLA antigens in couple with repeated abortion, Clin. Immunol. Immunopath. 7:330 (1975).
61. Komlos, L. and Halbrecht, I., Repeated abortions and histocompatibility antigens. Can HLA antigen restricted gene close effects influence the feto-maternal relationship? Med. Hypotheses 5:901 (1979).
62. Purpma, M., Coghi, I., Micotra, M., Carapella, E., and Bottini, E., HLA Bw35 antigen and human reproduction, J. Med. Genet. 17:157 (1980).
63. Gerencer, M., Kastelan, A., Drazancic, A., Kerhin-Brkljacic, V., and Madjaric, M., The HLA antigens in women with recurrent abnormal pregnancies of unknown etiology, Tissue Antigens 12:223 (1978).
64. Taylor, C. and Faulk, W. P., Prevention of recurrent abortion with leucocyte transfusions, Lancet:68 (1980).
65. Beer, A. E., Quebbeman, J. F., Ayers, J. W. T., and Haines, R. F., Major histocompatibility complex antigens, maternal and paternal immune responses, and chronic habitual abortions in human, Amer. J. Obstet. Gynecol. 141:987 (1981).
66. Unander, M. H. and Olding, L. B., Easily suppressed lymphocytes and absence of cytotoxic antibody in three women with habitual abortion, Amer. J. Reprod. Immunol. 2:254 (1982).
67. Aoki, K., Katahira, T., Nakane, S., et al., Search for HLA, especially DR antigen-antibody system in the couples of the unexplained habitual abortions (in Japanese), Proceeding of 33rd General Meeting of Japan Society of Obstet. Gynecol. 113 (1981).
68. Vassilakos, P., Riotton, G., and Kajii, T., Hydatidiform mole: two entities. A morphologic and cytogenetic study with some clinical considerations, Amer. J. Obstet. Gynecol. 127:167 (1977).
69. Szulman, A. E. and Surti, U., The syndrome of hydatidiform mole, I. Cytogenetic and morphologic correlation, Amer. J. Obstet. Gynecol. 131:665 (1978).
70. Szulman, A. E. and Surti, U., The syndrome of hydatidiform mole, II. Morphologic evolution of the complete and partial mole, Amer. J. Obstet. Gynecol. 132:20 (1978).
71. Lewis, J. and Hertz, R., Effects of early embryectomy and hormonal therapy on the fate of the placenta in pregnant Rhesus monkey, Proc. Soc. Exptl. Biol. Med. 123:805 (1966).
72. Brewer, J. I. and Mazur, M. T., Gestational trophoblastic disease: morphology and pathogenesis, in: "Human Reproduction," K. Semm and L. Mettler, eds., Excerpta Medica, Amsterdam-Oxford-Princeton (1981), p. 398.

COMPLEMENT SYSTEM IN ABNORMAL PREGNANCY AND CHORIONIC NEOPLASIA: IMMUNOTHERAPY AND CHEMOTHERAPY OF CHORIONIC NEOPLASIA

Ryoki Ohkawa, Kimiyasu Ohkawa, Norio Tosaka,
Toshikatsu Ohhashi, Akira Hatano, and Tsutomu Ohkawa

Department of Gynecology and Obstetrics
Nippon Medical School, 1-1-5 Sendagi-cho
Bunkyo-ku, Tokyo, and
Department of Biochemistry
Kanazawa University School of Medicine
13-1 Takara-cho Kanazawa-shi
Ishikawa-ken
Japan

INTRODUCTION

In normal pregnancy the cellular immunity of the mother is generally suppressed, because the fetus must develop in the uterus. By this mechanism of cellular immunity, the fetus is not rejected. On the other hand, the suppressed cellular immunity seems to pose a danger for the mother during pregnancy. Is it possible that there is a compensatory mechanism for the suppressed cellular immunity? From the phylogenetic point of view, when cellular immunity is suppressed, the C_3 system of complement must be enhanced.

When the defense mechanism of the entire organism is examined from the phylogenetic point of view, the C_3 system of the complement system in the *Mollusca*, and only this system, undertakes the self-defense in the organism, as a vigilante corps. Self-defense by this mechanism alone, however, is low in efficiency and requires considerable cost. To increase the efficiency of the self-defense system, for example in the hagfish, cellular immunity has evolved. This in turn has led to a security maintenance mechanism and to the development of lymphocytes which specialize in recognizing both exogenous and endogenous foreign material as non-self, and in eliminating them. However, because lymphocytes react only at the site where such foreign bodies are present, the lymphocytes have

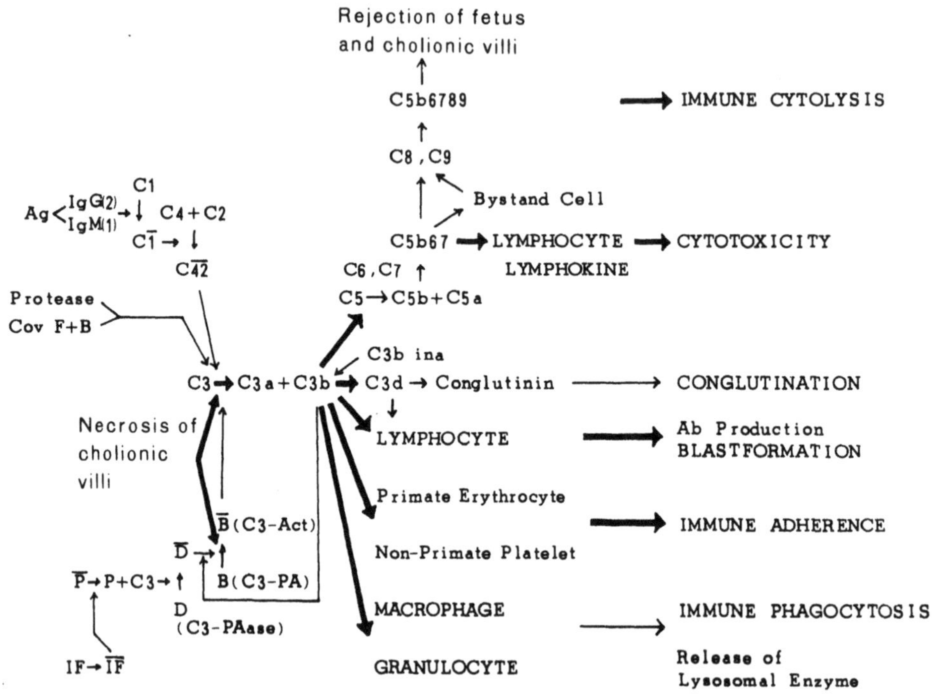

Fig. 1. Network of complement system.

to be mobilized from lymph nodes and spleen and gathered there. This response requires 24 to 48 hours. Since this delayed response is not entirely satisfactory, humoral immunity (the missile mechanism) has developed, as, for example, in the shark. Mammals possess all three of these defense mechanisms. Fig. 1 shows the complement network, with both the classical and alternate pathways. Teleologically, it can be envisioned that the alternate pathway first developed in the lower animals, and then the classical pathway added to it. The alternate pathway is also referred to as the C_3-shunt pathway. The alternate pathway can be activated with zymosan, polysaccharides (*e.g.*, TGDS), dextran sulfate, and other substances (*e.g.*, lipopolysaccharides of bacteria). When this activation takes place, and reaction proceeds to the formation of C_3---C_9, many chemical mediators are produced, leading to the activation of macrophages, granulocytes, lymphocytes, and eventually to the occurrence of cytotoxicity and immunocytolysis (1, 2).

In almost all cancer patients, delayed hypersensitivity is suppressed. It is important to intensify the suppressed cellular immune response of cancer patients by drugs that act on the complement system and activate the alternate pathway of complement. This results in the production of many chemical mediators and activation of macrophages and T lymphocytes. Therefore, the ability

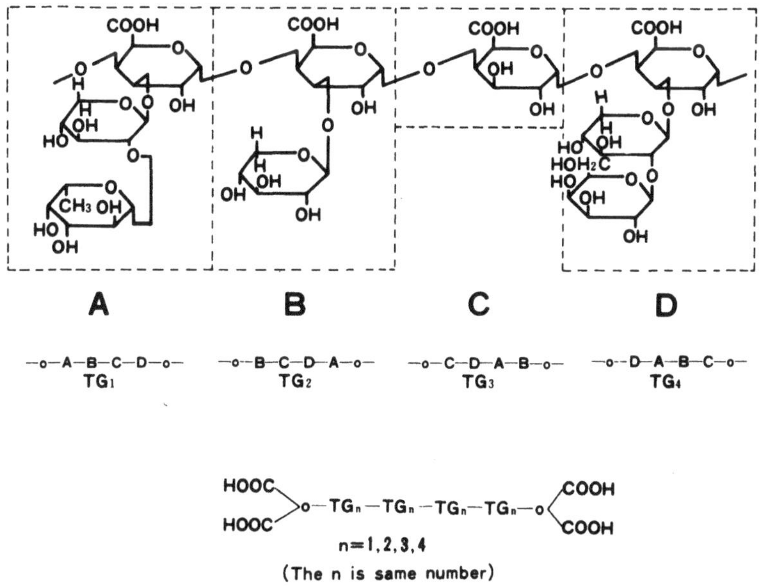

Fig. 2. The structure of pectin gum tragacanth.

to activate complement is important (1-4).

We previously showed that the acid polysaccharides produced by sulfation of oxidative degradation products of vegetable polysaccharides, such as pectin gum tragacanth (Fig. 2), activate the C_3 system of complement. TGDS is the product prepared from tragacanth gum. The molecular model of TGDS is shown in Fig. 3. We demonstrated in cancer patients as well as in animals that these polysaccharides had only low toxicity, but markedly activated the alternate pathway, resulting in enhancement of cellular immunity (5-7). The biochemical properties of these polysaccharides are summarized in Table 1.

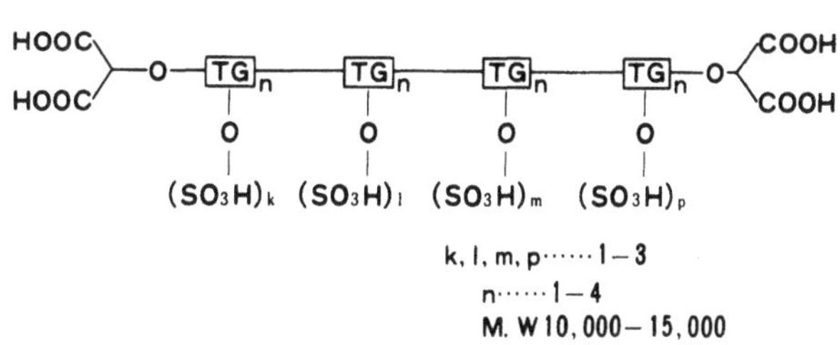

Fig. 3. Molecular model of TGDS.

Table 1. Biochemical Properties of These Polysaccharides (Heparinoid Substances)

1. Average molecular weight, 3000-5000.
2. Chelation of calcium, but not magnesium.
3. Inhibition of hyaluronidase.
4. Low anticoagulant activity.
5. Faster electrophoretic mobility than heparin (*i.e.*, greater negative charge).
6. Fibril formation with heat denatured collagen.
7. Mobilization of lymphocytes from thymus-dependent regions of lymph nodes and spleen following intravenous injection.
8. Local injection: increase in number of lymphocytes, plasma cells, and mast cells in connective tissue (or in stroma of cancer following increasing the number of fibroblasts).
9. Conversion of C_3-proactivator (G. B. G.) to C_3-activator (complex of G. B. G. and polysaccharides), resulting in activation of complement C_3 to C_{3b}. Consequently, non-immune activation of complement alternate pathway occurs, with release of a chemical mediator which induces chemotaxis of lymphocytes.
10. Marked enhancement of cellular immunity.
11. Low toxicity (LD_{50} = 1500-2500 mg/kg).

MATERIAL AND METHODS

The study group consisted of 491 cases of normal pregnancy, 250 cases of threatened abortion, 85 cases of hydatidiform mole, 22 cases of chorionic malignancy, 35 cases of severe toxemia, 11 cases of abruptio placentae, and 25 cases of normal gravida during labor.

Immunologic Examination

For the established hypersensitivity reaction, PPD, *Candida albicans*, and varidase were used as antigens. In the new delayed hypersensitivity reaction, DNCB, hemocyanin croton oil, and carraghenan were used. In the nonspecific skin reaction, PHA and Con A were used.

For measurement of factors involved in the classical pathway, CH_{50} was determined by a modification of Mayer's method. C_4 was measured by radial immunodiffusion.

Activation of Complement

In vitro activation of complement by chorionic villi was measured. Chorionic villi with or without contraction of the uterus were used. In the pregnant guinea pig experiment, contraction of the uterus was tested by anaphylatoxin caused by activation of complement.

Factors Involved in the Alternate Pathway ($Al\text{-}CH_{50}$)

Hemolytic activity was measured by hemolysis of rabbit erythrocytes. C_3 and C_3-proactivator were measured by radial immunodiffusion. As a measure of cell-mediated cytotoxicity, a modified Hellstrom assay was used, as outlined in Fig. 4.

Immunostimulation (Fig. 5)

For enhancement of delayed hypersensitivity, BCG, OK-432, and TGDS were used. For enhancement of complement activity, BCG and OK-432 were used. TGDS was used for complement activation and also for abrogation of blocking factor. For enhancement of cytotoxicity against cancer, TGDS and OK-432 were used.

TGDS was used by drip injection of 100 to 300 mg in 500 ml lactate G solution intravenously, or intramuscularly, every day. OK-432 was administered intradermally; 1 to 5 units were administered every 2 days. BCG was used by infusion in the skin.

Combination Chemotherapy

For combination chemotherapy, three to five courses with 8 anticancer drugs were used. Medication was for 3 days at 10-day intervals (Fig. 5).

Prevention of Malignant Transformation of Hydatidiform Mole

For this purpose, the methods of Table 2 were used.

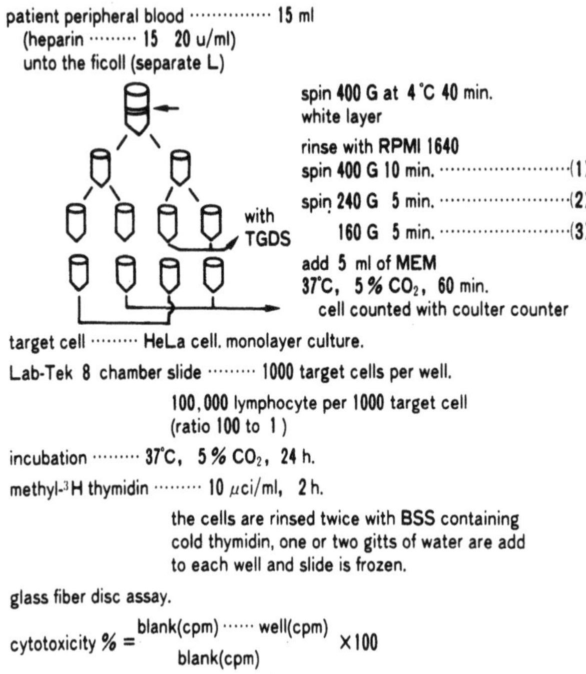

Fig. 4. Cell-mediated cytotoxicity assay.

A) IMMUNOTHERAPY

1. Semisynthesized acid Polysaccharides
   a) T.G.D.S. 50mg in oil/1ml
      20mg/2ml
   b) CH6S-S 50mg in oil/ml
2. B.C.G. 8mg
3. Drugs from streptococcus
   0.2–0.4u.
4. Tumor specific antigen is used in combination with these Immunostimulator.

C) ADDITIONAL THERAPY

1. Hyperalimentation
2. Lysozomelabilizer
   vitamin A 4500u
   dextran sulfate
3. Co-Enzym Q
4. Urokinase

B) CHEMOTHERAPY

Ac···ActinomycinD	0.5mg
Ad···Adryamycin	10mg
B ··· Bleomycin	5mg
En···Endoxan (Cyclophosphamide)	100mg
Es···Esquinon (Carboquone)	1mg
M_T···Methotorexate	15mg
M_{MT}···Mitomycin	2mg
T ··· Toyomycin (Clomomycin)	0.5mg
5Fu······	250mg

[Binblastin
Vinclistin]

a) Induction of Remission
   6-Polychemotherapy
   5×······1Kur
b) Maintenance
   5-Polychemotherapy
   5×······1Kur

Fig. 5. Drugs used in immunochemotherapy.

Table 2. Treatment of Chorionic Malignancy and Prevention of Malignant Change of Hydatidiform Mole

A. Immunotherapy

1. Enhancement of complement activity:
BCG
OK-432
TGDS

2. Abrogation of blocking factor; enhancement of and activation of complement following enhancement of delayed hypersensitivity:
TGDS, 100-200 mg/day
Dextran sulfate, 2000-4000 ng
Other plant polysaccharides
Lentinan, etc.

B. Polychemotherapy (in case of malignancy)

3 Days long every 10 days

RESULTS

In pregnancy, the skin reaction as cellular immunity decreased, as shown in Table 3. In cases of hydatidiform mole and chorionic malignancy, skin reactions were negative in almost all cases.

Complement profiles in pregnancy are shown in Table 4. Both the classical and alternate pathways were enhanced. Likewise, in threatened abortion patients with good prognosis, C_3-proactivator and hCG titer increased progressively (Fig. 6). In cases of hydatidiform mole, the alternate pathway decreased markedly. In cases of threatened abortion with poor prognosis, C_3-proactivator and alternate pathway activity were low (Fig. 7). Furthermore, C_3-proactivator activity decreased before the urinary hCG titer dropped. In 25 out of 28 cases of hydatidiform mole and in 5 cases of chorionic malignancy, alternate pathway and C_3-proactivator were markedly depressed. In cases of severe toxemia, C_3-proactivator and alternate pathway activity were low, especially in patients with apoplexia utero placentare (Table 4).

After evacuation of hydatidiform mole, the activity of the alternate pathway and of C_3-proactivator remain low for a long time. Activation of complement by chorion is shown in Fig. 8.

Table 3. Skin Test in Pregnancy

Antigen	Positive rate (percent): Pregnant, 20-40 years old	Positive rate (percent): Nonpregnant, 20-40 years old, healthy women
DNCB	65	100
Croton oil	55	95
Caraghenan	45	80
PPD	68	90
Varidase	65	89
PHA[a]	68	96
Con A	58	85
PWM	66	98

[a]Abbreviations: PHA, phytohemagglutinin; Con A, concanavalin A; PWM, pokeweed mitogen.

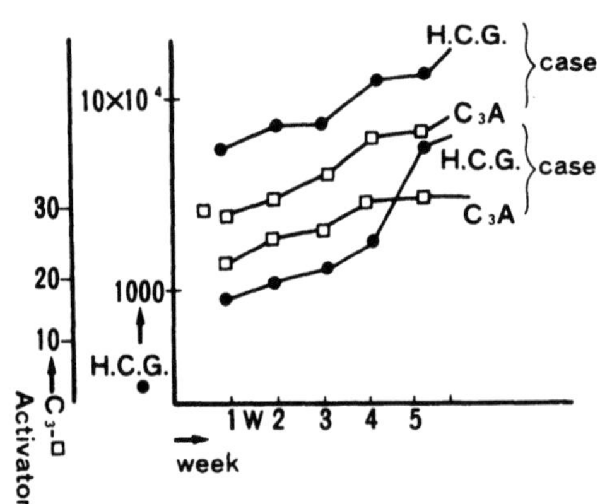

Fig. 6. C_3-activator and hCG levels in cases of threatened abortion with good prognosis.

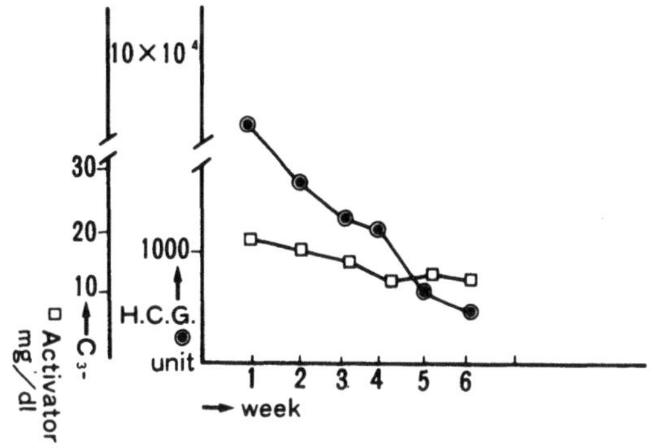

Fig. 7. C_3-activator and hCG levels in threatened abortion with poor prognosis.

Table 4. Complement Profiles in Pregnancy

Type of pregnancy	Cases	CH_{50}	C_3	C_3-activator	C4	Al-CH_{50}
Normal nonpregnant	20	40±2	66±3	18±2	32±3	18±1
Pregnancy						
1st Trimester	25	53±2	68±5	25±2	42±1	21±2
2nd Trimester	25	56±2	84±2	24±2	39±2	23±1
3rd Trimester	32	66±3	88±1	26±1	37±2	27±2
Threatened abortion						
Good prognosis	52	53±2	70±5	25±6	39±7	22±2
Poor prognosis	63	38±2	60±5	19±3	35±7	17±1
Hydatidiform mole	25	28±2	60±2	17±6	35±2	16±1
	3	45±2	67±2	24±1	38±1	21±2
Choriocarcinoma	5	29±1	55±1	16±1	35±1	16±2
Toxemia						
Severe	9	40±1	65±2	18±2	28±2	18±2
Mild	15	52±1	22±1	26±3	38±3	23±2
Apoplexy	2	27	50	13	24	

		CH_{50}	$AlCH_{50}$
Pregnancy IX 37°36		65.8 63.5	26.3 25.1
uterus contraction ⊖	IVM chorion (Myom. Op.)	61.0	24.6
	XM chorion Cesarean Sc.	59.5	23.1
uterus contraction ⊕	XM chorion	38.5	18.1
	Thr. Ab.	31.5	18.6
Chorion homozinet		30.1	17.1

Fig. 8. Anticomplement activity of chorion.

Complement activity in the tenth month of pregnancy is 65.8 unit for CH_{50}, and 26.3 unit for Al-CH_{50}. After the serum (1 ml) was mixed with 0.5 g fresh chorion (without uterus contraction), CH_{50} was 61.0 unit, and Al-CH_{50} was 24.6. Thus, the fresh chorion did not activate complement. On the other hand, when 0.5 g chorion (with contraction of uterus) was mixed in this serum, CH_{50} activity decreased to 38.5 unit, and Al-CH_{50} decreased to 18.1 unit. These results suggest that the aging chorion or necrotic chorion activate the alternate pathway. In 10 cases of hydatidiform mole and 9 cases of chorionic pregnancy, C_3-proactivator and Al-CH_{50} were both decreased. The same decrease was observed in chorionic malignancy; in 12 of 19 cases, neither C_3-proactivator nor Al-CH_{50} had attained normal levels 1 to 2 years following therapy. Table 5 shows that CH_{50} and Al-CH_{50} also decrease during labor.

That TGDS has the ability to activate the alternate pathway was demonstrated in experiments with guinea pigs (5). Into the abdominal cavity of 10 guinea pigs in the fourth week of pregnancy was injected 10 mg of TGDS. Abortion occurred in all 10 guinea pigs. This finding seems to be analogous to the situation in abruptio placentae.

Table 5. Activity of Alternate Pathway During Labor

Third trimester without labor pain	Labor stage			
	First	Second	Third	Puerperium
25.5 unit	19.7	19.1	19.0	30.1

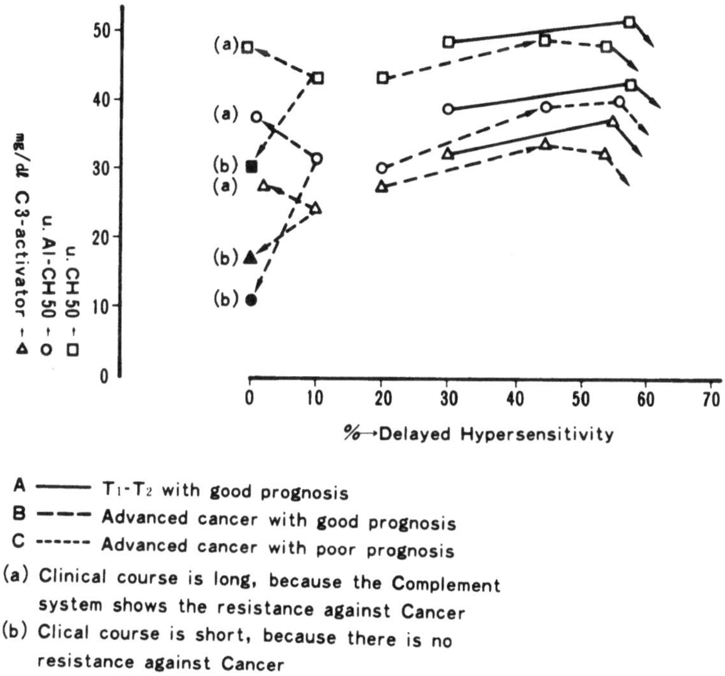

Fig. 9. Changes in complement and delayed hypersensitivity activity following immunochemotherapy of choriocarcinoma.

As shown in Fig. 9, trophoblastic cancer patients with good prognosis showed enhancement of delayed hypersensitivity (*i.e.*, positive skin reaction) in their clinical course. Furthermore, in the cell-mediated cytotoxicity assay, cytotoxicity of lymphocytes was enhanced by rinsing with TGDS in the presence of the patient's serum (Fig. 10, Tables 6 and 7). These results suggest that blocking factor will disappear by adding TGDS in the serum of the cancer patient.

Lymphocytes were rinsed with TGDS	(−)	(+)	(+)	(−)
	MEM FCS	MEM FCS	MEM Patient-serum	MEM Patient-serum
good	67.9%	62.3%	52.6%	33.5%
Poor	15.1%	40.0%	31.0%	5.0%

Fig. 10. Lymphocyte-mediated cytotoxicity in trophoblastic disease cases with good and poor prognosis. Serum from patients was added at a concentration of 10%.
MEM, culture medium; FCS, 10% fetal calf serum.

Table 6. Cytotoxicity Mediated by Lymphocytes With or Without Macrophages in Cases of Recurrent Cancer in Peripheral Blood (5 Cases)

	Time after operation		
Macrophages	2-3 Months	4-12 Months	>5 Years
Present	78%	45%	63%
Absent	8%	15%	21%

As shown in Table 6, cytotoxicity mediated by lymphocytes in the presence of macrophages is high, while that mediated by lymphocytes alone is very low. The function of the macrophages compensatorily enhances the cytotoxicity function of the lymphocytes.

Table 7. Cytotoxicity Mediated by Lymphocytes and Macrophages in 5 Cases of Recurrent Choriocarcinoma

	Lymphocytes rinsed with TGDS			
	-	+	-	+
	MEM FCS	MEM FCS	MEM Patient serum (10%)	MEM Patient serum (10%)
Lymphocytes plus macrophages	54%	54%	44%	37%
Lymphocytes only	18.5%	51%	46%	12.5%

MEM, culture medium; FCS, 10% fetal calf serum.

In 58 cases of hydatidiform mole studied, the skin test was negative in 90% of the patients. In addition, the activity of the alternate pathway decreased. In particular, C_3-proactivator decreased to 18.5 mg/dl. Skin reaction, as measured by the delayed hypersensitivity test, and complement decreased in all 35 cases of chorionic malignancy. In 8 cases of choriocarcinoma with lung metastasis, immunotherapy in conjunction with chemotherapy was markedly effective, and lung metastases completely disappeared.

DISCUSSION

In normal pregnancy, CH_{50} and Al-CH_{50} are significantly elevated and C_3, C_3-proactivator and C_4 were increased, whereas the skin test was depressed in 50% of the patients. We should consider that the suppression of cellular immunity is compensated by enhancement of alternate pathway, which is the primitive defense system. In threatened abortion with intrauterine fetal death, CH_{50}, Al-CH_{50}, and C_3-proactivator were decreased with the consumption of complement, because the necrotic chorionic villi activate the alternate pathway.

In cases of severe toxemia of pregnancy, especially abruptio placentae, CH_{50}, Al-CH_{50}, and C_3-proactivator were also decreased. In cases of hydatidiform mole and chorionic pregnancy, CH_{50} and Al-CH_{50} were depressed and the skin test (as measured by delayed hypersensitivity) was low. This phenomenon presents a risk to the patients, since the defense system is depressed.

At the onset of and during labor, CH_{50}, Al-CH_{50}, and C_3-proactivator decline, because the aging of the placenta activates the alternate pathway of complement. As a result, C_3-a (anaphylatoxin) is produced, which triggers the onset of labor. Fig. 11 shows how the polysaccharide of placenta, in which sialic acid is decreased, activates the alternate pathway.

In normal pregnancy, cellular immunity is suppressed, with compensatory enhancement of the pathway of complement. In cases of hydatidiform mole and chorionic malignancy, both skin reaction (measured as delayed hypersensitity reaction) and the alternate pathway of complement are suppressed, resulting in a poorer prognosis. In consideration of cellular immunity and activity of complement, chorionic malignancy and hydatidiform mole patients with low complement activity and decreased skin reaction must be treated by immunotherapy in addition to chemotherapy.

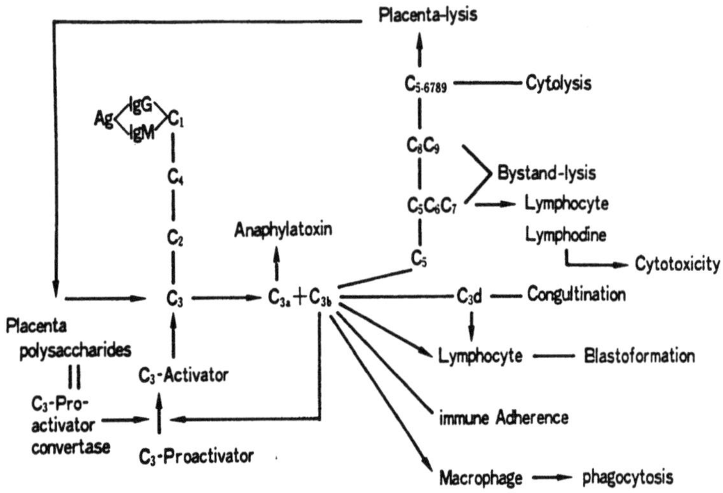

Fig. 11. The network of complement.

SUMMARY

In normal pregnancy, the activity of the alternate pathway elevates latently and compensatorily for the suppression of cellular immunity. Aging of the placenta becomes a trigger for the onset of labor and production of C_3-a. In cases of hydatidiform mole, abruptio placentae, threatened abortion, and chorionic malignancy, the activity of the complement system is depressed, especially that of C_3-activator and alternate pathway. This may in turn result from activation of complement by the pathologic lesion of the chorionic villi. In pathologic lesions of the placenta, activation of alternate pathway can lead to a number of diseases.

Immunotherapy is effective in the prevention of malignant transformation of hydatidiform mole. Immunotherapy and combination chemotherapy are markedly effective for treatment of metastatic chorionic malignancy.

REFERENCES

1. Baines, M. G., Studies of the complement level in normal pregnancy, Obstet. Gynecol. 43:806 (1974).
2. Fireman, P., et al., Development of human complement system, J. Immunology 103:25 (1969).
3. Platts-Mills, T. E. A., Ishizaka, K., Activation of alternative pathway of complement by rabbit erythrocytes, J. Immunology 113:348 (1974).

4. Nishioka, H., Infection, inflamation and immunity, 5:55 (1975).
5. Ohkawa, R., and Ohkawa, K., Immunotherapy and chemotherapy of ovarian cancer stage 3, World of Obstet. Gynecol. 55:34 (1982).
6. Ohkawa, R., Third Symposium of Complement 1 (1976).
7. Ohkawa, R., Physico. Biology and Physicochemistry 19:435 (1975).

PLACENTAL SENESCENCE

Tim Parmley

Department of Gynecologic Pathology
Johns Hopkins University
Baltimore, Maryland, USA

PLACENTAL AGING

There are no universally accepted definitions of inherent biologic aging. Consequently, it is currently impossible to state whether or not the placenta fits any such definition, *i.e.* ages. The question is further complicated by the possibility that the placenta does, in fact, age but has not reached readily recognizable old age by the end of its normal life span. The only analysis currently possible is to observe those things which are associated with aging in individuals and to see if they occur in the placenta.

Increased Incidence of Disease

So universal is the presence of disease in old age that one of the major stumbling blocks in providing a definition of aging has been the inability to separate the effects of disease from those of any intrinsic aging process (1). As term approaches, a variety of changes are seen in the placenta that have been viewed as pathological.

Intervillous thrombi most commonly consist of laminated plaques of fibrin which lie between and disperse the villi laterally. However, this is their late appearance. Earlier examples are red cell thrombi; significantly, many of the red cells are nucleated. Although there has been some debate on the point, these have been felt to represent fetal red cells (2). Therefore, it would seem that intervillous thrombi occur when fetal blood, interacting with maternal blood in the intervillous space, initiates clotting. The idea that these thrombi represent sites of fetal blood loss into the maternal circulation is supported by the fact that they may be correlated with the presence of fetal red cells in the maternal circulation (3), and with Rhesus isöimmunization (4).

Assuming that intervillous thrombi represent breaks in the trophoblastic membranes separating the fetal capillary from the intervillous space, are they to be viewed as disease, or as signs of age? Obviously, this is impossible to answer. It is not even immediately obvious how to state the question so that it is more scientific than philosophical.

Another type of ambiguity that may arise when one tries to assess the presence of disease in a mature placenta is illustrated by infarcts. A significant ischemic infarct would seem to be a reasonably good example of disease but, in fact, the disease seems to be maternal as most infarcts are due to maternal vascular disease or compromise, and do not reflect any intrinsic placental abnormality (4). On the other hand, fetal placental artery thrombosis resulting in local villous devascularization, is certainly an intrinsic placental process. Even in this case, however, the only known association is to maternal abnormality (5).

Even more confusing is the example of calcification. Increasing amounts of calcium may be deposited in the villous tissues as pregnancy progresses; this has long been thought to be pathological. After many attempts to correlate its presence with disease states, however, it has been possible only to suggest an association with a maternal serum calcium level (4).

Thus, these and other changes simulating disease appear in the placenta near term, but a precise view of their true biologic nature is not available. Consequently, all that can be said is that a variety of conditions tend to occur in the placenta nearing term and that these seem to be pathological but cannot, in fact, be proven to be placental disease.

Decreased Ability to Function

Although the extent to which it can be attributed to age rather than to disease is highly debatable, most observers accept that aged individuals experience some diminution in their capacity to function (6). In the placenta the evidence is contradictory.

The placenta has two primary functions that may be examined. It produces hormone products that alter maternal physiology to accomodate the developing pregnancy, and it transports material from the maternal to the fetal circulation and in the reverse direction. With respect to the first function, the problem is complicated. There is variation in the production of hormone by the placenta that may be physiologic rather than senescent. Chorionic gonadotropin production peaks between 70 and 90 days of gestation. By 110 to 130 days, it has declined to a level which is maintained to term (7). Chorionic somatomammotropin levels rise until term (8). Estrogen production appears to be complicated by the fact that it is not purely a placental function but in a normal pregnancy remains high after 36 weeks until term (9).

Progesterone production, which is more properly a pure placental function, may decrease just before term, but this point, too, is problematic. Although Csapo (10) has suggested in a series of studies that placental production of progesterone drops immediately prior to labor, this author has not been looking for senescent function but for the mechanism of the onset of labor. Of course, it is not intrinsically obvious that maturational or senescent changes in the placenta could not be involved in the initiation of labor.

With respect to transport, the available studies indicate decreased transport of sodium and water at term (11, 12). Unfortunately, little other information is available.

Aging Occurs After Growth and Development

In any given individual, aging occurs after an earlier period of growth and development. This aging is adaptive, in that the individual becomes more capable of functioning and reproducing. This process is characterized early on, by growth that results from cell division. Indeed, a large proportion of the total cell population may be dividing. However, development and maturation of the individual is associated with differentiation and maturation of the cells comprising that individual. After cell maturation has progressed to a point, most cells do not appear to divide any further but to grow, if at all only by hypertrophy. Fully mature individuals contain populations of cells that continue to divide, of course, but numerically these are a smaller percentage of the total cell population than is the case for an immature individual, and they constitute mechanisms for repair and replacement of mature populations, not for additional growth.

Certainly the placenta goes through a dramatic process of growth and development. The question is whether it is still growing and developing at term, rather than having turned the corner and begun to age (13). The evidence is equivocal. Certainly a higher percentage of its total cell population is engaging in proliferation at 10 weeks of gestational age than at term, and certainly growth is dramatically slowed at term, or possibly ceases, but there is evidence that minimal growth continues. There is certainly evidence that minimal cell proliferation continues, but this may represent repair or replacement proliferation rather than growth (14).

Differentiation of the vast majority of the trophoblasts is certainly a feature of the term placenta in contrast to that of the first trimester. Cytotrophoblast is present, but is much less prominent, and evidence of its continued proliferation is very rare. The trophoblast displays a large number of vasculo-syncytial membranes which appear to be specific responses to increased transport needs (15), and an increasing number of syncytial knots which appear to be sequestered senescent nuclei. These may represent the same sort of senescent nuclei seen in the most superficial cells of the squamous epithelium of the well-estrogenized vagina, but they could also be functional structures, since they have been observed to join with other knots on adjacent villi to form struts which may be adaptive (16). Thus, the placenta certainly grows and matures; whether or not it ages remains a question. It is appropriate to remember at this point that the process of getting old is different than the process of being old, and if the placenta at term is not old, it does not mean that it does not engage in the process of getting old, but only that its life is usually sacrificed before it progresses very far.

Specific Aging Studies

Specific attempts to detect placental aging have been few. In 1961 Hayflick and Moorehead (17) demonstrated that human fibroblasts treated in a standardized way would replicate a certain number of times in culture and then cease to replicate, and die. Hayflick further suggested (17) that the number of generations required before death of the culture occurs is inversely related to the age of the donor. When this type of experiment was performed (18) using placental tissues and fetal skin from a 13-week pregnancy, it was demonstrated that the fetal skin culture survived for approximately 20 generations longer than the placental one. When an attempt was made to follow up on this work by documenting decreased capacity to repair DNA in placental tissue, the decrease could not be shown (19). The first study is afflicted by the failure to distinguish trophoblast from stroma in the material cultured; interpretation of the latter is hampered by the consideration that, as mentioned above, the tissues could be in the process of getting old after 36 weeks, but of not having become very old.

An additional attempt to detect placental aging involves a search for "aging pigments" (lipofuchsin). These are a chemically heterogeneous group of compounds that accumulate in all fixed, post-mitotic cells in proportion to the chronologic age of that cell. This relationship has been carefully documented in the human myocardium by Strehler (20), who demonstrated an increase of 0.6% per decade in the fraction of the myocardium occupied by the pigment. These pigments are believed to result from the peroxidation of intracellular lipids by free radical-oxygen byproducts of respiration. As the pigments are insoluble, they accumulate in the cell. Because they are fluorescent, fluorescence microscopy is a convenient method for detecting them. When the fluorescent microscope was used to search for this material in placenta, it was first noted in placentas as young as 32 weeks, but was almost universally present in those older than 36 weeks (21). It was absent from the placenta of a term anencephalic, the significance of which is unclear. It was often present in the trophoblast of the membranes, so these cells must continue to respire until term. The fact that the pigment was found only in the trophoblast suggests that this is the only potential site of placental aging.

SUMMARY

As the nature of any intrinsic biologic aging process or even of its existence independent of disease is unknown, it is not possible to state whether or not the placenta gets old. As term approaches, the placenta accumulates a variety of lesions which seem pathological. In most cases, however, it is not certain that they represent intrinsic disease in the sense that older people tend to develop cancer or atherosclerosis. Several placental functions decrease near term, but it is not possible to attribute these to aging. In fact, some may represent adaptive additional maturation. A variety of laboratory phenomena seen in aging cells may be detected in the placenta but again, their significance is uncertain.

In short, the placenta looks and acts as if it grows old. That is clinically important and probably all the clinician needs to know, but whether or not it truly grows old remains a mystery, an important point for the biologist. For if the placenta truly ages, then the embryo and its placenta represent genetically identical tissues which age at different rates. Such a model might give us much more specific information about our limits than a currently popular reference, the 90th Psalm.

REFERENCES

1. Weisfeldt, M. A. and Abben, R., Presbycardia, The Johns Hopkins Medical Journal 149:203 (1981).
2. Bernischke, K. and Driscoll, S. G., Placenta, in: "Handbuch der Speziellen Pathologischen Anatomie Und Histologie, Springer-Verlag, New York (1967), p. 279.
3. Banti Devi, Jennison, R. F., and Langley, F. A., Significance of placental pathology in transplacental haemorrhage, J. Clin. Pathol. 21:322 (1968).
4. Fox H., "Pathology of the Placenta," W. B. Saunders Co., Philadelphia (1978), pps. 122-139.
5. Fox, H., Thrombosis of fetal arteries in the human placenta, J. Obstet. Gynecol. Brit. Commonwealth 73:961 (1966).

6. Strehler, B. L., "Time, Cells, and Aging," Second Ed., Academic Press, New York (1977), p. 125.
7. Teoh, J., J. Obstet. Gynecol. Brit. Commonwealth 74:77 (1967).
8. Spellacy, W. N., Buhi, W. C., and Birk, S. A., The effectiveness of human placental lactogen measurements as an adjunct in decreasing perinatal mortality, Amer. J. Obstet. Gynecol. 121:835 (1975).
9. Frandsen, V. A. and Stakemann, G., The urinary excretion of oestriol during the early months of pregnancy, Acta Endocrinol. 44:196 (1963).
10. Csapo, A. I., Knobil, E., von der Molen, H. J., and Wiest, W. G., Peripheral plasma progesterone levels during human pregnancy and labor, Amer. J. Obstet. Gynecol. 110:631 (1971).
11. Hellman, L. M., Flexner, L. B., Wilde, W. S., Vosburgh, G. J., and Proctor, N. K., The permeability of the human placenta to water and the supply of water to the human fetus as determined with deuterium oxide, Amer. J. Obstet. Gynecol. 56:861 (1948).
12. Flexner, L. B., Cowie, D. B., Hellman, L. M., Wilde, W. S., and Vosburgh, G. J., The permeability of the human placenta to sodium in normal and abnormal pregnancies and the supply of sodium to the human fetus as determined with radioactive sodium, Amer. J. Obstet. Gynecol. 55:469 (1948).
13. Teasdale, F., Gestational changes in the functional structure of the human placenta in relation to fetal growth: a morphometric study, Amer. J. Obstet. Gynecol. 137:560 (1980).
14. Fox, H., The placenta as a model for organ aging, in: "Placenta, A Neglected Experimental Animal," P. Beaconsfield and C. Villee, ed., Pergamon Press, New York (1979), p. 365.
15. Fox, H., The incidence and significance of vasculo-syncytial membranes in the human placenta, J. Obstet. Gynecol. Brit. Commonwealth 74:28 (1967).
16. Jones, C. P. J. and Fox, H., Syncytial knots and intervillous bridges in the human placenta: an ultrastructural study, J. Anat. 125:275 (1977).
17. Hayflick, L., The cell biology of human aging, New Engl. J. Med. 295:1302 (1976).
18. Vincent, R. A., Jr., Huang, P. C., and Parmley, T. H., Proliferative capacity of cell cultures derived from the human placenta, In Vitro 12:649 (1976).
19. Lekfowitz, D., Johnson, R. C., Faulk, W. P., and Vincent, R. A., Unscheduled DNA synthesis in mixed-cell primary cultures of eleven-week and term human placentae, J. Supramolec. Struct. 8:Abstract 214 (1978).
20. Strehler, B. L., Mark, D. D., Mildvan, A. S., and Gee, M. V., Rate and magnitude of age pigment accumulation in the human myocardium, J. Gerontology 14:430 (1959).
21. Parmley, T. H., Gupta, P. K., and Walker, M. A., "Aging" pigments in term human placenta, Amer. J. Obstet. Gynecol. 139:760 (1981).

GENETIC ORIGIN OF TROPHOBLAST NEOPLASMS

Morphologic and structural patterns in trophoblastic neoplasms span the spectrum of complete and partial hydatidiform moles, hydatid changes in the trophoblast, and choriocarcinoma without villous structures. While the genetic origin of hydatidiform moles was first reported by Kajii and Ohama, the authors of the following chapters have contributed significantly to the understanding of genetic factors in hydatidiform moles. The results from the first editor's laboratory documented the genesis of a 46,XX hydatidiform mole. Significant progress has been made toward elucidating the origin of genetic information in the hydatidiform moles and choriocarcinoma. Careful study of this field using new technology may provide important further information on the etiology of these neoplasms. Particularly important will be the application of techniques currently being utilized by molecular biologists to probe the human oncogenes. These newly discovered DNA sequences transform normal cells into neoplasms. Geneticists have become aware of the fact that through translocation, genes move and change positions within individual chromosomes and among different chromosomes. The recent discoveries that have shown translocations in Burkitt's Lymphoma, in which the human cellular oncogene C-myc is joined to one of the immunoglobulin loci characteristically found in this lymphoma, points the way for new research in the genetic origin of human neoplasia. Careful genetic studies of maternal and paternal chromosome contributions to trophoblast neoplasms may provide new information regarding possible translocation of genetic material that could represent initiation events in the genesis of these neoplasms.

COMPLETE AND PARTIAL HYDATIDIFORM MOLES: CYTOGENETIC AND MORPHOLOGICAL ASPECTS

A. E. Szulman and Urvashi Surti

Department of Pathology
Magee-Womens Hospital and
School of Medicine
University of Pittsburgh
Pittsburgh, Pennsylvania, USA

INTRODUCTION

Although records of molar pregnancies reach back to antiquity, the fetal origin of hydatidiform moles was established only at the end of the last century. The elucidation of the relationship with choriocarcinoma as well as the occurrence of nongestational cancers followed during the next decade (1). Several generations later, many of the mysteries still remain, but new insights in the field of trophoblastic disease are now being gained rapidly, mainly through the study of the chromosomal composition of hydatidiform moles. The latter inquiry into correlation with morphology has allowed the delineation of at least two distinct molar syndromes: the complete, diploid, androgenetic mole of a 46,XX or 46,XY karyotype without an embryo/fetus; and the partial mole with a fetus and a 69,XXY, XXX, or XYY karyotype. Only the classic, complete mole retains at present a known association with chorionic cancer.

Cytogenetics employs the several new techniques of chromosome banding. Aided by the study of biochemical (enzyme) and HLA antigenic polymorphisms, it was used to establish the parental origin of the chromosomes and the chromosomal make-up of a molar conceptus. The results in this area have correlated well with the distinctive gross and microscopic appearances of the metamorphosed placenta in the two syndromes. The latter have been established by the study of moles in their early stages of development that permitted a reconstruction of the morphologic evolution of the placenta, and gave an insight into the fate of the embryo-fetus in the two respective syndromes.

The state of knowledge prior to the application of cytogenetics and of the newer morphologic data is summarized in the writings of Hertig (2), Bagshawe (3), and Park (4), where all the clinico-pathological elements of "hydatidiform moles" are comprehensively described. This field of inquiry, however, had suffered from a lack of a common definition as to what constituted a "hydatidiform mole", and allowed for a variety of pathological conceptuses to be grouped together, often only on the strength of grossly visible and more or less generalized edema of the placental villi. The morphological definition of a hydatidiform mole that has been gaining wide acceptance (5), and one employed in our laboratory, is based upon the long-maintained suggestion of W. W. Park (4), stating that the fundamental attribute of a mole - and one significantly reflected in choriocarcinoma - is the hyperplasia of the trophoblast. In this definition the edema of the placental villi, by itself, is deemed to be of secondary importance. Nevertheless, true hydatidiform change, as seen in complete and partial moles, is a specific process that leads to central villous cistern formation (6, 7). This contrasts the simple nonspecific swelling and degeneration of stroma typical of common spontaneous abortions. Conceptuses with such hydropic villous change have not been found associated with choriocarcinoma or residual trophoblastic disease (4, 8) to a degree higher than that of other nonmolar gestations.

The presence or absence of an embryo/fetus has proved another diagnostic element. Fetal survival or death (including its gestational timing) serve well as an additional criterion by which to distinguish the two kinds of mole. In the classic complete mole the embryo dies very early, at a stage of a few millimeters and before establishment of its placental circulation. Therefore, the villous vessels are always devoid of (nucleated) erythrocytes. The partial mole, on the contrary, gives evidence of the embryo's existence, past or present. The identification of the embryo/fetus itself, in a fresh or macerated state, is established by an analysis of the villous capillaries which hold and preserve the fetal erythrocytes long after fetal death.

CYTOGENETICS OF COMPLETE AND PARTIAL MOLES

With the development of chromosomal banding techniques, individual chromosomes can be recognized. In addition, some of the heritable morphologic differences between homologous chromosomes can be identified with greater certainty than before. These differences remain within the normal phenotypic repertoire and are not associated with any known pathology. They serve as markers in pedigree analysis to determine parental origin of the extra chromosomes in trisomy, triploidy, and also in identifying maternal cell contamination in amniotic fluid cultures for prenatal diagnosis (9). With the use of quinacrine banding technique, Kajii and

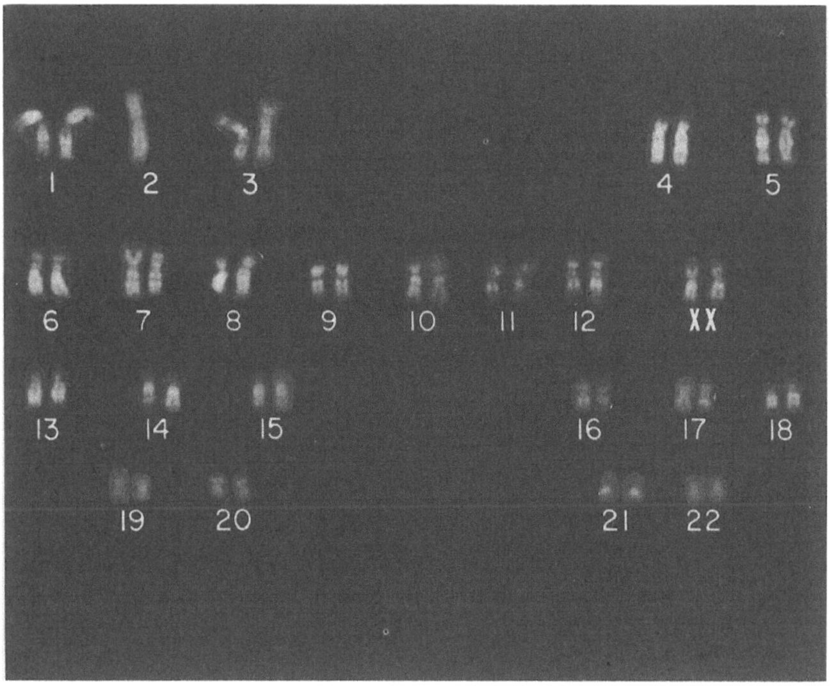

Fig. 1. A karyotype of a diploid androgenetic complete mole. The 46,XX chromosomes were stained using quinacrine banding technique. The polymorphic markers are identical for each chromosomal pair (3, 4, 13, 14, 15, 21, 22) and referable exclusively to one set of paternal chromosomes (X 1,900).

Ohama (10) clearly demonstrated that the familiar complete mole, known for its propensity toward carcinoma, was an androgenetic parthenogenone, *i.e.*, a conceptus whose chromosomes were derived totally from the father in the absence of the maternal chromosomes, and that one haploid set of paternal chromosomes was present in duplicate in the molar cells (Fig. 1). The above findings were soon confirmed by others, some of whom used enzyme polymorphisms along with chromosomal markers and analysis of HLA antigens to differentiate between paternal meiosis II error and post-meiotic duplication of a haploid sperm (11-13). Thus, the commonly shared view was established that the complete mole with a 46,XX karyotype results from a fertilization of an "empty egg" by a spermatozoon containing a post-meiotic set of 23,X chromosomes which duplicates without cytokinesis to give the requisite 46,XX chromosomes (Fig. 2). A spermatozoon carrying a set of 23,Y chromosomes would result in a nonviable zygote of 46,XY. This left the problem of the few, but

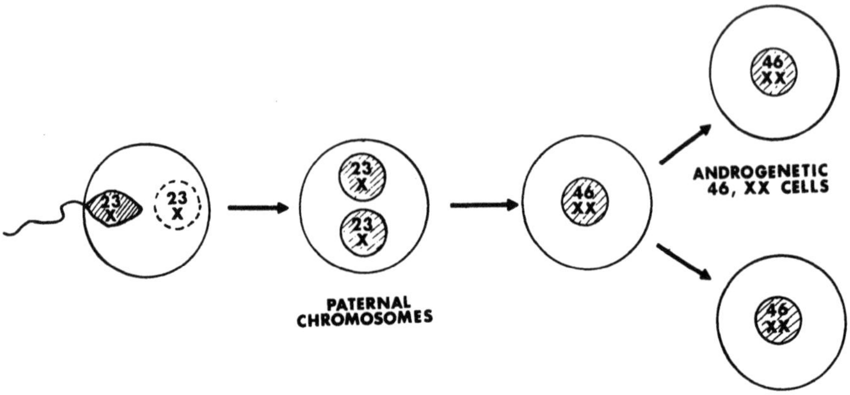

Fig. 2. Paternal origin of complete classical mole (46,XX). The diagram illustrates the penetration of an "empty egg" (nucleus inactivated or absent) by a single sperm which duplicates its haploid set to give a total of 46,XX chromosomes.

well authenticated complete moles of 46,XY karyotype, morphologically and clinically undistinguishable from the common 46,XX variety. Studied by means of chromosomal banding and enzyme polymorphisms (14-17), they were found to originate by the fertilization of an "empty egg" by two sperms, one carring the X and the other the Y chromosome. While the YY zygotes can be written off as nonviable, the XX dispermic moles are still waiting to be discovered. The monospermic and the dispermic moles are totally paternally derived and represent a total allograft in the maternal organism.

The partial moles represent a large subpopulation of triploid conceptuses and were studied by the same methods of chromosomal and biochemical polymorphisms as the complete moles (20-23). Triploidy is a condition wherein there is an extra set of parental 23 chromosomes (Fig. 3). Most often it is derived from the father, either through fertilization by a spermatozoon that failed to undergo the reduction division (paternal meiosis-I error), or by two separate spermatozoa. Significantly fewer cases are associated with an ovum that contains the whole maternal genome (maternal meiosis-I error), while meiosis-II errors in either parent make only an insignificant contribution.

CLINICO-PATHOLOGICAL PROFILES OF THE TWO MOLAR SYNDROMES

It has long been known that moles are morphologically heterogeneous. Although the complete mole and the partial mole or mole with a fetus had been described by many authors (2, 18), their separate characters were formally established only recently (6, 7, 12, 19-23).

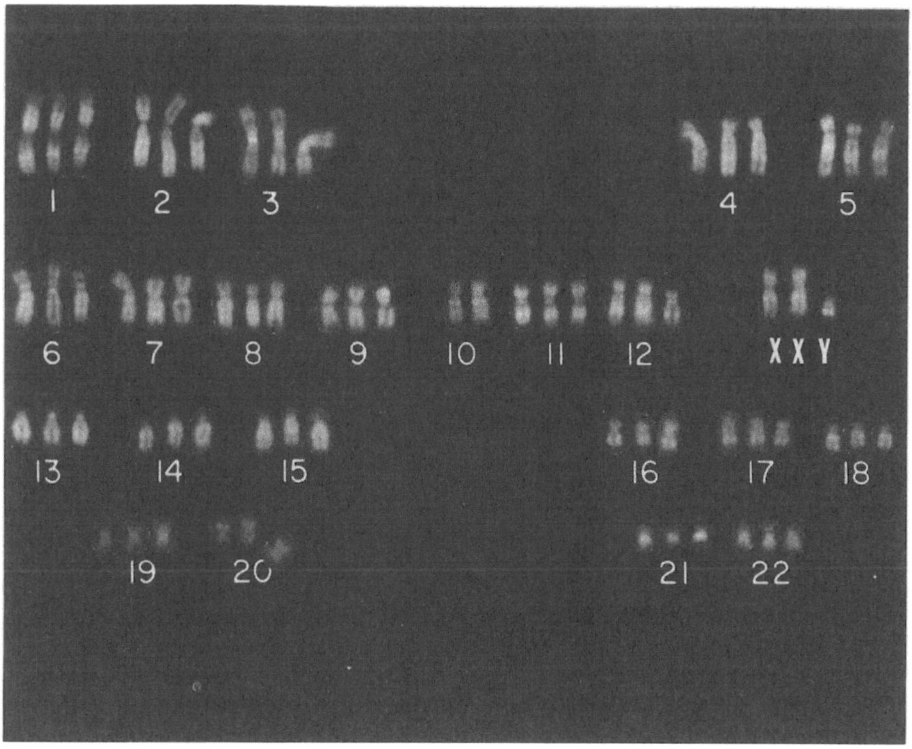

Fig. 3. A triploid karyotype (69,XXY) illustrating the presence of three instead of two sets of chromosomes in a partial mole (origin-dispermy). Quinacrine banding allows for a study of the parental origin of many of the chromosomes (X 1,700).

Since it seems obvious that the mole is genetically programmed at fertilization, its phenotype should come to early morphologic expression with the formation of villi during the third post-fertilization week. In keeping with this idea is the fact that complete moles seen in our laboratory could be identified among the earliest specimens derived from elective abortions at four weeks post-fertilization age. Such early and later specimens show a general swelling of the villi with cistern formation and a trophoblastic hyperplasia affecting both layers (Figs. 4 and 5). Other morphologic changes include random necrobiosis of the mesenchymal cells, formation of empty vessels, often filled with debris derived from degenerating endothelium, and absence of fetal (nucleated) erythrocytes. Since placental growth goes on throughout the life of the mole, the formation of new villi with young vasculogenic mesenchyme

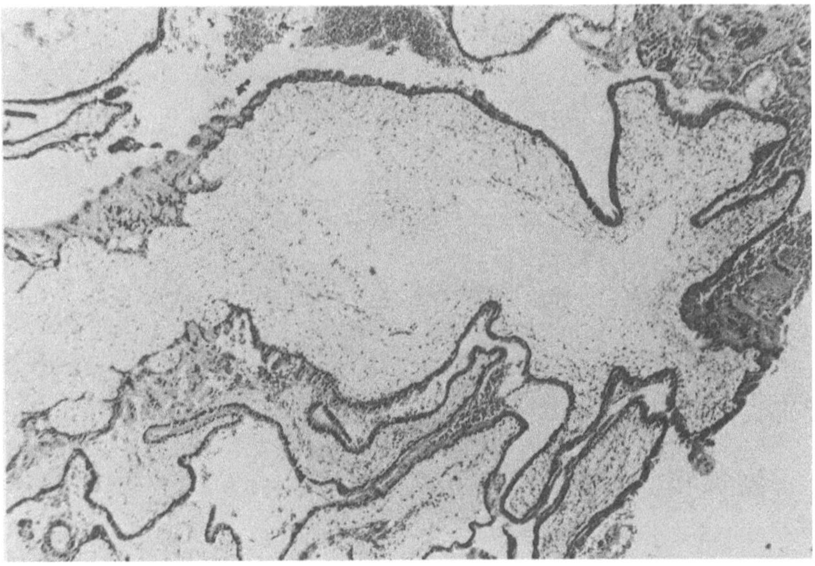

Fig. 4. Complete hydatidiform mole, 10.5 weeks menstrual age. Various stages of edema of the villi are shown. Cistern formation is shown in the villus in the center of the photograph. Moderate trophoblastic hyperplasia is evident (X 45).

and cistern formation continue as a staggered process. The morphology described here holds equally for the 46,XX and 46,XY moles.

A complete mole with a fetus is represented by only two known examples. Its morphology is that of the complete 46,XX or 46,XY variety, except for the presence of an ascertainable fetus. One case, a product of an elective abortion, presented well-preserved fetal parts and had a karyotype of 46,XX. The other (spontaneous) abortus showed fetal blood in the villous vessels, attesting to fetal survival beyond 6-7 weeks menstrual age, and whose 46 chromosomes were of normal father/mother derivation (6, 21).

The partial hydatidiform moles can be assumed to be virtually exclusively of triploid karyotype. Most, if not all, are of diandric origin, *i.e.*, contain one maternal and two paternal haploid sets with all three viable sex chromosome configurations (XXY, XXX, and XYY) possible (21, 22). While partial moles turn out to be triploid, not all triploids need to be partial moles. In a study of two separate populations of spontaneous abortions with a triploid karyotype, 15 to 20% were nonmolar conceptuses. A control series of several hundred abortions with normal and abnormal karyotypes yielded no cases with partial-molar morphology (20, 22).

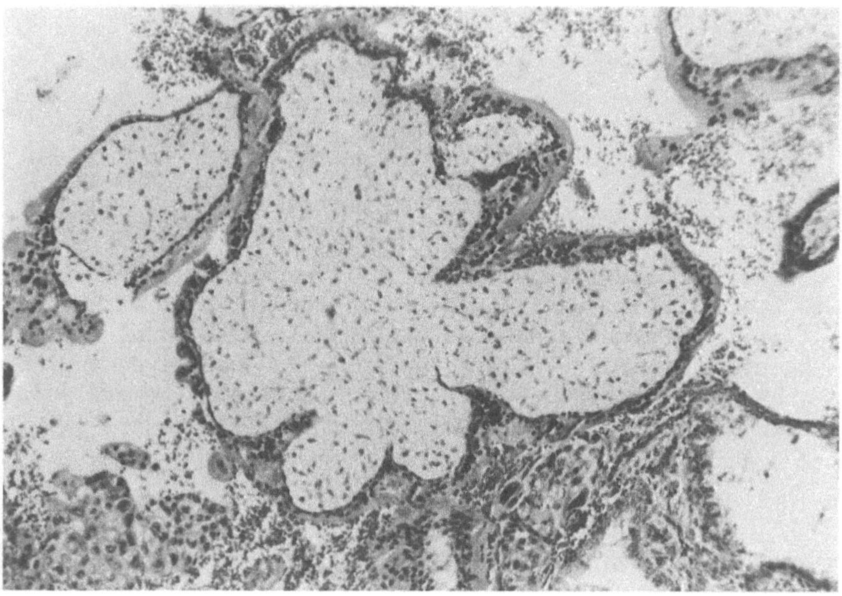

Fig. 5. The same complete mole as in Fig. 4. The villus has generalized edema, focal necrobiosis of stromal mesenchymal cells, and marked hyperplasia of both layers of confluent trophoblast (X 110).

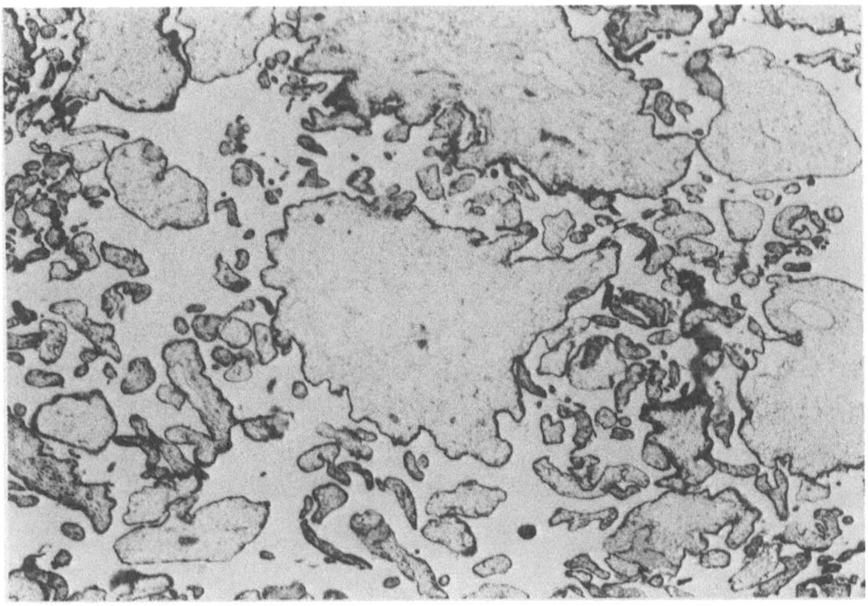

Fig. 6. Partial hydatidiform mole, of 12 weeks menstrual age, with live fetus. General view of edematous villi with early cistern formation and patent vessels with fetal erythrocytes. "Small villi" apparently are uninvolved in the hydatidiform process. Focal trophoblastic hyperplasia is inconspicuous at this magnification (X 30).

The morphology of the partial mole (6, 7, 20) represents a mosaic of seemingly normal small villi and villi that slowly replicate the sequence of fluid accumulation from edema to cistern formation, as seen in complete moles (Figs. 6 and 7). In cases past 18-20 weeks gestational age, a peculiar type of cistern, with a maze-like outline, is sometimes seen (20). If the fetus is alive the vessels contain fetal blood both in the normal and in the edematous villi, including those with cisterns. Irrespective of the fate of the fetus, there is a crinkling or scalloping of the villous outlines from the earliest stages, quite characteristic and unique for triploid partial moles. This process is apt to become exaggerated by the fibrosis following fetal death, but it is often the most striking feature upon general view (Fig. 8). Another highly characteristic feature is stromal trophoblastic inclusions (24), found also in a small (1-2%) proportion of abortuses with trisomy 16.

The trophoblastic hyperplasia of partial moles has been ignored or overlooked altogether by many authors. It is most often inconspicuous, with only occasional cases displaying a gross degree

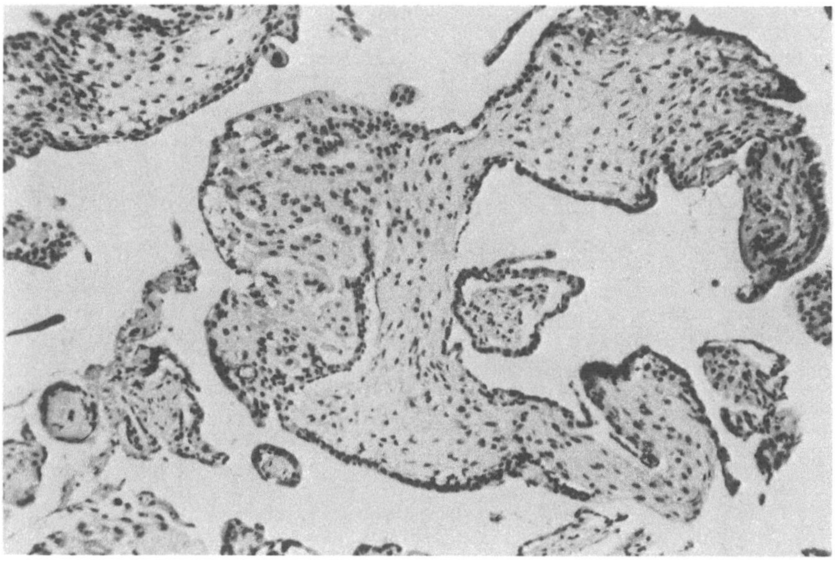

Fig. 7. Partial mole, of 12.5 weeks menstrual age. A medium-sized villus with mild edema and conspicuous syncytial trophoblastic hyperplasia is shown (X 110).

equal to that of complete moles. The increased levels of hCG found in partial mole patients reflect this trophoblastic overactivity. Usually the hyperplasia is confined to the syncytiotrophoblast with much vacuolization that is normally seen in placentas during implantation. Only few cases evince cytotrophoblastic involvement (20), which is apparently of no clinical consequence.

The mosaic-like pattern of the partial mole calls for a wide placental sampling. The usual one or two routine blocks taken for pathologic examination often prove inadequate. Cistern formation can be inconspicuous, especially in older moles and in retrospective studies, with a limited number of histologic slides, may be difficult to demonstrate.

The triploid fetus most frequently dies at 8-9 weeks menstrual age. In this case the loss of vessels and fibrosis of the villous mesenchyme proceed, both in the core of the small unaffected villi, and in the peripheral wall of the cisterns. This is a common picture, since early fetal death is the rule and survival beyond the first trimester, an exception.

While the partial mole seems to represent a dilute version of the complete molar syndrome in both morphology and in many clinical aspects (25), the most important clinical question is of the

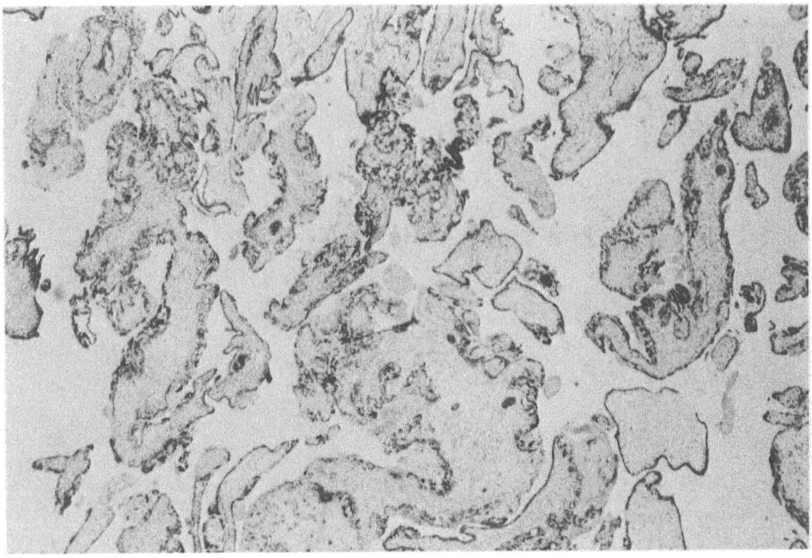

Fig. 8. Partial mole, from "missed abortion" at 18 weeks menstrual age; long-standing fetal death. Note the scalloped outline of villi, trophoblastic inclusions and foci of moderate trophoblastic hyperplasia. The villous stroma is fibrosed and avascular owing to fetal demise several weeks earlier (X 30).

association of the former with residual trophoblastic disease. The trophoblastic hyperplasia, high hCG levels, and their sometimes slow return to normal, create a legitimate suspicion, strengthened by several reports where post-evacuation hCG curves warranted chemotherapy (26-28). Overt proven choriocarcinoma has not been reported to date. The pathological lesions associated with the patient's abnormal recovery remain unknown, since present diagnostic and therapeutic practices yield no material for the pathologist. It remains a strong possibility, however, that the abnormal, "proliferative" sequelae of the partial mole most often represent undue deportation and/or persistence of the trophoblast in the maternal organism (25), analogous to molar embolization to the lungs and other organs described for the complete mole (1, 29, 30). These are considered nonmalignant processes explicable in terms of two unique circumstances: the normal, maternal systemic deportation of trophoblast, and the trophoblast's capability of penetrating maternal vessels and tissues (31). That the classic mole and its "invasive mole" variant are not malignant is strongly suggested by experiments on nude, immunologically inactive mice used as hosts for transplants from complete moles, invasive moles, and choriocarcinoma in which only the latter behaved as a malignant tumor killing the host (32).

Similar experiments might cast light upon the putative malignant propensity of partial moles.

REFERENCES

1. Ober, W. B., Historical perspectives on trophoblast and its tumors, Ann. N. Y. Acad. Sci. 80:3 (1959).
2. Hertig, A. T., "Human Trophoblast," Charles C. Thomas, Springfield, Illinois (1968).
3. Bagshawe, K. D., "Choriocarcinoma: The Clinical Biology of the Trophoblast and Its Tumours," Arnold, London (1969).
4. Park, W. W., "Choriocarcinoma: A Study of Its Pathology," Heinemann, London (1971).
5. Fox, H., "Pathology of the Placenta," W. B. Saunders Co., New York, New York (1978), p. 382.
6. Szulman, A. E. and Surti, U., The syndromes of hydatidiform mole. I. Cytogenetic and morphologic correlations, Amer. J. Obstet. Gynecol. 131:665 (1978).
7. Szulman, A. E. and Surti, U., The syndromes of hydatidiform mole. II. Morphologic evolution of the complete and partial mole, Amer. J. Obstet. Gynecol. 132:20 (1978).
8. Elston, C. W., The histopathology of trophoblastic tumours, J. Clin. Pathol. 29 (Suppl., Royal College of Pathology 10): 111 (1976).
9. Jacobs, P. A., Human chromosome heteromorphisms (variants), Progr. Med. Genetics 2:252 (1977).
10. Kajii, T. and Ohama, K., Androgenetic origin of hydatidiform mole, Nature 268:633 (1977).
11. Jacobs, P. A., Wilson, C., Sprenkle, J., et al., Mechanism of origin of complete hydatidiform moles, Nature 286:714 (1980).
12. Lawler, D., Povey, T., Fisher, A., and Pickthall, J., Genetic studies on hydatidiform mole II. The origin of complete moles, Ann. Human Genetics 46:232 (1982).
13. Yamashita, K., Wake, N., Tsuneo, A., et al., A further HLA study of hydatidiform moles, Gynecol. Oncol. 11:238 (1981).
14. Surti, U., Szulman, A., and O'Brien, S., Complete (classic) hydatidiform mole, with 46,XY daryotype, of paternal origin, Human Genetics 51:153 (1979).
15. Ohama, K., Kajii, T., Okamoto, E., et al., Dispermic origin of XY hydatidiform moles, Nature 292:551 (1981).
16. Surti, U., Szulman, A. E., and O'Brien, S., Dispermic origin and clinical outcome of three complete hydatidiform moles with 46,XY karyotype, Amer. J. Obstet. Gynecol. 144:84 (1982).
17. Pattillo, R. A., Sasaki, S., Katayama, K. P., Roessler, M., and Mattingly, R. F., Genesis of 46,XY hydatidiform mole, Amer. J. Obstet. Gynecol. 141:104 (1981).
18. Beischer, N. A., Hydatidiform mole with co-existent foetus, J. Obstet. Gynaecol. Brit. Emp. 68:231 (1961).

19. Vassilakos, P., Riotton, G., and Kajii, T., Hydatidiform mole: Two entities, Amer. J. Obstet. Gynecol. 127:167 (1977).
20. Szulman, A. E., Phillippe, E., Boue, J. G., and Boue, A., Human triploidy: Association with partial hydatidiform moles and nonmolar conceptuses, Human Pathology 12:1016 (1981).
21. Jacobs, P. A., Szulman, A. E., Hunt, P., et al., Complete and partial hydatidiform mole in Hawaii, Brit. J. Obstet. Gynecol. 89:258 (1982).
22. Jacobs, P. A., Szulman, A. E., Funkhouser, J., et al., Human triploidy: Relationship between parental origin of chromosomes and development of partial mole in the placenta, Ann. Human Genetics 46:233 (1982).
23. Lawler, D., Fisher, R. A., Pickthall, et al., Origin of hydatidiform moles, I: Origin of partial moles, Cancer Gen. and Cytogenetics 5:309 (1982).
24. Philippe, E., "Pathologic Placentaire," Masson and Cre, Paris (1974).
25. Szulman, A. E. and Surti, U., The clinicopathologic profile of the partial hydatidiform mole, Obstet. Gynecol. 59:597 (1982).
26. Szulman, A. E., Surti, U., and Berman, M., Patient with partial mole requiring chemotherapy, Lancet 2:1009 (1978).
27. Berkowitz, R. S., Goldstein, D. P., Marean, A. R., et al., Proliferative sequelae after evacuation of partial hydatidiform mole, Lancet 2:804 (1979).
28. Szulman, A. E., Ma, H., K., Wong, L. C., and Hsu, C., Residual trophoblastic disease in association with partial hydatidiform mole, Obstet. Gynecol. 57:392 (1981).
29. Bagshawe, K. D., Wilson, H., Dublon, et al., Follow-up after hydatidiform mole, J. Obstet. Gynecol. Brit. Cmwth. 80:461 (1973).
30. Ring, A. M., The concept of benign metastasizing hydatidiform moles, Amer. J. Clin. Pathol. 58:111.J (1972).
31. Johnson, T., Comstock, C., and Anderson, D., Benign gestational trophoblastic disease metastatic to pleura: Unusual cause of hemothorax, Obstet. Gynecol. 53:509 (1979).
32. Kato, M., Tanaka, K., and Takeuchi, S., The nature of trophoblastic disease initiated by transplantation into immunosuppressed animal, Amer. J. Obstet. Gynecol. 142:497 (1982).

GENETIC STUDIES ON HYDATIDIFORM MOLES

Sylvia D. Lawler

Section of Human Genetics
Institute of Cancer Research
Royal Marsden Hospital
Fulham Road, London, SW3 6JJ
United Kingdom

INTRODUCTION

In this article the term gestational trophoblastic tumor is used to describe both invasive mole and choriocarcinoma and thus includes a nonmalignant and a malignant condition. This difficulty with nomenclature arises because when patients being treated with chemotherapy for a gestational trophoblastic tumor are studied, a histological diagnosis is not available in the majority of cases.

HYDATIDIFORM MOLE: HISTORY AND SEX

Hydatidiform mole was known to the ancients; the term "hydatid" was first used by Aetius of Amida in the 6th century A.D. (1). Later, the vesicles were interpreted as living embryos. According to Rather (2), in the second edition of Paré's Ouvres (Paris, 1579) may be found the story of Countess Margaret of Cracow, who is reported to have given birth to 36 live infants on January 20, 1269. The achievements of the Countess of Cracow were surpassed by those of the Countess Margaret of Flanders, "who brought forth at one birth 365 infants of whom 182 were solemnly baptized John and 182 Elizabeth, and the odd one after much ecclesiastical debate was adjudged a hermaphrodite and accordingly buried without baptism." Although the origin of the story of the Countess of Flanders is a subject for debate (2), it nevertheless illustrates that interest in the sex of hydatidiform moles goes back for 700 years.

Sex Chromatin

The presence of a chromatin body in the resting cells of mammalian females was first described by Barr and Bertram (3) in the neurones of cats. The technique of nuclear sexing was rapidly applied to the elucidation of sex chromosomal abnormalities in man. The sex chromatin body represents one of the two X chromosomes in a normal female cell in the resting phase. The maximum number of sex chromatin masses in a cell is one less than the number of X chromosomes. The sex chromatin is not expressed in every cell of a normal tissue, so that the chromatin body at the nuclear membrane may only be observed in 30 to 50 percent of suitable nuclei. Sex chromatin has been detected in trophoblastic cells by the twelfth day after fertilization in human embryos (4).

The Sex of Hydatidiform Moles

Park (5) was the first pathologist to make a systematic observation of the presence of sex chromatin in hydatidiform moles. The results of a number of studies from different parts of the world are shown in Table 1.

The results in Table 1 give an overall frequency of sex chromatin-positive cases of hydatidiform mole of 90%. Thus, it has been known for more than 20 years that, on the basis of the presence of sex chromatin, the majority of hydatidiform moles are of female sex. Nevertheless, it was clear that a sex chromatin body was not present in every case and that a minority (*circa* 10%) of hydatidiform moles can therefore be assumed to be of male sex.

Table 1. Sex Chromatin Studies in Hydatidiform Moles, 1957-1969

Reference	Locality	Total cases	Sex chromatin-positive cases (No.)
Park (5)	United Kingdom	22	16
Serr (6)	United Kingdom	5	4
Klinger *et al.* (7)	Switzerland	9	9
Wagner (8)	Germany	9	7
Stolte (9)	Holland	3	3
Tominaga and Page (10)	USA	18	17
Baggish *et al.* (11)	Singapore, 70 USA, 20	90	87
Loke and Borland (12)	Malaya, Kuala Lumpur	105	92

Table 2. Chromosome Studies of Hydatidiform Moles and Similar Lesions

Source	Locality	Total no. of cases	Chromosome findings	No. of cases
Stolte *et al.* (13) Hydatidiform moles	Holland	3	Diploid range	3
Harnden (14) Hydatidiform moles	United Kingdom	2	46,XX	2
Sasaki *et al.* (15) Hydatidiform moles	Japan	6	Diploid range	2
			46,XX	3
			46,XY	1
Makino *et al.* (16) Chorionic lesions	Japan	9	46,XX	9
Makino *et al.* (17) Chorionic lesions	Japan	3	69,XXY	3
Makino *et al.* (18) Chorionic lesions	Japan	19	46,XX	18
			46,?	1
Szulman (19) Spontaneous abortions	USA	1	69,XXY	1
Bourgoin *et al.* (20) Hydatidiform moles	France	4	46,XX	3
			46,XY	1
Carr (21) Spontaneous abortions	Canada	4	46,XX	2
			46,XY	1
			46,XXY	1
Klinger *et al.* (22) Hydatidiform moles	Europe	6	46,XX	4
			46,XY	1
			69,XXX	1
Boué *et al.* (23) Spontaneous abortions	France	3	69,XXX	2
			69,XXY	1
Carr (24) Spontaneous abortions	Canada	12	Diploid range	2
			Triploid range	1
			46,XX	1
			69,XXX	3
			69,XXY	4
			92,XXXX	1

Sex Chromosomes of Hydatidiform Moles

In 1956, Tjio and Levan (25) demonstrated that the number of chromosomes in man was 46. This observation was a prelude to a great deal of activity in defining the chromosomal abnormalities associated with clinically recognized constitutional abnormalities.

As shown in Table 2, the first studies of the chromosomes of hydatidiform moles were made in the 1960s. In Table 2 an attempt has been made to define how the cases were ascertained. The assignment of hydatidiform mole or chorionic lesions is given to series where the collection of hydatidiform moles was the primary objective. Those series in which the cases appear to have been ascertained through a systematic study of spontaneous abortion are marked accordingly; in some of these series, for example that of Carr (24), the histological appearances were distinguished from those expected of a frank hydatidiform mole.

Some interesting points emerge in the data collected between 1960 and 1969, when the sex chromosome complements and ploidy of the samples are considered in relation to the method of ascertainment (Table 3). Firstly, in considering the diploid (46 chromosomes) cases, the majority (42 of 46) were found in the series designated as hydatidiform mole or chorionic lesion. Secondly, the majority of these were of female sex (42 of 46), thus confirming the earlier work on the sex of hydatidiform moles. On the other hand, most of the cases of triploidy (69 chromosomes) were found in the cases ascertained in series of spontaneous abortions (12 out of 16 cases). Thus triploids, with features of hydatidiform mole, were more likely to be found among spontaneous abortions than among

Table 3. Cases (1960-1969) of Hydatidiform Moles and Similar Lesions with Defined Sex Chromosomal Complement Subdivided According to Ascertainment

Method of ascertainment	Sex chromosomes (No. of cases) XX	XY	XXX	XXY	XXXX	Total
Hydatidiform moles or chorionic lesions	39	3	1	3	0	46
Spontaneous abortion series	3	1	5	7	1	17
Total	42	4	6	10	1	63

Table 4. Chromosomal Findings in 75 Cases of Hydatidiform Mole (26).

Karyotype	56 Partial moles	19 Complete moles
Tetraploid	1	0
Triploid	22	0
Trisomic	17	0
46,XX	2	10
46,XY	7	0
Not known	7	9

cases examined because the diagnosis of hydatidiform mole was suspected. The sex chromosome complement of the triploids is also of interest in that, even though numbers are small, there appears to be an excess of XXY, the ratio of XXY to XXX being 10:6.

There was a lull in publication on chromosomes in trophoblastic disease during the early 1970s. In 1977, Vassilakos and associates (26) were the first to describe the two entities of hydatidiform mole based on morphological and cytogenetic studies. They had a series of 811 spontaneous abortions and 1097 induced abortions. Among these they identified 75 specimens (65 spontaneous abortions, 10 induced abortions) with gross swellings of the chorionic villi, of which they classified 56 as partial mole and 19 as complete mole, based on gross morphology and histopathology. Partial moles were associated with a fetus, cord, and/or amniotic membrane. In most cases the villi did not exceed 5 mm, and normal villi were also present. Histologically, partial moles were characterized by the absence of marked trophoblastic hyperplasia and the presence of fetal blood vessels. Complete moles were characterized by the absence of embryo, cord, or amniotic membrane, and marked trophoblastic hyperplasia and anaplasia. The chromosome findings in these two types of mole are shown in Table 4.

Firstly, the greater number of partial than complete moles in the series of Vassilakos and co-workers (26) may be due to the fact that the majority (65 out of 75) of the cases were found among spontaneous abortions. Secondly, their findings confirm the excess of 46,XX among complete moles, and the association of triploidy with partial moles. But in this series a high proportion of trisomic cases was described as partial mole on the basis of morphology and histology.

In the following year, further evidence of the two entities of hydatidiform mole, both on pathological and cytogenetic grounds, was published by Szulman and Surti (27). They did a cytogenetic and morphological analysis of 23 hydatidiform moles and divided them into at least two syndromes: 1) the syndrome of complete (classical) mole which was without an ascertainable embryo/fetus, and of diploid karyotype showing progressive fluid engorgement of the villi as well as a gross, haphazardly distributed trophoblastic hyperplasia; and 2) the syndrome of partial (incomplete) mole with evidence of fetal presence, a triploid chromosome constitution, and showing slowly progressing hydatidiform swelling in the presence of functioning villous capillaries. Trophoblastic immaturity was constant and focal hyperplasia, inconspicuous but present. They found all 7 of 11 diploid cases of complete mole where sex chromosomes could be defined to be 46,XX, and 11 out of 12 cases of partial mole to be triploid; the sex chromosome complement was XXY in 5 triploids testable.

ANDROGENETIC ORIGIN OF COMPLETE MOLE

In 1977, by using chromosomal polymorphisms, Kajii and Ohama (28) established that the chromosomes in seven cases of complete mole were entirely paternal in origin. In seven 46,XX moles, two Spanish and five Japanese in origin, and the parents, the fluorescent banding polymorphisms for seven pairs of chromosomes were studied. All of the 49 pairs of homologous chromosomes showed homozygous banding patterns in the moles. In 26 pairs of chromosomes it could be demonstrated that neither of the maternal homologues was transmitted to the mole. In 20 of the 26 pairs a paternal chromosome was shown to be inherited in duplicate by the mole. These results showed that complete moles are androgenetic in origin. Androgenesis is the development of an ovum under the influence of the nucleus of a sperm, the egg nucleus either absent or inactivated. Kajii and Ohama (28) reasoned that their chromosome findings were compatible with either fertilization by a diploid sperm due to nondivision at second meiotic division or fertilization by a haploid sperm followed by duplication of its chromosome and nondivision at first "blastomere" meiosis. Because a cell must have at least one X chromosome to survive, the predominance of XX was accounted for by the nonviability of a YY conceptus. These observations were subsequently confirmed by Wake and associates (29) and by Jacobs *et al.* (30). The duplicated paternal chromosomes identified by their polymorphisms in these studies are shown in Table 5.

Thus, by 1978, on the basis of cytogenetic findings, the androgenetic origin of complete moles was accepted and up until that time they were all homozygous. In 1979, Lawler and co-workers (31) first described the use of biochemical markers in the elucidation of the genetic origin of moles. They used the phosphoglucomutase 1 (PGM_1), acid phosphatase 1 (ACP_1), adenylate kinase 1 (AK_1), glyoxalase 1 (GLO), and phosphoglycolate phosphatase (PGP) systems

Table 5. Paternal Origin of Chromosomes in Complete Hydatidiform Moles

Reference	Duplicated paternal chromosome
Kajii and Ohama (28)	
Case 1	3, 14, 21
Case 2	21, 22
Case 3	14, 21, 22
Case 4	13, 14, 15
Case 5	4, 13, 14, 21
Case 6	13, 14, 15
Case 7	15, 22
Wake *et al.* (29)	
Case 1	13, 21
Case 2	21
Case 3	3, 13, 15, 22
Jacobs *et al.* (30)	
Case 1	3, 19, 13
Case 2	3, 13, 15, 22
Case 5	1, 21, 22

in the moles, the patients, and their husbands. On molar tissue, three additional markers were used: phosphoglucomutase 3 (PGM_3), glutamic oxaloacetic transaminase (GOT_2), and placental alkaline phosphatase (PL). Of the eleven complete moles examined, all results were compatible with exclusively paternal origin. In at least seven moles, a maternal contribution was excluded by at least one marker. The results suggested that complete moles arise from a duplicated haploid sperm rather than from a failure of meiosis II.

Thus, up to 1979, studies of cytogenetic and biochemical polymorphisms showed that complete moles were androgenetic, female, homozygous, and favored origin by a duplicated haploid sperm. When, in 1979, Surti and colleagues (32) described a complete XY mole of paternal origin, it became apparent that all cases of complete mole were not homozygous. The cytogenetic and biochemical markers used in this case did not allow the origin by error at first paternal meiosis or dispermy to be distinguished. In a series of 24 complete moles, in which chromosomal polymorphisms and the PGM_1 marker were studied, Jacobs and associates (33) found two atypical cases. One, 46,XX, was found to be the product of a normal conception because it contained both a maternal and a paternal genome. The other was 46,XY, but the origin could not be determined because the results of the genetic studies were compatible with either a normal conception or fusion of two sperm with an empty egg, although they excluded fertilization by a diploid sperm. Recent studies show that the origin of 46,XY complete moles is most likely to be by dispermy (34).

The genomic DNA in complete moles is paternal in origin, and so the question arises as to the origin of mitochondrial DNA (mtDNA) which is known to be maternally derived in man (35). Wallace and associates (36) have determined the parental origin of mtDNA using restriction endonuclease site polymorphisms, to study mtDNA in 12 complete moles. They found that the parents of three moles were informative and that in all these cases the mtDNA was maternally derived.

THE ORIGIN OF PARTIAL MOLES

In their studies of molar conceptuses, examined because the diagnosis of hydatidiform mole had already been made on clinical grounds, Lawler and co-workers (31, 37) found that those with a histological diagnosis of partial mole were triploid when examined cytogenetically.

Triploidy can arise from failure at the first or second meiotic division. This produces a diploid gamete that, after fertilization, results in a triploid zygote, by digyny (an extra maternal set), or diandry (an extra paternal set). Alternatively, a normal haploid ovum may be fertilized by two normal haploid sperms, leading to triploidy by dispermy.

As shown in Table 6, Lawler and colleagues (37) summarized the results of the investigations of the genetic origin of 51 previously published cases of spontaneous triploid abortion. Among the partial moles studied by Lawler *et al.* (37), diandry was proved to be the mechanism of origin in six cases and in a seventh, digyny could not be excluded. In all of these cases, origin by dispermy was possible and it was proven in four. Thus, triploid partial moles ascertained because of a diagnosis of mole are most likely to have a dispermic origin. So also are triploids found among spontaneous abortions, although in these cases origin by digyny has been proved in 24% of cases (Table 6).

So the question is, if all partial moles are triploid, are all spontaneously aborted triploids also partial moles? Jacobs and co-workers (38) have studied the question of the relationship between parental origin of the additional haploid complement and the development of partial mole. They ascertained 106 triploids during a study of 1500 consecutive spontaneous abortions in one maternity hospital in Honolulu. The mechanism of origin of the additional

Table 6. The Origin of 51 Triploid Abortuses Aged Less than 30 Weeks

Diandry 39	17 Dispermy
	15 Error at pat I or dispermy
	7 Error at pat II or dispermy
Digyny 12	5 Error at mat I
	3 Error at mat II
	3 Error at mat I or II
	1 Fusion of two eggs?

Sources of material:

1 Case	Schinzel *et al.* (39)	(Switzerland)
1 Case	Kunze *et al.* (40)	(Germany)
4 Cases	Lauritsen (41)	(Denmark)
10 Cases	Kajii and Niikawa (42)	(Japan)
8 Cases	Couillin *et al.* (43)	(France)
20 Cases	Jacobs *et al.* (44)	(Hawaii)
7 Cases	Brennan and Carr (45)	(Canada)

haploid complement was determined by studying chromosomal polymorphisms. Subsequently, the histopathological diagnosis was made independently as a blind study. Twenty-one of the cases had been reported previously (44). Among these 106 triploid spontaneous abortions, 74 were diagnosed histologically as partial mole, 2 as complete moles, and 16 were not hydatidiform moles. Fourteen cases were excluded from the pathological study because of an inadequate sample. The mechanism of origin of the additional haploid chromosome complement was established in 78 cases; 57 (73%) were found to be paternally derived and 21 (27%) maternally derived. All 54 paternally derived triploids, with adequate material for a histological diagnosis, were found to have the microscopical features of partial mole, whereas only 3 of 15 triploids with an extra maternal chromosome complement turned out to be histologically partial moles. The three maternally derived partial moles arose from an error at the first division of maternal meiosis. Jacobs and colleagues (38) further showed that not only was the histological appearance of a triploid conceptus correlated with the origin of the extra chromosome complement, but also with gestational age. The mean gestational age of the paternally derived triploids was 122 days, whereas that of maternally derived triploids was 74 days.

RELATIVE FREQUENCY OF COMPLETE AND PARTIAL MOLES

As indicated in the historical section of this review, the relative frequency of partial to complete mole depends on how the cases are ascertained. This still holds true in more recent studies when the diagnosis of the type of mole was made more precisely. Thus, among the hydatidiform moles found in a study of spontaneous abortions in Hawaii, Jacobs and colleagues (46) reported a higher number of partial (88 cases) than complete moles (40 cases), whereas in a series of patients ascertained because a molar pregnancy had been diagnosed, Fisher and co-workers (47) reported a higher frequency of complete than partial moles (50 compared to 16).

MOLE WITH TWIN

Beischer (48) reviewed 92 cases of molar pregnancy associated with fetus and identified 30 cases of dizygotic twin pregnancies in which there was a normal placenta associated with a fetus and a separate molar mass. Since 1966, about 15 more cases of mole with coexistent fetus, and one case of a triplet pregnancy where there was a separate molar mass and two normal placentae (49), have been reported. Fisher and associates (47) have recently reported a twin pregnancy with complete hydatidiform mole in which the fetus was shown to be 46,XY and to have a chromosomal contribution from both parents. The molar tissue was XX and proved to be androgenetic in origin.

CHEMOTHERAPY AND GESTATIONAL TROPHOBLASTIC TUMORS

In the United Kingdom, about 10% of patients who have a hydatidiform mole subsequently require treatment with chemotherapy for persistent trophoblastic activity (50). Since the entities of partial and complete mole were defined, the question arose as to which type is the more likely to be associated with the risk of progression to a gestational trophoblastic tumor. At first it was thought that partial moles did not show persistence of trophoblastic activity after evacuation (51). Now, although it is believed that treatment is required more frequently after complete mole, patients with partial mole who have subsequently required chemotherapy have been described (52, 53). In my department, a prospective study of hydatidiform moles is in progress in which, in addition to histopathology, whenever possible chromosomal polymorphisms and, in collaboration with Dr. S. Povey of the Medical Research Council UK Human Biochemical Genetics Unit, biochemical markers are studied (54). At the end of September 1982, 94 moles had been entered into the study, of which 74 (79%) were complete and 20 (21%) were partial. At the time of this writing (January 1983), none of the patients who had had a partial mole have required chemotherapy, whereas 12 of

Table 7. Summary of Genetics in 74 Cases of Complete Mole (Up to 30 September 1982)

	Number of cases with no further treatment after evacuation	Number of cases having chemotherapy after evacuation
Total	62	12
Tested for genetic markers	37	7
Male parent heterozygous	26	5
Homozygous moles	35	7
Homozygous moles with exclusion of maternal contribution	19	5
Heterozygous mole	2	0
Heterozygous mole with exclusion of maternal contribution	1	0

the patients with complete mole have required such treatment. Although in these data the trend for partial moles not to require treatment is apparent, the difference is not statistically significant at the 1 in 20 level ($\chi^2 = 3.7$). A summary of the genetics of the 74 cases of complete mole is given in Table 7, from which it can be seen that in our series up to the present time, there are no obvious differences between the cases requiring chemotherapy and those that do not. Only two heterozygous moles were detected, so the observation that neither have required treatment cannot yet be assessed. This prospective study is continuing. Surti and co-workers (34) have described three cases of 46,XY complete moles in which the origin was by dispermy. These authors referred to another 15 cases of complete mole with 46,XY karyotype, and of the 18 known cases, 10 had been followed up and two had required treatment for lung metastases, whereas the other 8 had a benign course. Clearly, more information is required on heterozygous moles. For example, can they be XX?

SUMMARY AND CONCLUSIONS

Using an historical approach, this article describes how genetic studies have elucidated the two entities into which the syndrome of hydatidiform mole can now be divided. Partial moles are triploid, have a maternal chromosomal set, and are associated with the presence of a fetus. Complete moles lack a fetus and are always diploid and androgenetic in origin, having two sets of paternal chromosomes. They are most often XX and homozygous, the most likely origin being by duplication of a haploid sperm. About 4% of complete moles have been shown to by XY and heterozygous, the most likely origin being by dispermy. The frequency of partial and complete mole observed depends on the method of ascertainment. Among spontaneous abortions, partial moles are more common than complete moles, but among cases having an elective termination of pregnancy because of a prior diagnosis of hydatidiform mole, complete mole is the more common. Patients with either type of mole may require treatment for persistent trophoblastic activity. More prospective studies of cases in which the type of mole has been confirmed by genetic studies are required in order to find out whether (a) patients with complete moles are more likely than those with partial moles to require treatment for persistence of trophoblastic activity after evacuation; and (b) heterozygous complete moles have a different prognosis from the point of view of malignant sequelae than homozygous complete moles.

ACKNOWLEDGEMENTS

The research on hydatidiform mole done in my laboratories is financed by the Medical Research Council (MRC) UK and the Cancer Research Campaign UK. I am grateful to my co-workers, Rosemary A. Fisher, D. M. Sheppard, and Veronica Pickthall, and for the collaboration of Dr. Sue Povey, MRC Human Biochemical Genetics Research Unit, London, UK.

REFERENCES

1. Ober, W. B. and Fass, O. S., The early history of choriocarcinoma, J. Hist. Med. 16:49 (1961).
2. Rather, L. J., Ambroise Paré, The Countess Margaret, multiple births, and hydatidiform moles, Bull. N. Y. Acad. Med. 47:508 (1971).
3. Barr, M. L. and Bertram, E. G., A morphological distinction between neurones of the male and female, and the behaviour of the nucleolar satellite during accelerated nucleoprotein synthesis, Nature 163:676 (1949).

4. Miller, O. J., The sex chromosome anomalies, Amer. J. Obstet. Gynecol. 90:1078 (1964).
5. Park, W. W., The occurrence of sex chromatin in chorionepitheliomas and hydatidiform moles, J. Path. Bact. 74:197 (1957).
6. Serr, D. M., in discussion in: "Symposium on Nuclear Sex," D. R. Smith and W. M. Davidson, eds., William Heinemann, London (1958), p. 175.
7. Klinger, H. P., Ludwig, K. S., Schwarzacher, H. G., and Hauser, G. A., Neue Ergebnisse der Sex-Chromatin-Forschung an Placenta und Eihäuten, Gynaecologia 146:328 (1958).
8. Wagner, D., Zur Frage der chromosomalen Geschlechtsbestimmung bei Frühaborten und Tubargraviditäten, Beburtsh. Grauenheilk. 18:1460 (1958).
9. Stolte, L. A. M., Chromosomal disorders in hydatidiform mole, Nederl. Tydschr. verlosk. 60:418 (1960).
10. Tominaga, T. and Page, E. W., Sex chromatin of trophoblastic tumors, Amer. J. Obstet. Gynecol. 96:305 (1966).
11. Baggish, M. S., Woodruff, J. D., Tow, S. H., and Jones, H. W., Sex chromatin pattern in hydatidiform mole, Amer. J. Obstet. Gynecol. 102:362 (1968).
12. Loke, Y. W. and Borland, R., A histological study of chromatin positive and negative hydatidiform moles, Brit. J. Cancer 23:554 (1969).
13. Stolte, L. A. M., van Kessel, H. I. A. M., Seelen, J. C., and Tijdink, G. A. J., Chromosomes in hydatidiform moles, Lancet ii:1144 (1960).
14. Harnden, D. G., Congenital abnormalities with apparently normal chromosome complement, in: "Human Chromosomal Abnormalities," W. M. Davidson and D. R. Smith, eds., Staples, London (1961).
15. Sasaki, M., Fukuschima, T., and Makino, S., Some aspects of the chromosome constitution of hydatidiform moles and normal chorionic villi, Gann 53:101 (1962).
16. Makino, S., Sasaki, M. S., and Fukuschima, T., Preliminary notes on the chromosomes of human chorionic lesions, Proc. Japan Acad. 39:54 (1963).
17. Makino, S., Sasaki, M. S., and Fukuschima, T., Triploid chromosome constitution in human chorionic lesions, Lancet ii:1213 (1964).
18. Makino, S., Sasaki, M. S., and Fukuschima, T., Cytological studies of tumours: XLI. Chromosomal instability in human chorionic lesions, Okajimas Fol. Anat. Jap. 40:439 (1965).
19. Szulman, A. E., Chromosomal aberrations in spontaneous human abortions, New Engl. J. Med. 272:811 (1965).
20. Bourgoin, P., Baylet, R., Ballon, C., and Grattepanche, H., Exploration d'une hypothèse sur l'êtiopathogênie des môles hydatiformes. Etude chromosomique, Rev. Franc. Gynec. Obstet. 60:673 (1965).
21. Carr, D. H., Chromosome studies in spontaneous abortions, Obstet. Gynecol. 26:308 (1965).

22. Klinger, H. P., Atkin, N. B., and Weiss, J., Results of sex chromatin and chromosome studies in hydatidiform moles, Bull. WHO 34:781 (1966).
23. Boûe, J. J., Boûe, A., and Lazar, P., Les aberrations chromosomiques dans les avortements, Ann. Genet. (Paris) 10:179 (1967).
24. Carr, D. H., Cytogenetics and the pathology of hydatidiform degeneration, Obstet. Gynecol. 33:33 (1969).
25. Tjio, J. H. and Levan, A., The chromosome number of man, Hereditas 42:1 (1956).
26. Vassilakos, P., Riotten, G., and Kajii, T., Hydatidiform mole: two entities. A morphologic and cytogenetic study with some clinical considerations, Amer. J. Obstet. Gynecol. 127:167 (1977).
27. Szulman, A. E. and Surti, U., The syndromes of hydatidiform mole. 1. Cytogenetic and morphologic correlations, Amer. J. Obstet. Gynecol. 131:665 (1978).
28. Kajii, T. and Ohama, K., Androgenetic origin of hydatidiform mole, Nature 268:633 (1977).
29. Wake, N., Takagi, N., and Sasaki, M., Androgenesis as a cause of hydatidiform mole, J. Natl. Cancer Inst. 60:51 (1978).
30. Jacobs, P. A., Hassold, T. J., Matsuyama, A. M., and Newlands, I. M., Chromosome constitution of gestational trophoblastic disease, Lancet ii:49 (1978).
31. Lawler, S. D., Pickthall, V. J., Fisher, R. A., Povey, S., Wyn Evans, M., and Szulman, A. E., Genetic studies of complete and partial hydatidiform moles, Lancet ii:580 (1979).
32. Surti, U., Szulman, A. E., and O'Brien, S., Complete (classic) hydatidiform mole with 46,XY karyotype of paternal origin, Human Genetics 51:153 (1979).
33. Jacobs, P. A. Wilson, C. M., Sprenkle, J. A., Rosenheim, N. B., and Migeon, B. R., Mechanism of origin of complete hydatidiform moles, Nature 286:714 (1980).
34. Surti, U., Szulman, A. E., and O'Brien, S., Dispermic origin and clinical outcome of three complete hydatidiform moles with 46,XY karyotype, Amer. J. Obstet. Gynecol. 144:85 (1982).
35. Giles, R. E., Blanc, H., Cann, H. M., and Wallace, D. C., Maternal inheritance of human mitochondrial DNA, Proc. Natl. Acad. Sci. USA 77:6715 (1980).
36. Wallace, D. C., Surti, U., Adams, C. W., and Szulman, A. E., Complete moles have paternal chromosomes but maternal mitochondrial DNA, Hum. Genet. 61:145 (1982).
37. Lawler, S. D., Fisher, R. A., Pickthall, V. J., Povey, S., and Wyn Evans, M., Genetic studies on hydatidiform moles. 1. The origin of partial moles, Cancer Genet. Cytogenet. 5:309 (1982).
38. Jacobs, P. A., Szulman, A. E., Funkhauser, J., Matsuura, J. S., and Wilson, C. C., Human triploidy: relationship between parental origin of the additional haploid complement and development of partial hydatidiform mole, Ann. Hum. Genet. 46:223 (1982).

39. Schinzel, A., Hayashi, K., Schmid, W., Knecht, B., Tuschy, G., and Boltshauser, E., Triploidie als Ursache von Schwangerschafts gestose in 2 Trimonen, Arch. Gynak. 218:113 (1975).
40. Kunze, J., Oldigs, H. D., and Tolksdorf, M., Identification of the triploid genome by the C-banding method, Europ. J. Pediat. 123:111 (1976).
41. Lauritsen, J. G., Aetiology of spontaneous abortion. A cytogenetic and epidemiological study of 288 abortuses and their parents, Acta Obstet. Gynecol. Scand. (Suppl. 52):1 (1976).
42. Kajii, T. and Niikawa, N., Origin of triploidy and tetraploidy in man: 11 cases with chromosome markers, Cytogenet. Cell Genet. 18:109 (1977).
43. Couillin, P., Hors, J., Boué, J., and Boué, A., Identification of the origin of triploidy by HLA markers, Hum. Genet. 41:35.
44. Jacobs, P. A., Angell, R. R., Buchanan, I. M., and Hassold, T. J., The origin of human triploids, Ann. Hum. Genet. 42:49 (1978).
45. Brennan, B. G. and Carr, D. H., Parental origin of triploidy and D and G trisomy in spontaneous abortions, J. Med. Genet. 16:287 (1979).
46. Jacobs, P. A., Szulman, A. E., Hunt, P. A., Matsuura, J. S., and Wilson, C. C., Complete and partial hydatidiform mole in Hawaii: cytogenetics, morphology and epidemiology, Brit. J. Obstet. Gynecol. 89:258 (1982).
47. Fisher, R. A., Sheppard, D. M., and Lawler, S. D., Twin pregnancy with complete hydatidiform mole (46,XX) and fetus (46,XY): genetic origin proved by analysis of chromosome polymorphisms, Brit. Med. J. 284:1218 (1982).
48. Beischer, N. A., Hydatidiform mole with co-existent foetus, Aus. N. Z. J. Obstet. Gynaecol. 6:127 (1966).
49. Sauerbrei, E. E., Salem, S., and Fayle, B., Coexistent hydatidiform mole and live fetus in the second trimester, Radiology 135:415 (1980).
50. Bagshawe, K. D. and Lawler, S. D., Choriocarcinoma, in: "Cancer Epidemiology and Prevention," D. Schottenfeld and J. F. Fraumeni, eds., W. B. Saunders, Philadelphia (1982), p. 916.
51. Vassilakos, P. and Kajii, T., Hydatidiform mole: two entities, Lancet i:259 (1976).
52. Stone, M. and Bagshawe, K. D., Hydatidiform mole: two entities, Lancet i:535 (1976).
53. Szulman, A. E., Surti, U., and Berman, M., Patient with partial mole requiring chemotherapy, Lancet ii:1099 (1978).
54. Lawler, S. D., Povey, S., Fisher, R. A., and Pickthall, V. J., Genetic studies on hydatidiform moles. II. The origin of complete moles, Ann. Hum. Genet. 46:209 (1982).

EPIDEMIOLOGIC ASPECTS OF TROPHOBLASTIC NEOPLASMS

The reported high incidence of trophoblastic neoplasms in the developing world, including the Far East, Africa, India, etc., may bear upon nutritional, genetic, hormonal, or chemical influences. The following chapters will outline some unique aspects of the disease process in various parts of the world. Synthesis of hCG, a sensitive tumor marker, provides the most advantageous asset in diagnosis and treatment of trophoblastic neoplasms. Because of this tumor marker, immediate diagnostic and monitoring surveillance is available for patients bearing these tumors. The potential for final tumor cell kill upon effective surgical or chemotherapeutic maneuvers is possible because of this marker. Without doubt, the high cure rate and effective follow-up of this disease process is the result of sensitive methods of hCG determination.

EPIDEMIOLOGY OF GESTATIONAL TROPHOBLASTIC NEOPLASM AT THE DR. CIPTO MANGUNKUSUMO HOSPITAL, JAKARTA, INDONESIA

M. Farid Aziz, Nugroho Kampono, Endy Muhardin Moegni, Sjahrul Sjamsuddin, Budianto Barnas, and Ratna Suprapti Samil

Medical Faculty University of Indonesia/
Dr. Cipto Mangunkusumo Hospital
Department of Obstetrics and Gynaecology
Subdivision of Oncology
Jakarta, Indonesia

INTRODUCTION

The incidence of molar pregnancy is much higher among oriental people than among white people, the cause of which is not yet known. The majority of gestational trophoblastic tumors are preceded by molar pregnancy, hence the number of patients who have developed gestational trophoblastic disease is higher among oriental people than among white people (1).

The incidence of gestational trophoblastic neoplasm in Indonesia has seldom been mentioned in foreign literature, although the incidence is reasonably high, even higher than in neighboring countries. The purpose of this paper is to give an epidemiological view of the gestational trophoblastic neoplasm, recorded at the Dr. Cipto Mangunkusumo Hospital. The general hospital functions as the teaching and referral hospital in the capital city of the Republic of Indonesia, which has a population of more than 6.7 million. The population of the entire country is 150 million.

MATERIALS AND METHODS

The data were compiled from all hydatidiform mole patients hospitalized in the Department of Obstetrics and Gynaecology, Medical Faculty University of Indonesia/Dr. Cipto Mangunkusumo Hospital, during the period 1977-1981.

The diagnosis of hydatidiform mole was confirmed through histological findings. Some of the moles emanated from abortions, while others came from ectopic pregnancies or normal deliveries. The majority of malignant trophoblastic diseases originated from hydatidiform moles which degenerated into malignancies during the follow-up period. The diagnosis of trophoblastic disease was based on clinical examinations supported by immuno-agglutination studies, chest X-ray, pelvic arteriography, and histological examination following curettage and hysterectomy. In the medical report were recorded patient's age, pregnancy, parity, blood group, gestational age, uterine size, and medical development during the follow-up period.

RESULTS

Incidence

The number of hydatidiform mole and malignant trophoblastic disease patients from 1977 to 1981 were 406 and 169, respectively. During the same period there were 31,280 pregnancies and 23,153 deliveries. Hence, the incidence of hydatidiform mole was 1 per 77 pregnancies (1 per 57 deliveries), and the incidence of malignant trophoblastic disease, 1 per 185 pregnancies (1 per 137 deliveries). Of the 406 hydatidiform moles that were followed, 93 (22.9%) progressed into malignancy (Tables 1 and 2).

Age

In the total population at risk, the highest frequency of hydatidiform mole occurred in women 24 years of age or younger ($P<0.05$). The tendency for hydatidiform moles to change into malignancy increased with advanced age and became obvious at 40 (Table 2).

Table 1. Incidence of Molar Pregnancy and Malignant Trophoblastic Disease

Number				Incidence		
Mole	MTD[a]	Pregnancies	Deliveries	Mole	MTD	
406	169	31,280	23,153	1:77	1:185	(Pregnancies)
				1:57	1:137	(Deliveries)

[a]MTD, malignant trophoblastic disease

Table 2. Distribution of Cases of Molar Pregnancy and Post-Molar Malignancy by Maternal Age

Age	Population at risk	Mole cases	Moles becoming malignant	
			No.	%
<20	83,197 (9.5)[a]	57 (14.0)	8	14.0
20-24	167,843 (19.2)	129 (31.8)	24	18.0
25-29	183,262 (20.9)	97 (23.9)	22	22.7
30-34	156,796 (17.9)	40 (9.9)	12	30.0
36-39	132,413 (15.1)	39 (9.6)	12	30.7
≥40	151,456 (17.3)	44 (10.8)	15	34.9
Overall	874,967 (100)	406 (100)	93	22.9

[a]Numbers in parenthesis represent percent frequency distribution.

Parity

In the total population at risk, women with parous 1 or less ran a greater risk of getting hydatidiform mole than women of higher parity ($P<0.05$). The tendency for hydatidiform moles to become malignant, however, was not influenced by parity (Table 3).

Blood Group

Women with either blood group A or B had a slightly greater tendency toward getting hydatidiform mole than women with blood groups O or AB. On the other hand, in patients with blood groups O or B, there was a greater tendency for hydatidiform moles to progress into malignancy (Table 4).

Table 3. Distribution of Cases of Molar Pregnancy and Post-Molar Malignancy by Parity

Parity	Population at risk	Mole cases	Moles becoming malignant No.	Moles becoming malignant %
0-1	265,840 (32.7)[a]	166 (40.4)	31	18.7
2	139,673 (17.2)	58 (14.3)	18	31.0
3	115,685 (14.2)	38 (9.4)	5	13.2
4	92,755 (11.4)	31 (7.6)	6	19.4
≥5	199,988 (24.6)	113 (27.8)	33	29.2
Overall	813,941 (100)	406 (100)	93	22.9

[a]Numbers in parenthesis represent percent frequency distribution.

Gestational Age and Uterine Size

Gestational age did not influence the change into either malignancy or metastasis. Most malignancies occurred when the uterine size was larger than that of a 20-week pregnancy. There was no relationship between uterine size and occurrence of metastasis (Tables 5 and 6).

Previous Pregnancies

The majority of malignant trophoblastic diseases originated from hydatidiform moles (76.4%). The remainder originated from abortions (12.4%), ectopic pregnancies (1.2%), or normal deliveries (9.5%). The non-hydatidiform mole category had the tendency for metastasis, although this was not significant ($P>0.05$)(Table 7).

The Histology of Hydatidiform Mole

According to the classification of Hertig-Mansell, hydatidiform mole in stages II and III runs a greater risk of becoming malignant

Table 4. Distribution of Cases of Post-Molar Malignancy by Blood Group

Blood group	Population at risk[a]	Mole cases	Moles becoming malignant No.	Moles becoming malignant %
A	(25.02)[b]	92 (26.8)[b]	17	18.5
B	(24.48)	93 (27.1)	26	27.9
AB	(6.48)	20 (5.8)	4	20.0
O	(40.52)	138 (40.2)	36	26.1

[a]Frequency distribution in Jakarta.
[b]Numbers in parenthesis represent percent frequency distribution.

Table 5. Distribution of Post-Molar Malignancies and Nonmalignant Mole Cases by Gestational Age

Age in weeks	Total cases	Nonmalignant No.	Malignancies No.	%	Metastatic	% Metastatic
≤8	62	45	17	27.4	7	41.2
9-12	124	89	35	28.2	6	17.1
13-16	115	95	20	17.4	8	40.0
17-20	60	49	11	18.3	1	9.1
21-24	29	22	7	24.1	1	14.3
≥25	16	15	1	6.3	0	0.0
Overall	406	315	91	22.4	23	25.0

Table 6. Distribution of Post-Molar Malignancies and Nonmalignant Mole Cases by Uterine Size

Uterine size (Weeks)	Total cases	Nonmalignant (No.)	Malignancies No.	%	Metastatic	% Metastatic
≤8	5	5	0	0.0	0	0.0
9-12	21	17	4	19.0	1	25.0
13-16	52	44	8	15.4	1	12.5
17-20	55	48	7	12.7	3	42.9
21-24	65	46	19	29.2	4	21.1
≥25	26	19	7	26.9	1	14.3
Overall	224	179	45	20.1	10	22.2

Table 7. Distribution of Post-Molar Malignancies by Origin of Pregnancy

Origin of pregnancy	Total cases	Nonmetastatic (No.)	Metastatic No.	Metastatic %
Hydatidiform mole	130 (76.4)[a]	86	44	33.8
Abortion	21 (12.4)	13	8	38.0
Ectopic pregnancy	2 (1.2)	1	1	50.0
Normal pregnancy	16 (9.5)	6	10	62.5
Overall	169 (100)	106	63	37.2

[a]Numbers in parenthesis represent percent frequency distribution.

Table 8. Distribution of Cases of Molar Pregnancy and Post-Molar Malignancy by Histological Classification

Histological classification	Mole cases	Malignancies No.	Malignancies %
I	180	25	13.9
II	110	25	22.7
III	78	20	25.6

than in stage I. This difference becomes significant ($P<0.05$) when stage I is compared with a combination of stages II and III (Table 8).

DISCUSSION

Incidence

There are in Indonesia 285 hospitals of various classes which are managed by the government. In 1981, the number of cases of hydatidiform mole, recorded from 154 of these hospitals, was 2,136. There were 156,806 pregnancies in the same year, giving an incidence of hydatidiform mole of 1:73. This incidence is essentially the same as the incidence of hydatidiform mole in the Dr. Cipto Mangunkusumo Hospital, Jakarta, during the period from 1977-1981 (Tables 1 and 9). About 22% of the hydatidiform moles progressed into malignancy. This figure is much higher than has been reported before by Prawirohardjo and co-workers (11) in 1957 in the same hospital, although the socio-economic condition during the period 1977-1981 was considerably improved compared to 25 years earlier. There are probably other factors besides nutrition that influence this change into malignancy.

Age Factor

The influence of age towards the incidence of hydatidiform mole varies in different reports. Some workers found a higher risk in the age group of 14-25 years (4, 12, 13), while others reported the greatest risk in the group in the thirties (9), or in the age group of over 40 years (10, 14). Morrow and colleagues (15) found that trophoblastic disease was not prevalent in any particular age group. In our investigation, the age group of 24 years or younger was more

Table 9. Incidence of Molar Pregnancy in Various Countries

Country (city)	Date	Incidence	Reference
Alaska	1978	1:157 Deliveries	2
Nigeria (Ibadan)	1978	1:205 Pregnancies	3
Iran	1978	1:314 Pregnancies	4
Taiwan	1978	1:188 Deliveries	5
Malaysia (Kuala Lumpur)	1965	1:341 Pregnancies	6
USA	1958	1:1438 Deliveries	7
Taiwan	1963	1:125 Deliveries	8
Mexico	1963	1:200 Pregnancies	9
USA	1968	1:1450 Pregnancies	10
Indonesia (Jakarta)	1982	1:77 Pregnancies	Present report

at risk for getting hydatidiform mole, and the risk of the mole becoming malignant increased with age (Table 2).

The Factor of Parity and Pregnancy

This disease if frequently found among patients with low parity, *e.g.*, multipara (5) or para primipara and secundigravide in particular in the 20th and 30th years of age (9). This correlates with our results (Table 3). The reverse situation, however, has also been reported, with most frequent occurrence in multiparous women (5, 7). Again, Morrow *et al.* (15) found no significant difference between the different pregnancy groups.

According to Bagshawe and Begent (13), the influence of pregnancy cannot be observed if it is not related to age. The risk of getting hydatidiform mole will increase with advanced age. Hence, the risk of changing into invasive mole and choriocarcinoma will also increase proportionally when advanced age is connected with the number of previous pregnancies.

The Factor of Blood Group

Blood group ABO can influence either the formation of hydatidiform mole or the progression of hydatidiform mole into malignancy. A shift in the ABO blood group can occur, from blood group O in the wife (6, 16) and toward blood group O in the husband (16). A woman of blood group A who marries a man with blood group O has a 10 percent higher chance of getting choriocarcinoma than a woman of blood group A who marries a man with blood group A. A woman with blood group AB has a poor prognosis (16).

In our investigation the influence of blood group ABO was not so clear, although there was a tendency for moles to occur more frequently in patients with blood groups A or B. On the other hand, change into malignancy was more frequent in women with blood groups B or O (Table 4).

Gestational Age and Uterine Size

Complications that lead to trophoblastic disease are more frequent during early pregnancy than in later pregnancy. Trophoblastic disease was more probable during the gestational age of 12 weeks or less, compared to 16 weeks or greater ($P<0.05$). By contrast, metastasis occurred more often during advanced age of pregnancy (15). Similarly, the occurrence of trophoblastic disease increases as the size of the uterus becomes larger (14, 15).

The frequency of trophoblastic disease in molar pregnancies with a uterine size of 16 weeks or less was significantly different ($P<0.02$) when compared with the frequency at a larger uterine size (15). On the other hand, Martaadisubrata (14) concluded that malignancy will become more frequent when the uterine size is larger than 28 weeks. According to Martaadisubrata (14), uterine size seems to be more important than gestational age in the progression of hydatidiform mole into malignancy. This was also suggested in our investigation (Tables 5 and 6). The tendency to become malignant increased with uterine size, becoming greatest after the uterus reached a size of at least 20 weeks. The frequency of metastasis, however, was not influenced by uterine size. Gestational age had no influence on the change into malignancy.

Previous Pregnancy

Hydatidiform mole patients run a greater risk of malignancy than patients with abortion or normal pregnancy. Ten to 20 percent of hydatidiform moles progressed into malignancy. According to other reports, about half of all trophoblastic malignancies originate from hydatidiform mole, whereas 25 percent originate from abortion, 22.5 percent from normal delivery, and 2.5 percent from ectopic pregnancy (16). As shown in Table 7, we found a higher proportion, of more than 75 percent, originating from hydatidiform mole.

The Histology of Hydatidiform Mole

The histologic picture of hydatidiform mole can be predicted in advance (17), as shown in Table 8. Therefore, preventive measures of medication can be initiated early.

SUMMARY

This retrospective research was conducted in the Department of Obstetrics and Gynaecology of the Dr. Cipto Mangunkusumo Hospital, Jakarta, covering the period between 1977 and 1981. The incidence of hydatidiform mole was 1 in 77 pregnancies. The incidence of malignant trophoblastic disease was 1 in 185 pregnancies. Of the 406 cases of hydatidiform mole, 22.9% became malignant. Patients of 24 years of age or younger had a higher risk of getting hydatidiform mole ($P<0.05$) compared to older patients. The risk of becoming malignant increased with age and became evident after 40 years of age. Parity 1 or less was associated with a higher risk of getting hydatidiform mole ($P<0.05$), but had no influence on hydatidiform mole becoming malignant. The influence of blood group was not so clear, although there was a tendency for moles to occur more frequently in patients with blood groups A or B. By contrast, there was a tendency for the change into malignancy to occur more frequently in women with blood groups B or O. Gestational age had no influence towards the change into malignancy or metastasis. Uterine size (greater than 20 weeks gestation) correlated with the progression of hydatidiform mole into malignancy. However, subsequent metastasis was not influenced by the size of the uterus. It was found that 76.4% of malignant trophoblastic diseases originated from hydatidiform moles, 12.4% from abortions, 9.5% from normal deliveries, and 1.2% from ectopic pregnancies. Non-hydatidiform moles had a slightly greater risk for metastasis, although this was not significant. Hydatidiform mole in histologic stages II or III (Hertig-Mansell classification) had a significantly greater tendency ($P<0.05$) to become malignant than in stage I.

REFERENCES

1. Ma, H. and Wong, L. C., Gestational trophoblastic disease in Hong Kong, in: "Seminars in Oncology - Gestational Trophoblastic Disease," J. W. Yarbro, R. S. Bornstein, and M. J. Mastrangelo, eds., Grune & Stratton, New York (1982), Vol. 9, No. 2, p. 224.
2. Martin, P. M., High frequency of hydatidiform mole in native Alaskans, Int. J. Gynecol. Obstet. 15:395 (1978).

3. Ogunbode, O., Benign hydatidiform mole in Ibadan, Nigeria, Int. J. Gynecol. Obstet. 15:387 (1978).
4. Janvey, J. and Sajadi, H., Hydatidiform mole in southern Iran: a statistical survey of 113 cases, Int. J. Gynecol. Obstet. 15:390 (1978).
5. Tat, N. H., Current status of trophoblastic disease in Taiwan, Modern Medicine of Asia 15:50 (1979).
6. Llewellyn-Jones, D., Trophoblastic tumours. Geographical incidence and possible aetiological factors, J. Obstet. Gynecol. Brit. Cwlth. 72:242 (1965).
7. Schelpert, J. W., Hydatidiform mole. A survey of 66 cases at Hartford Hospital, Amer. J. Obstet. Gynecol. 76:883 (1958).
8. Wei, P. and Ouyang, P. C., Trophoblastic disease in Taiwan, Amer. J. Obstet. Gynecol. 85:844 (1963).
9. Marques-Monter, H., De La Vega, G. A., Robles, M., Bolio-Cicero, A., Epidemiology and pathology of hydatidiform mole in the General Hospital of Mexico, Amer. J. Obstet. Gynecol. 85: 856 (1963).
10. Yen, S. and MacMahon, B., Epidemiologic features of trophoblastic disease, Amer. J. Obstet. Gynecol. 101:126 (1968).
11. Prawirohardjo, S., Martiono, K. S., and Tjokronegoro, S., Hydatidiform mole and chorio carcinoma in Indonesia, in: "Racial Peculiarities in Obstetrics and Gynecology. Asiatic Congress of Obstetrics and Gynecology, Tokyo, Japan," The Japanese Obstetrical and Gynecological Society, Tokyo (1957), p. 112.
12. Morrow, C. P. and Townsend, D.E, "Synopsis of Gynecologic Oncology," 2nd Edition, John Wiley & Sons, New York (1981) p. 327.
13. Bagshawe, K. D. and Begent, R. H. J., Trophoblastic tumors: clinical features and management, in: "Gynecologic Oncology. Fundamental Principles and Practice," Coppleson, ed., Churchill-Livingstone, London (1981), p. 757.
14. Martaadisoebrata, D., "Problematik penyakit trofoblas ditinjau segi epidemiologi serta pengelolannya," Disertasi, Universitas Pajajaran, Bandung (1980).
15. Morrow, C. P., Kletzky, O. A., Disaia, P. J., Townsend, D. E., Mishell, D. R., and Nakamura, R. M., Clinical and laboratory correlates of molar pregnancy and trophoblastic disease, Amer. J. Obstet. Gynecol. 128:424 (1977).
16. Barber, H. R. K., "Manual of Gynecologic Oncology," J. B. Lipincott Co., Philadelphia (1980).
17. Barnas, B., Hubungan klasifikasi histologik mola hydatidosa dengan penyakit trofoblas ganas, Skripsi Bagian Obstetri dan Ginekologi, FKUI/RSCM (1981).

EPIDEMIOLOGIC ASPECTS OF GESTATIONAL TROPHOBLASTIC DISEASES IN IBADAN, NIGERIA

T. A. Junaid

Department of Pathology
University College Hospital and
College of Medicine
University of Ibadan
Ibadan, Nigeria

INTRODUCTION

Acosta-Sison and other Asian workers (1, 2) first called world attention to the unusually high frequency of gestational trophoblastic disease - hydatidiform mole and choriocarcinoma - in their region. In 1959 the Joint Project of American and Asian physicians confirmed the geographic variation in incidence (3). In the early and mid-sixties, Hendrickse in Ibadan, Nigeria (4), Oettle in Southern Africa (5), and Dodin (6) in Madagascar (now Malagasy) raised the possibility that similar lesions were encountered more frequently by physicians working in Africa than by their colleagues in Europe or North America.

The present communication explores this possibility further, and highlights aspects of hydatidiform mole and choriocarcinoma that are primarily of epidemiologic interest.

MATERIALS AND METHODS

Data from patients were obtained from the Cancer Registry of the Department of Pathology, University College Hospital and the College of Medicine, University of Ibadan, Ibadan, Nigeria. Essential clinical information was supplied in hospital records and on request forms accompanying histopathological specimens from outlying hospitals. Only cases with histologically confirmed diagnoses were included in this report.

Clinical information supplied was incomplete in several cases and this accounts for the varying number of subjects analyzed for the different epidemiologic parameters.

RESULTS

Age

The age distribution of 172 patients with hydatidiform mole is shown in Table 1. Molar gestation is most common in the third decade. The youngest patient was 16 years and the oldest, 55 years. When this distribution is compared to that obtained for mothers in the same communities (7), there is an excess of older women (35 years and older) in the molar group (Table 2). Tables 3 and 4 show similar trends in patients with choriocarcinoma.

Parity

The parity distribution in delivered mothers and patients with gestational trophoblastic disease is depicted in Table 5. Both hydatidiform mole and choriocarcinoma show a significant association with parity in excess of 3. Nine patients who had choriocarcinoma were primiparous, while one patient had had 15 previous deliveries before developing choriocarcinoma.

Frequency

In our materials, hydatidiform mole accounted for 1:329 deliveries at University College Hospital, while choriocarcinoma showed

Table 1. Age Distribution in 172 Patients with Hydatidiform Mole

Age in years	No. of patients	Percentage
11-20	26	15.1
21-25	47	27.3
26-30	48	27.9
31-35	29	16.9
36-40	15	
41-45	3	12.8
46-50	3	
51-55	1	
Total	172	100

Table 2. Age Distribution of Delivered Mothers and 172 Patients with Hydatidiform Mole

Age (years)	Delivered mother (3076 total)	Hydatidiform mole (172 total)
24	30%	30.8%
25-34	61%	47.7%
≥35	9%	21.5%

showed a frequency of 1:473 deliveries or 1:270 necropsies.

Seasonal Variation

Table 6 summarizes the monthly distribution of hydatidiform mole, choriocarcinoma, and normal deliveries in the hospital. Both normal delivery and choriocarcinoma show a comparable frequency throughout the year, while hydatidiform mole shows a gradual fall in frequency over the year. The pattern shown by hydatidiform mole shows a significant departure from that of normal delivery ($P<0.025$).

Antecedent Pregnancy in Choriocarcinoma

Data on antecedent pregnancies were obtained from 145 patients. Twenty-two of these had hydatidiform mole which was confirmed

Table 3. Age Distribution in 191 Patients with Choriocarcinoma

Age in years	No. of patients	Percentage
Under 20	8	4.2
20-24	30	15.7
25-29	54	28.3
30-34	36	18.8
35-39	30	15.7
40-44	19	9.9
45-49	11	5.8
50 and older	3	1.6
Total	191	100

Table 4. Age Distribution in Delivered Mothers and 191 Patients with Choriocarcinoma

Age (years)	A Delivered mother (3076 total)	B Choriocarcinoma (191 total)
24	30%	19.9%
25-34	61%	47.1%
$\geq$35[a]	9%	33.0%

[a]Patients $\geq$35: Group A *vs* Group B, $P<0.01$.

Table 5. Parity Distribution in Delivered Mothers and Patients with Choriocarcinoma and Hydatidiform Mole

Subjects			Percentage with parity					
Group	Category	No.	0	1	2	3	4	$\geq$5
A	Delivered mother	3076	23	23	25	16	7	6
B	Choriocarcinoma	102	8.8	11.8	19.6	15.7	12.7	29.4
C	Hydatidiform mole	89	17.1	12.4	15.7	20.2	11.3	21.3

A *vs* B: $P<0.001$ with parity in excess of 3.
A *vs* C: $P<0.01$ with parity in excess of 3.
Nine primiparas and one patient with 15 previous deliveries had choriocarcinoma.

Table 6. Seasonal Distribution of Hydatidiform Mole, Choriocarcinoma, and Normal Deliveries in University College Hospital, Ibadan, Nigeria

		Percent distribution		
Subject	No.	Jan.-April	May-Aug.	Sept.-Dec.
Hydatidiform mole	318	45	30	25
Choriocarcinoma	139	33.1	34.5	32.4
Normal deliveries	27,558	33.3	33.7	33

Mole *vs* normal deliveries: $P<0.025$.

Table 7. Antecedent Pregnancy in 145 Patients with Choriocarcinoma

Antecedent pregnancy	No. of cases	Percentage
Hydatidiform mole	22	15.2
Normal delivery (birth)	37	25.5
Abortion	86	59.3
Total	145	100

histologically, while 123 recalled the form of pregnancy as shown in Table 7.

ABO Blood Group and Hemoglobin Type

Data obtained for patients with gestational trophoblastic disease showed fewer patients with blood groups A, B, and AB, and an excess with group O, but this was not significantly different from the the frequency in the control population (Table 8). Similarly, no significant variation in hemoglobin type was observed in 207 patients with gestational trophoblastic disease (Table 9).

Table 8. Blood Group Distribution in 260 Patients with Gestational Trophoblastic Disease and in Control Subjects

	Patients			Normal subjects	
	Observed				
Blood group	No.	Percent	No. expected	No.	Percent
A	48	18.5	55.4	5,544	21.3
B	52	20.0	60.6	6,064	23.3
AB	5	1.9	10.7	1,015	3.9
O	155	59.6	133.9	13,404	51.5
Total	260	100		26,027	100

Table 9. Distribution of Hemoglobin Types in 207 Patients with Gestational Trophoblastic Disease Compared with Normal Subjects

Hemoglobin type	Patients			Normal subjects	
	Observed				
	No.	Percent	No. expected	No.	Percent
A	146	70.5	136.6	1,980	66
A+C	12	5.8	12	174	5.8
A+S	48	23.2	53	768	25.6
S+C	1	0.5	1.7	24	0.8
S	0	0	3.5	51	1.7
C	0	0	0.6	3	0.1
Total	207	100		3,000	99.9

$0.7<P<0.5$

Geographic Distribution

Seventy percent of patients came from within 100 miles of the hospital while 30% were from different areas of Nigeria. This distribution was not different from that recorded for all patients attending the hospital.

Infections

Serological examinations performed on sera of patients with gestational trophoblastic disease showed no significant association with hepatitis B antigen, toxoplasmosis, or Epstein-Barr virus. Also, no correlation was found between the high incidence of tuberculosis in Ibadan autopsy materials and gestational trophoblastic disease.

DISCUSSION

Determining the incidence of any disease is a formidable task, even in developed countries where national and biostatistical data such as census figures and population structures are available for national and regional planning. In most of Africa such basic information is unavailable; where it exists, it is little more than informed (more often, uninformed) guesses. For instance, the population of Nigeria, Africa's most densely populated country, may be any figure between 60 and 120 million.

Secondly, attempts at finding an accurate incidence of gestational trophoblastic disease face greater problems in both developed and developing countries, since this group of diseases is related to the specific state of conception. It is doubtful if the exact number of women who have conceived at a particular time is known in any human community. It is largely because of this seemingly insurmountable obstacle that figures on the frequency of gestational trophoblastic disease have been based on births, deliveries, pregnancies, or necropsies, usually for small communities (9).

Our data, although biased since University College Hospital is a known reference center, reflect a high frequency of hydatidiform mole and choriocarcinoma in our material. They also suggest that gestational trophoblast disease may be more common in Ibadan, Nigeria, than in Europe or North America (9). Hendrickse (10) reported an estimated frequency of 1:2518 pregnancies for choriocarcinoma.

Both hydatidiform mole and choriocarcinoma show significant association with maternal age at 35 years or older and with parity above 3. Parity increases with age and as maternal age has been associated with a greater frequency of hydatidiform mole in some series (11), it is possible that age and parity may contribute independently to the development of gestational trophoblastic disease. However, this separation was not possible with our data which, contrary to the data of others, failed to show a significant association between hydatidiform mole and low maternal age (11).

Reports from different countries have shown that the majority of cases of choriocarcinoma follow abnormal pregnancies, mainly hydatidiform mole (Table 10). On the surface, our data on antecedent pregnancy would seem to contradict this. However, there is little doubt that abortion is over-represented in the total number, principally because such aborted materials were not subjected to histopathological examination since most patients only came or were referred to University College Hospital when the "abortions" became complicated. Both hydatidiform mole and choriocarcinoma are commonly seen in Ibadan, unlike in South Africa where there appears to be a lower incidence of hydatidiform mole (5).

Somewhat intriguing but not explained is the seeming variation in the seasonal frequency of hydatidiform mole compared to normal delivery and choriocarcinoma. The decline in frequency of molar abortions during the wet months of the year is a finding for which we have not found an explanation.

Negative correlation was found between gestational trophoblastic disease, the sickle cell gene, and ABO blood groups. The latter finding is contrary to the experience of other workers who reported an excess of group A and a deficit of group O for patients with choriocarcinoma (12, 13). Our data are being re-examined as it has

Table 10. Antecedent Pregnancy of Choriocarcinoma in Selected Studies

Location	Cases (No.)	Antecedent pregnancy (% distribution) Mole	Birth	Abortion and ectopic preg.	Unknown	Ref.
Uganda	26	50	15	35	0	15
Hong Kong	41	44	24	31	0	16
Taiwan	22	82	5	14	0	17
Israel	32	41	34	19	6	18
United Kingdom	101	34	37	30	0	19
Ibadan, Nigeria	145	15	26	59	0	This study

become obvious that separation of gestational trophoblastic disease into hydatidiform mole and choriocarcinoma was less than satisfactory in the early period of the study.

CONCLUSION

Although it would appear that gestational trophoblastic disease is commonly encountered in Ibadan, no correlation between it and the high prevalence of such infections as tuberculosis, infective hepatitis, and toxoplasmosis in our environment has been demonstrated. At present it is not clear whether the exceedingly high frequency of nonfamilial dizygotic twinning in western Nigeria has any bearing on the seemingly high frequency of gestational trophoblastic disease, both of which may represent abnormalities of reproductive function (14).

REFERENCES

1. Acosta-Sison, H., Trophoblastic or chorionic tumours as observed in the Philippines, in: "Choriocarcinoma, Transactions of a Conference of the International Union Against Cancer," J. F. Holland and M. M. Hreshchyshyn, eds., Springer-Verlag, Berlin (1967), p. 33.
2. Wei, P. Y. and Ouyang, P. C., Trophoblastic disease in Taiwan, Amer. J. Obstet. Gynecol. 85:844 (1963).

3. Joint project for study of choriocarcinoma and hydatidiform mole in Asia. Geographic variation in the occurrence of hydatidiform mole and choriocarcinoma, Ann. N. Y. Acad. Sci. 80:178 (1954).
4. Hendrickse, J. P. de V., Cockshott, W. P., Evans, K. T., and Barton, C. J., Pelvic angiography in the diagnosis of malignant trophoblastic disease, New Engl. J. Med. 271:859 (1964).
5. Oettle, A. G., Cancer in Africa, especially in regions south of the Sahara, J. Natl. Cancer Inst. 33:383 (1964).
6. Dodin, A., Randrianarivo, P., and Brygoo, E. R., Hydatidiform moles and chorionic epitheliomas in Madagascar, Arch. Inst. Pasteur Madagascar 32:67 (1963).
7. Nylander, P. P. S., Maternal age and parity distribution in rural and urban communities in western Nigeria, Afr. J. Med. Sci. 1:285 (1970).
8. Esan, G. T. F., The thalassaemia syndromes in Nigeria, Brit. J. Haem. 19:47 (1970).
9. Park, W. W., "Choriocarcinoma - A Study of Its Pathology," William Heineman, Ltd., London (1971), pps. 114, 123.
10. Hendrickse, J. P. de V., I. E. A. Scientific meeting, Ibadan (1970).
11. Matalon, M. and Modan, B., Epidemiologic aspects of hydatidiform mole in Israel, Amer. J. Obstet. Gynecol. 112:107 (1972).
12. Bagshawe, K. D., Rawlings, G., Pike, M. C., and Lawler, S. O., The ABO blood group in trophoblastic neoplasia, Lancet 1: 553 (1971).
13. Dawood, M. Y., Teoh, E. S., and Ratnam, S. S., ABO blood group in trophoblastic disease, J. Obstet. Gyn. Brit. Commonwealth 78:918 (1971).
14. De George, Hydatidiform mole in other pregnancies of mothers of twins, Amer. J. Obstet. Gynecol. 108:369 (1970).
15. Leighton, P. C., Trophoblastic disease in Uganda, Amer. J. Obstet. Gynecol. 117:341 (1973).
16. Chan, D. P., Chorion epithelioma: a study of 41 cases, Brit. Med. J. 5310:953 (1962).
17. Hsu, C. T., Chen, T. U., Chiu, W. H., Yang, C. C., Lai, C. H., Changcheng, C. H., Tung, P. H., and Chen, C. C., Some aspects of trophoblastic diseases peculiar to Taiwan, Amer. J. Obstet. Gynecol. 90:308 (1964).
18. Matalon, M., Paz, B., Modan, M., and Modan, B., Malignant trophoblastic disorders. Epidemiologic aspects and relationship to hydatidiform mole, Amer. J. Obstet. Gynecol. 112:101 (1972).
19. Bagshawe, K. D., Risk and prognostic factors in trophoblastic neoplasia, Cancer 38:1373 (1976).

EPIDEMIOLOGY OF TROPHOBLAST DISEASE IN AFRICA - LAGOS

Akin Agboola and O. O. Abudu

University of Lagos
Department of Obstetrics and Gynaecology
College of Medicine
P.M.B. 12003
Lagos, Nigeria

INTRODUCTION

Trophoblast neoplasm is a common disease in Nigeria and this has been confirmed by previous workers (1, 2, 3). Choriocarcinoma is the third most common cancer in Nigeria, after cancer of the cervix and of the breast. Having realized the significance of this tumor, which fortunately is invariably curable if treated promptly, much attention is now focused on its epidemiology. Although racial incidence of this disease is undisputed, its etiology has in the past been linked with external factors including viral (4), chemical (5), dietary (6, 7), and genetic (8, 9). It has also been suggested (9) that trophoblastic neoplasms may be attributed to immune mechanisms.

MATERIALS AND METHODS

An analysis of the 42 cases admitted to the Department of Obstetrics and Gynaecology of the Lagos University Teaching Hospital over the two-year period of 1980-1981, and managed by the authors, was carried out.

All cases of hydatidiform mole were managed conservatively by evacuating the mole, while the choriocarcinoma patients were treated with chemotherapy. Since October, 1981, the unit has used the W.H.O. protocol regime in the management of choriocarcinoma. This regime consists of using either intramuscular injections of methotrexate plus folinic acid, or methotrexate plus folinic acid and actinomycin.

RESULTS

There was a total of 26 cases of hydatidiform mole during the study period. The total number of deliveries was 4,787, giving an institutional incidence of 1 in 184 deliveries. The age distribution of the patients was 19-42 years, with a mean of 27 years and a median of 26 years. The study group is summarized in Table 1.

The parity distribution of the patients was 0-6 with a mean of 2.6 and a median of 2 (Table 2). The incidence of previous abortion was recorded in 19 cases as shown in Table 3.

The clinical features of the patients are shown in Table 4. Of interest were the six cases who presented with pseudo-toxemia, and another case with eclampsia. Of these seven patients, five were found to have large abdomen. The management of the patients is illustrated in Table 5. The complications encountered included severe hemorrhage in 10 patients and sepsis in one patient.

Table 1. Relationship of Hydatidiform Mole with Age

Age group	No. of cases
15-19	1
20-24	7
25-29	10
30-34	5
35-39	2
40-44	1

Table 2. Relationship of Hydatidiform Mole with Parity

Parity	No. of cases
0	4
1	6
2	6
3	2
4	4
5	0
6	4

Table 3. Incidence of Previous Abortion in Hydatidiform Mole Patients

No. of abortions	No. of cases
1	16
2	2
3	1
	Total 19 (73%)

The policy of our unit is to follow up each patient after treatment for a period of one year before allowing her to start another pregnancy. Table 6 illustrates the problems encountered with this group of patients.

Table 4. Presenting Symptoms in Patients with Hydatidiform Mole

Symptom	No. of cases
Vaginal bleeding	28 (69%)
Abdominal pain	10 (38%)
Passage of vesicles	18 (69%)
Hyperemesis	5 (19%)
Pseudo-toxemia	6 (27%)
Eclampsia	1 (4%)
Large for dates	8 (31%)
Small for dates	4 (15%)
Enlarged cystic ovaries	7 (27%)
Bilateral	4
Unilateral	3

Table 5. Management of Hydatidiform Mole

Procedure	No. of cases	
Evacuation of uterus	13	
Induction	7	
Oxytocin		5
Prostaglandins		2
Evacuation followed by hysterectomy	1	
Primary D & C	5	

There was only one patient whose condition progressed to choriocarcinoma, for a progression rate of 4 percent. This occurred within 3 months of evacuation of the mole and subsequent to hysterectomy performed because of the patient's age. During the same two-year period, 16 cases of choriocarcinoma were admitted to the unit, giving an institutional incidence of 1 in 299 deliveries. The age distribution of the patients was 21 to 42 years, with a mean of 30 years, a mode of 21 to 30, and a median of 29 years.

The parity distribution of the choriocarcinoma patients was 0-12 with a mean of 3.7, a mode of 3, and a median of 3. The gravidity distribution was 1-13 with a mean of 5.25 and a median of 5.

Table 6. Follow-Up of Patients with Hydatidiform Mole

Status	No. of cases
Pregnant within one year	6 (23%)
Satisfactory	10 (38.5%)
Defaulted	10 (38.5%)

Table 7. ABO Blood Groups in Choriocarcinoma

Blood Group	No. of cases
O	5
A	2
B	1
AB	0
Total recorded cases	8

Table 8. Antecedent Pregnancy in Choriocarcinoma

Antecedent pregnancy	No. of cases
Abortion	6
Hydatidiform mole	3
Term pregnancy	2
Ectopic pregnancy	0

Table 9. Presenting Symptoms in Choriocarcinoma

Presenting symptom	No. of cases
Vaginal bleeding	10
Abdominal mass	2
Abdominal pain	1
Amenorrhea	1
Headache	1
Vomiting	1
Cough	1

Table 10. Outcome of Choriocarcinoma Patients

Outcome	No. of cases
Survived	5
Died	5
Lost to follow-up	6

The ABO blood group determination was recorded in only 8 cases of choriocarcinoma and is summarized in Table 7. The antecedent pregnancy is as shown in Table 8. The interval between the end of the antecedent pregnancy and diagnosis or treatment was 2 to 15 months, with a mean of 8.1 months.

The presenting symptoms in the choriocarcinoma patients are shown in Table 9. The duration of symptoms before diagnosis or management was 1 to 15 months, with an overall mean of 5.5 months. However, the duration of symptoms prior to the diagnosis of choriocarcinoma was twice as long for patients who ultimately succumbed (mean duration, 8 months) than for patients who survived (mean duration, 4 months).

The courses of chemotherapy received by the patients ranged from 4 to 8, with a mean of 5.4. The outcome of the patients is shown in Table 10. The duration of stay in hospital was 4 to 8 months, with a mean of 6.3 months.

The factors of parity, gravidity, antecedent pregnancy, and interval between end of antecedent pregnancy and diagnosis or treatment were compared in the patients who survived and those who succumbed. These are summarized in Table 11.

DISCUSSION

The incidence of trophoblast neoplasm in Lagos is most probably higher than formerly thought, when the institutional incidence of 1 in 184 deliveries for hydatidiform mole and 1 in 299 deliveries for choriocarcinoma is compared with a previous report (3). This may, in fact, represent the trend for the whole country.

The age and parity distribution of our patients with hydatidiform mole have not altered significantly since the last report (3). There was, however, an association between the occurrence of hydatidiform mole and age, in that 65 percent of our patients belonged to the 20-29 age group. Forty-six percent of the patients were also

Table 11. Comparison of Patients Who Survived Choriocarcinoma with Patients Who Succumbed

Parameter	Survived	Succumbed
Mean parity	2.4	6.0
Mean gravidity	5.2	6.2
Antecedent pregnancy	5	5
Abortion	3	2
Hydatidiform mole	3	1
Term pregnancy	2	1
Ectopic pregnancy	0	0
Months until diagnosis/treatment	6.8	9.4

of parity 1 or 2. This association has also been reported by other authors (6). However, no association between choriocarcinoma and age, parity or gravidity was observed from our present series, although such an association has been noted in Kenya (11).

It was interesting that 27 percent of our patients with hydatidiform mole had pseudotoxemia and one of them, eclamptic seisure. The mandatory one-year follow-up of patients with hydatidiform mole presented some problems which are not unfamiliar in a developing country. A high percentage (38.5%) defaulted after one or two initial visits; efforts to trace them invariably proved abortive. Twenty-three percent of the patients became pregnant prior to the expiration of the follow-up period, and their pregnancies were allowed to proceed. In all of them, pregnancy and labor were uneventful.

In our series of choriocarcinoma cases, abortion was found to be the most common antecedent pregnancy. This differs from the findings of a previous report (3), and suggests that the incidence of choriocarcinoma in relation to antecedent pregnancy is probably not constant even for a given locality.

The relationship of choriocarcinoma with ABO blood groups has not been clear from this study, since the record in this aspect was incomplete. It may be necessary to pursue this aspect of epidemiological study further to reach a probable conclusion.

A mortality rate of 31 percent was an improvement over the poor figure of 54 percent obtained from a previous review (3). The explanation for the relatively poor survival rate may be related to some prognostic indices. Unavailability of cytotoxic drugs when required was also another major contributory factor.

It was remarkable that patients who died from choriocarcinoma were of a higher parity than those who survived (Table 11). Gravidity was less significant in this comparison. It has been suggested that this group of women probably has weakened immunobiological response (11).

The factors of parity, antecedent pregnancy, interval between the end of antecedent pregnancy and diagnosis or treatment, and duration of symptoms before diagnosis may be more applicable as prognostic indices for choriocarcinoma in Nigeria. Parity, rather than gravidity as has been employed by some authors, may be more appropriate in our own locality as demonstrated by this study.

There is surely a need to create an increased awareness of the symptoms of this disease in this country and also to improve the existing poor referral system by the general medical practitioners. It is also hoped that a collaborative study will be undertaken in this country with a view to study especially the epidemiology of this disease. Provision of adequate funds for radioimmunoassays and, more importantly, for the purchase of chemotherapeutic drugs is a necessity if a developing country like Nigeria is to combat this disease effectively and reduce the relatively high mortality rate.

SUMMARY

Trophoblast neoplasm cases at the Lagos University Teaching Hospital in the two-year period, 1980-1981, have been reviewed. An apparent increased incidence of 1 in 184 deliveries for hydatidiform mole and 1 in 299 deliveries for choriocarcinoma has been noted when compared with a previous review. An association of hydatidiform mole with age and parity was observed in this study. Among patients with hydatidiform mole, 27 percent also had pseudotoxemia and in one case this progressed to eclampsia. In the case of choriocarcinoma, increased parity appears to be associated with a higher mortality. The relatively higher mortality of 31 percent from this study could be related to the long duration of symptoms before diagnosis and treatment, and a plea is made to the general medical practitioners for a better referral system, although the need to create an increased awareness of the clinical symptoms of this disease in the community is also very much desirable. A collaborative study of the epidemiology of this disease in Nigeria is advocated.

REFERENCES

1. de V. Hendrickse, J. P., Cockshott, W. P., Evans, K. T. E., and Barton, C. J., New Engl. J. Med. 271:859 (1964).
2. Ogunbode, O., Benign hydatidiform mole in Ibadan, Nigeria, Int. J. Gynecol. Obstet. 15:387 (1978).
3. Agboola, A., Trophoblastic neoplasia in an African urban population, J. Natl. Med. Assoc. 71:935 (1979).
4. Barr, S. J., More hydatidiform mole? Brit. Med. J. 2:707 (1977).
5. Calvert, J. P., More hydatidiform mole? Brit. Med. J. 2:578 (1977).
6. Javey, H. and Sajadi, H., Hydatidiform mole in southern Iran: a statistical survey of 113 cases, Int. J. Gynecol. Obstet.15: 390 (1978).
7. Novak, E. R. and Woodruff, J.D., "Gynaecologic and Obstetric Pathology," Edition 7, W. B. Saunders, Philadelphia (1974), p. 599.
8. Iliya, F. A., Williamson, S., and Azar, H. A., Choriocarcinoma in the Near East: consanguinity as a possible etiology factor, Cancer 20:144 (1967).
9. Bagshawe, K. D., ABO Blood groups in trophoblastic neoplasia, Lancet 1:553 (1971).
10. W.H.O. Special program of research, development and research training in human reproduction: task force on gestational trophoblastic disease (1979)(Unpublished).
11. Makokha, A. E. and Mati, J. K. G., Choriocarcinoma at Kenyatta National Hospital, 1973-79, J. Obstet. Gynecol. East Cent. Africa 1:27 (1982).

HUMAN CHORIONIC GONADOTROPIN

In addition to trophoblastic hCG, nontrophoblast sources of this hormone in nontrophoblastic tumors is becoming of increasing interest clinically. Alpha and beta subunits of hCG represent trophoblast and nontrophoblast tumor markers which are finding greater application. Significant new work is in progress in this area. New horizons in hCG detection and differentiation of trophoblast and nontrophoblast sources represent an important diagnostic discernment for current clinical monitoring.

From the time when bioassays were the only means of hormone detection until the present, when sensitive radioimmunoassays are available, the cornerstone of trophoblast disease diagnosis and treatment has been the ever-challenging glycoprotein, human chorionic gonadotropin. The chapters to follow will address in depth some of the unique aspects of structure and function of this hormone, its immunochemistry, new methods of detection, some of its electrophysiologic ramifications, its messenger RNA detection, and its clinical application. It can correctly be anticipated that this tumor marker will be the subject of even more intense investigation as more of its role in tumor metabolism unfolds.

IMMUNOCHEMISTRY OF HUMAN CHORIONIC GONADOTROPIN

R. E. Canfield, S. Birken, P. Ehrlich, and G. Armstrong

Departments of Medicine and Pathology
College of Physicians and Surgeons of
Columbia University
630 West 168th Street
New York, New York 10032

INTRODUCTION

In states of gestational trophoblastic disease, knowledge of the immunochemistry of human chorionic gonadotropin (hCG) is principally of value in relation to its use as a diagnostic tool and as a marker for the persistence of disease activity during chemotherapy (1, 2). Since these data are usually obtained through immunoassay of the hormone or its subunits, we have chosen to focus this review on that background information which relates to immunochemical recognition of the hormone. Numerous other summaries are available dealing with the biological role of the hormone and its action at target organ receptors (3-5).

CHEMISTRY OF hCG

Human chorionic gonadotropin is one of four glycoprotein hormones that are similar in structure in that they are comprised of two distinct subunits (α and β). Within a species the α-subunits have the same structure. The other three hormones are synthesized in the pituitary and are: luteinizing hormone (LH), follicle stimulating hormone (FSH), and thyroid stimulating hormone (TSH). Presumably, the target organ specificity resides in the different β-subunits. Interestingly, the β-subunit of hCG appears to exhibit a small amount of FSH and of TSH activity (6, 7).

Purification

Crude commercial preparations of hCG, concentrated from large pools of urine obtained from women during the first trimester of pregnancy, are the usual starting material for purification. Several different methods have been described (8, 9). In our laboratory we generally use a gel filtration step followed by ion exchange chromatography (10). hCG is heterogeneous in charge, owing to variations in sialic acid content, but it is possible to obtain highly purified material in approximately 50% yield and with a biological potency of 12,000 to 14,000 IU/mg (11). Preparations with higher potency, as measured by *in vivo* assays, have been reported (12), but these probably do not represent a greater degree of purity. Rather, they are produced by methods that select for hCG preparations with higher sialic acid content which conveys a longer *in vivo* circulating lifetime (and therefore greater potency) to the hormone.

Various attempts have been made to purify hCG from choriocarcinoma urine because of the generally high content of hCG in specimens obtained from untreated patients. There have been some claims that the hCG from this source has a greater intrinsic potency than that from pregnancy urine and, if this is correct, it may reflect a higher sialic acid content. On one occasion we undertook to examine the hCG isolated from choriocarcinoma urine and found that its amino acid content was chemically comparable to preparations from pregnancy urine (13).

The hormone's subunits have a high affinity for each other, but the bonding is noncovalent (14, 15). Therefore, they can be dissociated in urea and separated by ion exchange chromatography. A final gel filtration step takes advantage of the different exclusion volumes for each subunit in comparison with hCG (16). The purified subunits can be recombined under appropriate circumstances to restore a preparation of the native hormone with full biological potency (17).

Standard Preparations

For the past ten years, our laboratory, in collaboration with investigators at the National Institutes of Child Health and Human Development, has prepared a series of hCG reference standards for research use (18). These consist of hCG preparations with a potency of approximately 13,000 IU/mg, and purified α- and β-subunits with a potency that is approximately 0.1% that of the native hormone and presumably represents one part per thousand of contamination with native hCG. These may be obtained by writing to the Center for Population Research, NICHD, National Institutes of Health, Bethesda, Maryland. Preparations of hCG suitable for radiolabeling for immunoassay may be obtained from the National Pituitary Agency.

Protein Structure

The amino acid sequences of the α- and β-subunits were determined independently in our laboratory (19) and in that of Dr. Om P. Bahl (20, 21). Disagreements concerning the structure of the COOH-terminal regions of the β-subunit were subsequently resolved by additional studies (22, 23). These primary structures are illustrated in Fig. 1. In other studies, conducted in collaboration with the laboratory of Dr. Irving I. Boime, it was shown that each subunit is synthesized from a separate mRNA molecule and that precursor subunit forms containing the conventional hydrophobic polypeptide extension at the amino terminus existed for both hormones (24). The structures of these signal peptides have been determined (25). The structures of the α- and β-subunit genes have also been determined (26, 27). While only a single gene for the α-subunit was found (28), Fiddes reported finding eight different β-subunit gene locations in man (29). Whether or not the β-subunit genes have identical structures, and whether or not all of the genes are functional, is not yet known.

Carbohydrate Structure

There is good agreement that each subunit has two *N*-asparagine-linked carbohydrate side chains; their locations are shown in Fig. 1. The structures of these carbohydrate side chains are illustrated in Fig. 2 (30, 31). In addition, there are four *O*-serine-linked side chains in the COOH-terminal region of the β-subunit, and their structures are also illustrated in Fig. 2 (32).

β-Subunit COOH-Terminal Region

The β-subunits of the three pituitary glycoprotein hormones terminate in the vicinity of residues 114-126, but the hCGβ primary structure extends to position 145 with an amino acid sequence that is unique to this hormone and beginning at position 112. Fiddes (27) has proposed, based upon the structure of the β-subunit gene and its flanking regions, that this extension arose by virtue of a mutation in a terminator codon. Whatever its origin, that sequence of 34 amino acids serves as the largest structural feature of the hCG molecule to define an antigen which will give rise to antibodies that are unique for this hormone.

IMMUNOCHEMICAL RECOGNITION OF hCG

The specificity of the immune response when hCG is employed as antigen has evoked considerable interest, because of the many potential biological applications for the antibodies produced. The similarities between the structures of hLH and hCG lead to

α SUBUNIT

```
 1                                                       10
ALA - PRO - ASP - VAL - GLN - ASP - CYS - PRO - GLU - CYS - THR - LEU -
                                         20
GLN - GLU - ASP - PRO - PHE - PHE - SER - GLN - PRO - GLY - ALA - PRO -
                              30
ILE - LEU - GLX - CYS - MET - GLY - CYS - CYS - PHE - SER - ARG - ALA -
                  40
TYR - PRO - THR - PRO - LEU - ARG - SER - LYS - LYS - THR - MET - LEU -
       50        (CHO)                                            60
VAL - GLN - LYS - ASN - VAL - THR - SER - GLU - SER - THR - CYS - CYS -
                                                       70
VAL - ALA - LYS - SER - TYR - ASN - ARG - VAL - THR - VAL - MET - GLY -
                             (CHO)       80
GLY - PHE - LYS - VAL - GLU - ASN - HIS - THR - ALA - CYS - HIS - CYS -
                              90
SER - THR - CYS - TYR - TYR - HIS - LYS - SER
```

β SUBUNIT

```
 1                                                       10
SER - LYS - GLU - PRO - LEU - ARG - PRO - ARG - CYS - ARG - PRO - ILE -
(CHO)                                    20
ASN - ALA - THR - LEU - ALA - VAL - GLU - LYS - GLU - GLY - CYS - PRO -
                             (CHO)
VAL - CYS - ILE - THR - VAL - ASN - THR - THR - ILE - CYS - ALA - GLY -
                  40
TYR - CYS - PRO - THR - MET - THR - ARG - VAL - LEU - GLN - GLY - VAL -
       50                                                         60
LEU - PRO - ALA - LEU - PRO - GLN - VAL - VAL - CYS - ASN - TYR - ARG -
                                                       70
ASP - VAL - ARG - PHE - GLU - SER - ILE - ARG - LEU - PRO - GLY - CYS -
                                         80
PRO - ARG - GLY - VAL - ASN - PRO - VAL - VAL - SER - TYR - ALA - VAL -
                              90
ALA - LEU - SER - CYS - GLN - CYS - ALA - LEU - CYS - ARG - ARG - SER -
                  100
THR - THR - ASP - CYS - GLY - GLY - PRO - LYS - ASP - HIS - PRO - LEU -
       110                                                        120
THR - CYS - ASP - ASP - PRO - ARG - PHE - GLN - ASP - SER - SER - SER -
(CHO)                              (CHO)                 130      (CHO)
SER - LYS - ALA - PRO - PRO - PRO - SER - LEU - PRO - SER - PRO - SER -
                             (CHO)       140
ARG - LEU - PRO - GLY - PRO - SER - ASP - THR - PRO - ILE - LEU - PRO -
145
GLN
```

Fig. 1. Primary structures of the α- and β-subunits of hCG. Locations of carbohydrate chains are indicated by *CHO*.

cross-reactivity between these two molecules when either is employed for immunization and, therefore, to less specificity. One application that has received special emphasis is the development of antifertility vaccines (33-35). Considerable evidence exists in mammals to indicate that immunization with hCG can lead to

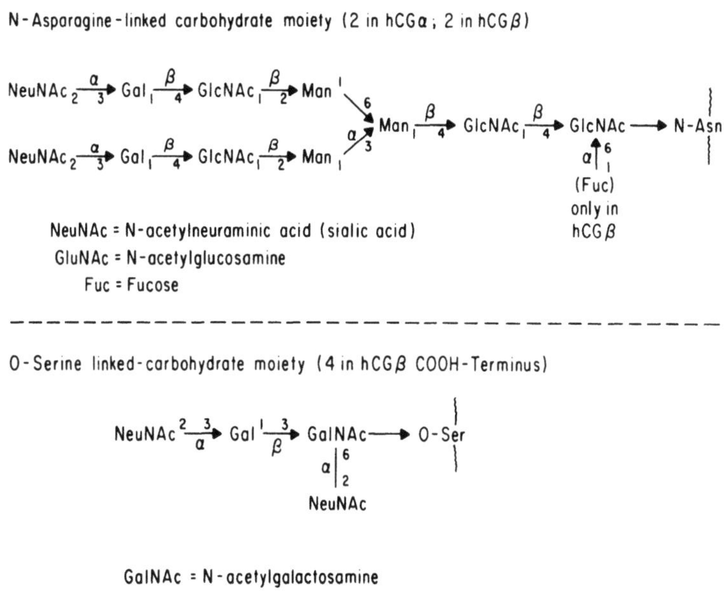

Fig. 2. Structures of carbohydrate groups attached to hCG. The upper part of the figure represents the complex carbohydrate moieties attached to asparagines 52 and 78 in hCGα, and 13 and 30 in hCGβ. The lower portion of the figure shows the small carbohydrate structures attached by *O*-serine linkages to the hCGβ COOH-terminal peptide. The structures shown are those proposed by Kessler *et al.* (30, 32). Endo *et al.* (31) proposed essentially the same *N*-asparagine-linked structures except for the finding of considerable heterogeneity in some moieties missing not only sialic acid but also some galactose and *N*-acetylglucosamine residues.

infertility (36-38), but there is concern about the possibility that cross-reactivity with luteinizing hormone could produce an immune complex disease. Another application is the use of antibodies to detect the minute quantities of hCG that are secreted following the first few days of implantation of the fertilized ovum or in patients with neoplasms that make hCG, where the ectopic hormone secretion serves as a tumor marker for chemotherapy. For example, a particularly vexing problem arises when clinical decisions about further surgery or chemotherapy following orchiectomy for testicular cancer, depend upon an equivocal report of a "trace" of hCG antigen in the patient's serum. Another application is the use of radiolabeled antibodies to hCG as a scanning agent when this hormone is synthesized ectopically by neoplastic tissue. In all these instances there is a need for immunochemical reagents that possess both sensitivity and specificity.

Antibodies can also be utilized to gather information about the conformation of regions at the surface of a protein (39). For example, dose-response curves employing antibodies that react with the hCG β-subunit give different reactions depending upon whether the epitope is present on the isolated subunit or combined with the α-subunit as in the case of the native hormone. These data confirm other results indicating that there is a change in conformation when the β-subunit combines with the α-subunit; knowledge of the epitopes would also identify the region of structural change. Immunologic surface mapping techniques can also be employed to ascertain whether a particular antigen gives rise to antibodies that block hormone binding at the receptor. This would be of particular importance in the design of immunogens for a fertility vaccine.

Injections of hCG have been employed in the treatment of infertility and hypogonadism in humans, as well as for some unsubstantiated clinical applications such as the treatment of obesity. Occasionally, during the course of these injections a patient develops an immune response to hCG despite a presumed state of immune tolerance for this molecule (40-43). Knowledge of the epitopes that give rise to these antibodies is also of considerable biological interest.

With these issues in view, we summarize below what is known about immunologic recognition of hCG.

Polyclonal Antibodies to hCG and Its Subunits

When hCG is employed as an immunogen, it almost invariably gives rise to antibodies that also exhibit a high degree of cross-reactivity with hLH. When the threshold for detection is deliberately set high, such as in a conventional pregnancy test in urine, the relatively small amount of hLH present becomes insignificant. In a well-established pregnancy then, the dose of antigen determines whether the test is positive or negative.

Shortly after we appreciated that hCG was made up of nonidentical subunits and had isolated some of each, Vaitukaitis, Ross and associates employed one of our β-subunit preparations as an immunogen. They discovered that, occasionally, it would give rise to antibodies that were highly selective for hCG or its β-subunit in comparison with hLH (44). The most celebrated of these was the SB-6 antiserum, and we refer here to all polyclonal anti-β-subunit antisera that exhibit this selectivity as being of the SB-6 type. Many others have confirmed their observations, and very sensitive anti-hCGβ antisera have made it possible to detect the hormone in serum specimens at a level of approximately 1 ng/ml (45).

We and others have attempted to learn something about the location of the epitopes that give rise to the SB-6 type antisera.

It is possible by selective proteolysis to cleave much of the COOH-terminal peptide of the β-subunit away from the disulfide-linked β-subunit core. When this is done, the immunoreactivity remains exclusively with the core, *i.e.*, the binding site does not contain any elements of the unique COOH-terminal peptide of the β-subunit. If the β-subunit is reduced and *S*-carboxymethylated, it loses its reactivity; in this case we can infer that the determinant is dependent on the conformation of the subunit.

Pandian and co-workers (46) produced sensitive, highly specific hCGβ antisera in rabbits by the use of an immunogen composed of nearly completely reduced and alkylated β-subunit which had been absorbed with immobilized antibodies to hLH. These antisera had high affinity for hCG (although not as high as SB-6), but exhibited less than 1% cross-reactivity with hLH. The antibodies were found not to be directed to the COOH-terminal peptide of the β-subunit, but rather were dependent on the remaining cystine-linked peptides in the partially reduced hCGβ immunogen. An alternative approach was applied by Swaminathan and Braunstein (47). These investigators absorbed an anti-native hCGβ antiserum with immobilized hLH and characterized the resultant hCG-specific antiserum with disulfide-bridged hCGβ peptides produced by partial reduction of hCGβ. They found that the hCGβ COOH-terminal peptides did not bind to the antibody, but that hCGβ peptides linked by cystines between 26 and 110, or between 23 and 72, were highly immunopotent. Birken and associates (48) have also shown that SB-6 and similar anti-hCGβ antisera do not contain antibodies reactive to the hCGβ COOH-terminus by use of hCGβ core fragments devoid of this peptide. Thus, the existence of two more antigenic sites unique to hCG has been demonstrated by several laboratories.

Polyclonal Antisera to the COOH-Terminal Region of hCGβ

The orientation of this glycopeptide region to the surface of hCG is unknown. Presumably, it is not an integral part of the elements that interact with the receptor, since it is totally lacking as a component of hLH, which has virtually full receptor reactivity. It seems likely that this polypeptide region lies across the surface of the molecule with its carbohydrate side chains adding further protection from proteolytic degradation. Ryan and Puett (49) have indicated that the amino acid sequence suggests a predisposition to a structure with a β turn in the region of each of the *O*-serine-linked oligosaccharide chains.

To the best of our knowledge, the COOH-terminal peptide region of the β-subunit of hCG has never been shown to give rise to antibodies when either hCG or its β-subunit were used as immunogens. Nevertheless, antibodies whose epitopes are confined to this unique structure should convey absolute specificity for reactions with hCG, and this type of antibody response can be forced by first isolating the COOH-terminal peptide (CTP) and then coupling it to a larger molecule to serve as an immunogen (48). We have devoted considerable study to the antigenic determinants that are involved in the immune response to these fragments (49, 50).

In general, the synthetic CTP polypeptide region, *i.e.*, without the carbohydrate side chains, gives rise to antisera that are of insufficient sensitivity for direct competitive binding assays. Chen and co-workers (51), in an elegant series of studies, have localized the principal determinants to the region of residues 130-145.

When the so-called native CTP is employed as the antigen, *i.e.*, with a full complement of carbohydrate, we have consistently obtained antisera that are more sensitive in reactions with hCG (52). Not only was the affinity of antibodies to hCG higher when CTP with sialic acid was the immunogen, but some antibodies displayed a stronger preference for native hCG, while desialylated hCG or synthetic CTP were very poor competitors.

Studies with Monoclonal Antibodies

The technique of fusing murine antibody-forming cells with a myeloma cell line to permit subsequent cloning of cells that secrete a single species of antibody molecule has made it possible to perform more precise immunochemical studies with hCG. Hundreds of cell lines that produce antibodies to hCG have been developed in many different laboratories for the purpose of assay development, but they also offer an opportunity to map some of the topographical features of the hormone. For example, we studied the capability of monoclonal antibodies to affect the binding of hCG to its receptor, and found that antibodies to some sites on both subunits were capable of doing this (53). Our results are summarized in Fig. 3. These data led to the inference that both the α- and the β-subunits are involved in interactions with the receptor. We also found that antibodies to at least one site on the β-subunit could bind to the hormone and not prevent the receptor interaction (and also bind to hCG when it occupies the receptor) leading to the conclusion that at least one antigenic site on the β-subunit remains exposed during its action. These distinctions are important in designing studies to evaluate potential immunogens for hCG vaccines, because it is unclear whether the action of the antibody in preventing (or terminating) an early pregnancy occurs through neutralization of the hormone or by setting off an inflammatory response at the surface of the fertilized ovum as a consequence of the hCG-antibody reaction triggering complement fixation (54).

Monoclonal antibodies have a high potential for improving hCG assays. They can be produced indefinitely in large quantities and employed to concentrate hCG from large volumes of biological fluids.

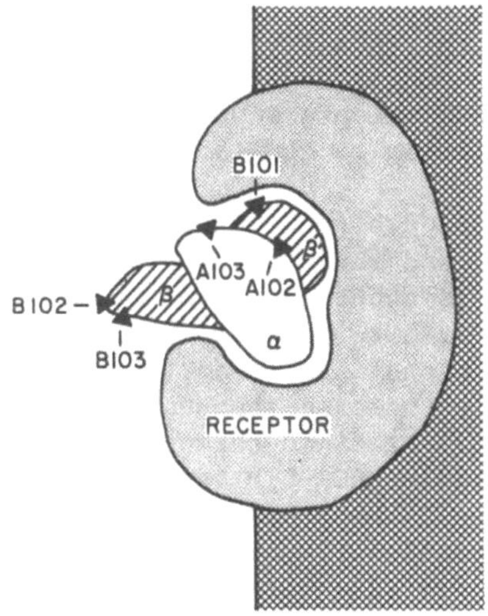

Fig. 3. Relative orientation on hCG of epitopes of monoclonal antibodies and receptor binding site. Monoclonal antibodies B102 and B103 did not inhibit hCG binding to the receptor and could bind to the hCG-receptor complex. Antibodies B101 and A102 inhibited hCG binding to receptor and could not bind to the hCG-receptor complex. Antibody A103 did not inhibit hCG binding to the receptor but could not bind the hCG-receptor complex. (Reproduced from reference 53, with permission of the Journal).

By selecting appropriate pairs of antibodies to construct sandwich assays, it is possible to design methods that will measure either whole hCG (*i.e.*, the presence of both α- and β-subunit epitopes) or the free subunit.

IMPROVEMENTS IN hCG ASSAY DESIGN

As noted earlier, the use of very sensitive polyclonal antisera to the β-subunit of hCG (usually raised in rabbits) has permitted the detection of hCG in plasma or serum at a concentration of approximately 1 ng/ml, and the selectivity of these antisera permit this measurement to occur in the presence of hLH (44, 45), as described above. Pandian and colleagues (46) have reported the development of a highly specific radioimmunoassay for βhCG using an antibody to the partially reduced and alkylated subunit. The actual claims for sensitivity of βhCG assays vary slightly, but in evaluating these claims it is important to distinguish between the lowest measurable value under optimal conditions and that which is the threshold of a reliably positive finding under routine diagnostic conditions. Sensitive assays have also been developed employing appropriate hCG receptors but they do not, in theory, have selectivity in relation to hLH (55).

The hCG molecule appears to be excreted into the urine in a relatively intact state and the available data suggest that the concentration in urine is about equal to that in plasma (56). Therefore, examination of a 24 hour urine specimen, which has been subjected to the conventional kaolin-acetone procedure to concentrate hCG, would greatly increase the sensitivity of the assay. Ayala and co-workers (57) examined this problem using both the SB-6 and the then-available hCGβ CTP antisera, and demonstrated that they could detect hCG in 24 hour urine specimens from normal individuals at levels as low as 2 ng/24 hours with SB-6, and 70 ng/24 hours with the anti-βCTP. These data were consistent with the observations of others that trace quantities of hCG can be detected in normal individuals (58, 59). Their results also pointed to two limitations in the conduct of these studies on urine specimens. The first limitation is that antisera generated against the hCG β-subunit not only contain antibodies that exhibit selectivity for native hCG over native hLH, but they also contain varying amounts of antibodies to denatured forms of hCG. The latter also react well with the denatured forms of hLH that exist in urine but not in blood. Thus, antibodies to the hCG β-subunit lose some of their selectivity when applied to assays of urine specimens, especially at very low hormone levels. The second limitation was that the antibodies to the CTP of hCGβ were incapable of detecting very low levels of hCG (in the range of SB-6 antibody sensitivity) due to their relatively low affinities, even though they possess the specificity to make this distinction.

The kaolin-acetone concentration procedure is cumbersome and not ideal for the processing of routine urine specimens for assay. One variation that was developed by Wehman *et al.* (60) was the use of affinity adsorption of hCG to concanavalin A-Sepharose. When this method of concentration was employed with some of our newer high-sensitivity antisera to the β-subunit CTP, it became possible to devise a routine assay for 3 ml of urine that was approximately equal in sensitivity to those assays that use hCG β-subunit antisera for measurement in serum (60). We are currently working on other improvements toward the goal of being able to measure less than 0.02 ng/ml in urine (20 ng/24 hours with a total volume of one liter). The value of such assays in the management of choriocarcinoma is illustrated in Fig. 4, where serial measurements of β-subunit CTP in urine concentrates from a patient undergoing chemotherapy for choriocarcinoma clearly demonstrated elevated hCG levels which were undetectable by conventional β-subunit radioimmunoassay for nearly six weeks (61).

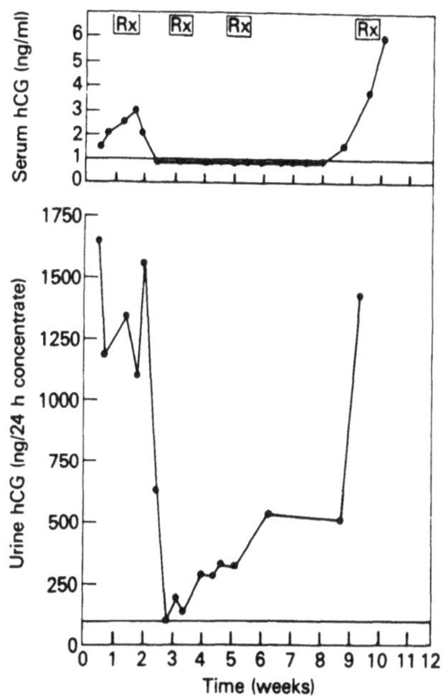

Fig. 4. Levels of hCG in serum and urine at various times in a 36 year-old woman who was undergoing chemotherapy for choriocarcinoma. The serum hCG level (upper panel) was determined in the conventional hCG β-subunit radioimmunoassay, and the urinary hCG level (lower panel) was determined by radioimmunoassay with the use of antiserum to the carboxyterminal peptide of hCGβ (antiserum R529). The interval, *Rx*, indicates a course of chemotherapy. (Reproduced from reference 61, with permission from the Journal).

We have generated a carbohydrate-sensitive β-subunit CTP antiserum (R141) to desialylated β-subunit CTP (residues 123-145) which distinguishes between native hCG and desialylated hCG. In collaboration with Dr. Bruce Nisula, examination of urine concentrates from a dozen choriocarcinoma patients indicated that half of them displayed immunoreactivity patterns indicating the presence of significant quantities of desialylated hCG, while normal pregnancy urine concentrates did not contain measurable asialo-hCG (62).

Nishimura and associates (63) have analyzed the carbohydrate content of hCG isolated from the urine of a choriocarcinoma patient and found it to be devoid of sialic acid, whereas hCG isolated from urine concentrates of pregnant women and a patient with hydatidiform mole had an 8.5% sialic acid content. In further studies of choriocarcinoma urine concentrates using our carbohydrate-sensitive antiserum R141, Amr *et al.* (64) have identified an asialo-carboxy-terminal hCGβ fragment in urine concentrates from choriocarcinoma patients. These fragments were not present in urine obtained from women during pregnancy or normal subjects who were given an intravenous infusion of highly purified hCG.

The finding that the urine of choriocarcinoma patients contains asialo-hCG and asialo-βCTP is suggestive of a defective sialylation mechanism in this malignant tissue. Furthermore, the possibility that these asialo forms of hCG are produced only by patients with malignant trophoblastic disease points to the possible use of antisera which are highly specific for asialo-hCG βCTP for the detection and management of these tumors.

These studies of the immunochemistry of hCG have provided us with a wide variety of antibodies to measure and characterize the nature of the hormone molecules that are secreted in different diseases. The next phase of our research will be oriented toward applying these results to clinical situations.

ACKNOWLEDGEMENTS

This work was supported by NIH Grants HD-15454 and RR-00645.

REFERENCES

1. Braunstein, G. D., Vaitukaitis, J. L., Carbone, P. P., and Ross, G. T., Ectopic production of human chorionic gonadotropin by neoplasms, _Ann. Intern. Med._ 78:39 (1973).
2. Braunstein, G. D., Human chorionic gonadotropin in non-trophoblastic tumros and tissues, _in_: "Recent Advances in Reproduction and Regulation of Fertility," G. P. Talwar, ed., Elsevier/North Holland Biomedical Press, Amsterdam (1979), p. 389.
3. Catt, K. J. and Dufau, M. L., Gonadotropin receptors and regulation of interstitial cell function in the testis, _in_: "Receptors and Hormone Action," L. Birnbaumer and B. W. O'Malley, eds., Academic Press, San Francisco (1978), p. 291.
4. Pierce, J. G. and Parsons, T. F., Glycoprotein hormones: structure and function, _Ann. Rev. Biochem._ 50:465 (1981).
5. Segal, S. J., ed., "Chorionic Gonadotropin," Plenum Press, New York (1980).
6. Nisula, B. C., Morgan, F. J., and Canfield, R. E., Evidence that chorionic gonadotropin has intrinsic thyrotropic activity, _Biochem. Biophys. Res. Commun._ 59:86 (1974).
7. Siris, E. S., Nisula, B. C., Catt, K. J., Horner, K., Birken, S., Canfield, R. E., and Ross, G. T., New evidence for intrinsic follicle stimulating hormone-like activity in human chorionic gonadotropin and luteinizing hormone, _Endocrinology_ 102:

8. Van Hell, H., Matthijsen, R., and Homan, J. D., Studies on human chorionic gonadotrophin, I: purification and some physico-chemical properties, Acta Endocrinol. 59:89 (1968).
9. Bahl, O. P., Human chirionic gonadotropin, I: purification and physicochemical properties, J. Biol. Chem. 244:567 (1969).
10. Canfield, R. E. and Morgan, F. J., Human chorionic gonadotropin (hCG). I: Purification and biochemical characterization, in: "Methods in Investigative and Diagnostic Endocrinology," S. A. Berson and R. S. Yalow, eds., North Holland Publishing Co., Amsterdam (1973), p. 727.
11. Morgan, F. J., Canfield, R. E., Vaitukaitis, J. L., and Ross, G. T., Properties of the subunits of human chorionic gonadotropin, Endocrinology 94:1601 (1974).
12. Van Hell, H., Goverde, B. C., Schuurs, A. H. W. M., DeJager, E., Matthijsen, R., and Homan, J. D. H., Purification, characterization and immunochemical properties of human chorionic gonadotropin, Nature 221:261 (1966).
13. Canfield, R. E., Agosto, G. M., and Bell, J. J., Studies of the chemistry of human chorionic gonadotrophin, in: "Gonadotrophins and Ovarian Development," W. R. Butt, A. C. Crooke, and M. Ryle, eds., E and S Livingstone, London (1970), p. 161.
14. Aloj, S., Edelhoch, H., Ingham, K. C., Morgan, F. J., Canfield, R. E., and Ross, G. T., The rate of dissociation and reassociation of the subunits of human chorionic gonadotropin, Arch. Biochem. Biophys. 159:497 (1973).
15. Strickland, T. W. and Puett, D., The kinetic and equilibrium parameters of subunit association and gonadotropin dissociation, J. Biol. Chem. 257:2954 (1982).
16. Morgan, F. J., Canfield, R. E., Vaitukaitis, J. L., and Ross, G. T., Preparation and characterization of the subunits of hCG, in: "Methods in Investigative and Diagnostic Endocrinology," S. A. Berson and R. S. Yalow, eds., A. S. P. Biological and Medical Press, North-Holland Publishing Company, Amsterdam, (1973), p. 733.
17. Morgan, F. J., Canfield, R. E., Vaitukaitis, J. L., and Ross, G. T., Properties of the subunits of human chorionic gonadotropin, Endocrinology 94:1601 (1974).
18. Storring, P. L., Gaines-Das, R. E., and Bangham, D. R., International reference preparation of human chorionic gonadotropin for immunoassay: potency estimates in various bioassay and protein binding assay systems, and International Reference Preparations of the α and β-subunits of human chorionic gonadotropin for immunoassay, J. Endocrinol. 84: 295 (1980).
19. Morgan, F. J., Birken, S., and Canfield, R. E., The amino acid sequence of human chorionic gonadotropin: the α subunit and β-subunit, J. Biol. Chem. 250:5247 _1975).
20. Bellisario, R., Carlsen, R. B., and Bahl, O. P., Human chorionic gonadotropin: linear amino acid sequence of the α subunit, J. Biol. Chem. 248:6797 (1973).

21. Carlsen, R. B., Bahl, O. P., and Swaminathan, N., Human chorionic gonadotropin: linear amino acid sequence of the β-subunit, J. Biol. Chem. 248:6810 (1973).
22. Keutmann, H. T. and Williams, R. M., Human chorionic gonadotropin. Amino acid sequence of the hormone-specific COOH-terminal region, J. Biol. Chem. 252:5395 (1977).
23. Birken, S. and Canfield, R. E., Isolation and amino acid sequence of COOH-terminal fragments from the β-subunit of human choriogonadotropin, J. Biol. Chem. 252:5386 (1977).
24. Daniels-McQueen, S., McWilliams, D., Birken, S., Canfield, R., Landefeld, T., and Boime, I., Identification of mRNAs encoding the alpha and beta subunits of human choriogonadotropin, J. Biol. Chem. 253:7109 (1978).
25. Birken, S., Fetherston, J., Canfield, R., and Boime, I., The amino acid sequences of the prepeptides contained in the alpha and beta subunits of human choriogonadotropin, J. Biol. Chem. 256:1816 (1981).
26. Fiddes, J. C. and Goodman, H. M., Isolation, cloning and sequence analysis of the cDNA for the α-subunit of human chorionic gonadotropin, Nature 281:351 (1979).
27. Fiddes, J. C. and Goodman, H. M., The cDNA for the β-subunit of human chorionic gonadotropin suggests evolution of a gene by readthrough into the 3'-untranslated region, Nature 286: 684 (1980).
28. Boothby, M., Ruddon, R. W., Anderson, C., McWilliams, D., and Boime, I., A single gonadotropin α-subunit gene in normal tissue and tumor-derived cell lines, J. Biol. Chem. 256: 5121 (1981).
29. Boorstein, W. R., Vamvakopoulos, N. C., and Fiddes, J. C., Human chorionic gonadotropin β-subunit is encoded by at least eight genes arranged in tandem and inverted pairs, Nature 300:419 (1982).
30. Kessler, M. J., Reddy, M. S., Shah, R. H., and Bahl, O. P., Structures of N-glycosidic carbohydrate units of human chorionic gonadotropin, J. Biol. Chem. 254:7901 (1979).
31. Endo, Y., Ashitaka, Y., Kobata, A., and Tojo, S., Structures of the asparagine-linked sugar chains of human chorionic gonadotropin, in: "Chorionic Gonadotropin," S. J. Segal, ed., Plenum Press, New York (1980), p. 127.
32. Kessler, M. J., Mise, T., Ghai, R. D., and Bahl, O. P., Structure and location of the O-glycosidic carbohydrate units of human chorionic gonadotropin, J. Biol. Chem. 254:7909 (1979).
33. Talwar, G. P., Sharma, N. C., Dubey, S. K., Salahuddin, M., Das, C., Ramakrishnan, S., Kumar, S., and Hingorani, V., Isoimmunization against human chorionic gonadotropin with conjugates of processed β-subunit of the hormone and tetanus toxoid, Proc. Natl. Acad. Sci. (USA) 73:218 (1976).

34. Stevens, V. C., Antifertility effects from immunizations with intact subunits and fragments of hCG, in: "Physiological Effects of Immunity Against Reproductive Hormones," R. G. Edwards and M. H. Johnson, eds., Cmbridge University Press, New York, NY (1976), p. 249.
35. Thanavala, Y. M., Hay, F. C., and Stevens, V. C., Affinity, cross-reactivity and biological effectiveness of rabbit antibodies against a synthetic 37 amino acid C-terminal peptide of human chorionic gonadotropin, Clin. Exp. Immunol. 39:112 (1980).
36. Stevens, V. C., Female contraception by immunization with hCG - prospects and status, in: "Immunization with Hormones in Reproductive Research," E. Nieschlag, ed., North-Holland Publishing Company, Amsterdam, The Netherlands (1975), p. 217.
37. Hearn, J. P., Immunization against pregnancy, Proc. Roy. Soc. London B 195:149 (1976).
38. Talwar, G. P., Ramakrishnan, S., Das, C., Dubey, S. K., Salahuddin, M., Shastri, N., Tandon, A., and Singh, Om., Anti-hCG immunization, in: "Recent Advances in Reproduction and Regulation of Fertility," G. P. Talwar, ed., Elsevier/North Holland Biomedical Press, Amsterdam, The Netherlands (1979), p. 453.
39. Sachs, D. H., Schechter, A. N., Eastlake, A., and Anfinsen, C. B., An immunologic approach to the conformational equilibria of polypeptides, Proc. Natl. Acad. Sci. (USA) 69:3790 (1972).
40. Sokol, R. Z., McClure, R. D., Peterson, M., and Swerdloff, R. S., Gonadotropin therapy failure secondary to human chorionic gonadotropin-induced antibodies, J. Clin. Endocrinol. Metab. 52:929 (1981).
41. Claustrat, B., David, L., Plauchu, H., Lebacq, E., and Franco, R., Frequence des anticorps antigonadotrophines dan les hypogonadismes d'origine centrale, Annales d'Endocrinologie (Paris) 36:337 (1975).
42. Healy, D. L., Fraser, I. S., Lee, V. W. K., Shearman, R. P., and Burger, H. G., Characteristics of an antiluteinizing hormone isoantibody produced during gonadotropin induction of ovulation, J. Clin. Endocrinol. Metab. 47:823 (1978).
43. Musch, K., Wolf, A. S., and Lauritzen, C., Antibodies to human chorionic gonadotropin in humans, Clin. Chim. Acta 113:95 (1981).
44. Vaitukaitis, J. L., Braunstein, G. D., and Ross, G. T., A radioimmunoassay which specifically measures hCG in the presence of hLH, Amer. J. Obstet. Gynecol. 113:751 (1972).
45. Vaitukaitis, J. L., Specific hormone chorionic gonadotropin assay, in: "Methods of Hormone Radioimmunoassay," 3rd Edition, B. M. Jaffe and H. R. Behrman, eds., Academic Press, New York, p. 817.

46. Pandian, M. R., Mitra, R., and Bahl, O. P., Immunological properties of the β-subunit of human chorionic gonadotropin (hCG). II. Properties of a hCG-specific antibody prepared against a chemical analog of the β-subunit, Endocrinology 107:1564 (1980).
47. Swaminathan, N. and Braunstein, G. D., Location of major antigenic sites of the β-subunit of human chorionic gonadotropin, Biochemistry 17:5832 (1978).
48. Birken, S., Canfield, R. E., Lauer, R., Agosto, G., and Gabel, M., Immunochemical determinants unique to human chorionic gonadotropin: importance of sialic acid for antisera generated to the human chorionic gonadotropin β-subunit COOH-terminal peptide, Endocrinology 106:1659 (1980).
49. Puett, D., Ryan, R. J., and Stevens, V. C., Circular dichroic and immunological properties of human choriogonadotropin-β carboxyl-terminal peptides, Int. J. Peptide Protein Res. 19:506 (1982).
50. Birken, S., Specific antisera to human choriogonadotropin, in: "Reproduction Processes and Contraception," K. McKerns, ed., Plenum Press, New York (1981), p. 523.
51. Matsuura, S., Chen, H-C., and Hodgen, G. D., Antibodies to the carboxy-terminal fragment of human chorionic gonadotropin β-subunit: characterization of antibody recognition sites using synthetic peptide analogues, Biochemistry 17:575 (1978).
52. Birken, S., Canfield, R., Agosto, G., and Lewis, J., Preparation and characterization of an improved beta COOH-terminal immunogen for generation of specific and sensitive antisera to human chorionic gonadotropin, Endocrinology 110: 1555 (1982).
53. Moyle, W. R., Ehrlich, P. H., and Canfield, R. E., Use of monoclonal antibodies to subunits of human chorionic gonadotropin to examine the orientation of the hormone in its complex with receptor, Proc. Natl. Acad. Sci. (USA) 79:2245 (1982).
54. Hearn, J. P., The immunobiology of chorionic gonadotropin, in: "Immunological Aspects of Reproduction and Fertility Control," J. P. Hearn, ed., University Park Press, Baltimore, MD (1980), p. 229.
55. Saxena, B. B., Saito, T., Saul, N., and Landesman, R., Radioreceptor assay of LH-hCG in urine: detection of the luteinizing hormone surge and pregnancy, Fertil. Steril. 28: 163 (1977).
56. Marshall, J. R., Hammond, C. B., Ross, G. T., Jacobsen, A., Rayford, P., and Odell, W. D., Plasma and urinary chorionic gonadotropin during early human pregnancy, Obstet. Gynecol. 32:760 (1968).
57. Ayala, A. R., Nisula, B. C., Chen, H-C., Hodgen, G. D., and Ross, G. T., Highly sensitive radioimmunoassay for chorionic gonadotropin in human urine, J. Clin. Endocrinol. Metab. 47: 767 (1978).

58. Chen, H-C., Hodgen, G. D., Matsuura, S., Lin, L. J., Gross, E., Reichert, L. E., Birken, S., Canfield, R. E., and Ross, G. T., Evidence for a gonadotropin from nonpregnant subjects that has physical, immunologic and biological similarities to human chorionic gonadotrophin, Proc. Natl. Acad. Sci. (USA) 73:2885 (1976).
59. Braunstein, G. D., Kamdar, V., Rasor, J., Swaminathan, N., and Wade, M. E., Widespread distribution of a chorionic gonadotropin-like substance in normal human tissues, J. Clin. Endocrinol. Metab. 49:917 (1979).
60. Wehmann, R. E., Harman, S. M., Birken, S., Canfield, R. E., and Nisula, B. C., Convenient radioimmunoassay for urinary human choriogonadotropin without interference by urinary human lutropin, Clin. Chem. 27:1997 (1981).
61. Wehmann, R. E., Ayala, A. R., Birken, S., Canfield, R. E., and Nisula, B. C., Improved monitoring of gestational trophoblastic neoplasia using a highly sensitive assay for urinary human chorionic gonadotropin, Amer. J. Obstet. Gynecol. 140:753 (1981).
62. Birken, S., Agosto, G., Canfield, R. E., Amr, S., and Nisula, B., Antisera sensitive to the carbohydrate in the COOH-terminal region of hCG beta: novel antibodies of clinical significance, Abstract 212, 63rd Annual Meeting of the Endocrine Society (1981).
63. Nishimura, R., Endo, Y., Tanabe, K., Ashitaka, Y., and Tojo, S., The biochemical properties of urinary human chorionic gonadotropin from the patients with trophoblastic disease, J. Endocrinol. Invest. 4:349 (1981).
64. Amr, S., Wehmann, R. E., Birken, S., Canfield, R. E., and Nisula, B. C., Characterization of a carboxyterminal peptide fragment of the human choriogonadotropin β-subunit excreted in the urine of a woman with choriocarcinoma, J. Clin. Invest. 71:329 (1983).

NEW HORIZONS IN hCG DETECTION

Robert Hussa and Laurence A. Cole

Department of Gynecology and Obstetrics
Medical College of Wisconsin
8700 W. Wisconsin Avenue
Milwaukee, Wisconsin 53226, USA

INTRODUCTION

This chapter will discuss nontrophoblastic hCG production, altered forms of hCG, and how these altered forms and other factors might lead to discordant results in hCG analyses. Finally, trends in clinical detection methods for hCG will be summarized.

NONTROPHOBLASTIC hCG PRODUCTION

Immunoreactive ectopic hCG is produced by nontrophoblastic tumors, nontrophoblastic normal tissues, and even microorganisms. This contrasts with eutopic hCG which is synthesized by the trophoblast, be it normal placenta, choriocarcinoma, or hydatidiform mole. There is an extensive and growing literature documenting the presence of hCG or its subunits in the serum of patients with nontrophoblastic neoplasms (Table 1)(1). The greatest incidence of positive hCG levels occurs in patients with gonadal, gynecologic, and pancreatic cancers. Among nongestational cancers, serum hCG determinations are particularly useful in testicular nonseminomatous germ-cell tumors. Ectopic hormone production is not limited to malignancy. Numerous reports have documented immunoreactivity of hCG or its subunits in normal nonpregnancy serum and urine, in extracts of normal nontrophoblastic tissues, and even in bacteria (Table 2). It is in the realm of nontrophoblastic hCG production that our laboratory has obtained evidence for a form of hCG that differs in structure from pregnancy urine hCG. The postulate will be developed that altered forms of hCG, in addition to other factors, can lead to discordant results in some hCG detection procedures.

Table 1. Incidence of Immunoreactive hCG in Sera of Cancer Patients

Tumor	Number examined		Number positive		Percent	
Testicular	1154		553		48	
Ovary (epithelial)	178		77		43	
Gynecologic	692		225		32	
Cervix		504		183		36
Vagina		6		2		33
Endometrium		167		38		23
Vulva		15		2		13
Prostate	74		7		10	
Breast	667		167		25	
Gastrointestinal	703		131		19	
Pancreas		60		23		38
Stomach		199		38		19
Liver		243		41		17
Large bowel/rectum		138		21		15
Esophagus		31		4		13
Small intestine		23		3		13
Biliary tract		9		1		11
Melanoma	210		40		19	
Lung	929		140		15	
Sarcoma	51		7		14	
Renal	126		7		6	
Hematopoietic	661		34		5	
Multiple myeloma		116		11		10
Leukemia		262		12		5
Lymphoma		283		11		4
Totals	5445		1388		26	
(Minus testicular tumors)	(4291)		(835)		(19.5)	

From Hussa (1), with permission.

Table 2. Widespread Occurrence of hCG-Like Substance

Source	Reference
Nontrophoblastic malignancies	Table 1
Bacteria	2-5
Normal human tissues	
Plasma and urine (nonpregnancy)	6-9
Testis	10, 11
Pituitary	8, 9, 11, 12
Liver, colon, stomach, lung, small intestine, adrenal, kidney, ovary	11, 13-15

Hypotheses for Nontrophoblastic hCG Production (Table 3)

To explain the production of hCG by nontrophoblastic malignancies, the most popular hypothesis for years has been derepression of the genes which code for hCG. The neoplastic process is accompanied by activation of some of these genes which are normally repressed, leading to production of normal peptides by tissues other than their natural sources. Alternatively, ectopic hCG production by nontrophoblastic tumors could represent eutopic secretion in which undifferentiated stem cells that normally produce hCG fail to differentiate. The relatively undifferentiated stem cells which are responsible for cell renewal in the different tissues may not have yet differentiated to the stage of repression of the hCG genome. In such a state of blocked ontogeny, a clone of cells might give rise to an hCG-secreting tumor. The presence of hCG-like material in normal human tissues, however, cannot be explained adequately on the basis of gene derepression or blocked ontogeny. This has led to the third suggestion, that most or all human cells synthesize the peptide portion of hCG, perhaps as a consequence of incomplete suppression of the genome responsible for hCG production. Some nontrophoblastic tissues, on the other hand, may be unable to synthesize the complete carbohydrate portion of the molecule, or may synthesize altered carbohydrate, resulting in a product that is cleared rapidly and/or is biologically inactive. To explain the production of hCG-like material in bacteria, hypotheses have been advanced that expression of the CG gene is a consequence of a natural process of DNA recombination. Since hCG is composed of two subunits, products of separate genes, plural recombination events would have to occur for the bacteria to secrete intact hCG.

Table 3. Hypotheses for Nontrophoblastic hCG Production

1.	Gene derepression
2.	Blocked ontogeny
3.	Incomplete suppression of hCG genome
4.	Natural DNA recombination
5.	Vestigial autocrine-isocrine secretion

From reference (1), with permission. Detailed references are given in Hussa (1).

The autocrine/isocrine hypothesis suggests that, early in evolution, polypeptides such as CG may have served growth-promoting or other functions for unicellular organisms. The term "autocrine" refers to an action on the cell of origin of the polypeptide, and "isocrine" to an action on neighboring cells of the same cell type (1). Sporn and Todaro (16) have suggested that autocrine secretion of growth-promoting or hormone-like peptides may actually mediate malignant transformation of cells. In this hypothesis, the ectopic production of low levels of vertebrate polypeptide hormones (including CG) by unicellular organisms, nonendocrine normal tissues and malignant tissues may represent a vestigial autocrine or isocrine secretion.

ALTERED FORMS OF hCG

As detailed elsewhere (1), a large number of malignant cell lines in tissue culture secrete hCG or one of its subunits. Some of the cell lines established in our laboratory are summarized in Table 4. The DoT and CaSki cell lines, each derived from cervical carcinoma, secrete the β-subunit of hCG, albeit in nanogram quantities.

Characterization of Ectopic hCGβ from Cervical Carcinoma

We were able to purify some of this ectopic β-subunit from cervical carcinoma culture fluids by affinity chromatography with low-affinity anti-hCGβ coupled to Sepharose (22). The β-subunit, in high purity, was eluted from the immunosorbent with guanidine HCl. To avoid heterogeneity due to differences in amounts of sialic

Table 4. Cell Lines Secreting hCG or Its Subunits

Cell line	Source	Date established in culture	Products hCG	α	β	Reference
BeWo	Choriocarcinoma	6-30-66	+	+	+	17
JAr	Choriocarcinoma	6-28-70	+	+	+	18
ElCo	Breast carcinoma	9-28-73	-	+	-	19
CaSki	Cervical carcinoma	11-19-74	-	-	+	20
DoT	Cervical carcinoma	12-5-74	-	-	+	21-24

acid, the affinity-purified ectopic hCGβ was desialylated by incubation with neuraminidase.

Figure 1 summarizes the behavior of standard hCGβ and affinity-purified ectopic hCGβ from cervical carcinoma cell culture fluid on DEAE-Sepharose ion-exchange chromatography. The column was eluted stepwise with increasing salt concentrations. Eluted fractions were analyzed by radioimmunoassay using two different antisera. The antiserum depicted by the solid line recognized the core, or internal, portion of the hCGβ molecule. The dashed line represents the results using an antiserum which recognized determinants on the carboxy-terminal peptide, or CTP, of the hCGβ molecule. Two observations are evident from this experiment. First, ectopic hCGβ is heterogeneous, and elutes as 6 major components, in contrast to standard hCGβ which eluted as a single major component. We reasoned that the heterogeneity of the ectopic hCGβ may result from differing degrees of sialylation. If so, removal of sialic acids by neuraminidase digestion should reduce ectopic hCGβ to a single component on ion-exchange chromatography. As shown on the right-hand panel of Fig. 1, however, desialylation resulted in two components. One form, ectopic hCGβ-I, co-eluted with the single species of desialylated standard hCGβ. The second component, ectopic hCGβ-II, eluted at higher salt concentrations (24). Thus, the heterogeneity in ectopic hCGβ cannot be explained solely on the basis of differing degrees of sialylation. The second major observation is that the different forms of ectopic hCGβ are recognized to differing extents by the two antisera. This can best be seen in the lower right-hand panel for the two forms of desialylated ectopic hCGβ. Ectopic form I, corresponding to desialylated standard hCGβ, is recognized equally by the core-directed antiserum (solid lines) and the CTP-directed antiserum (dashed lines).

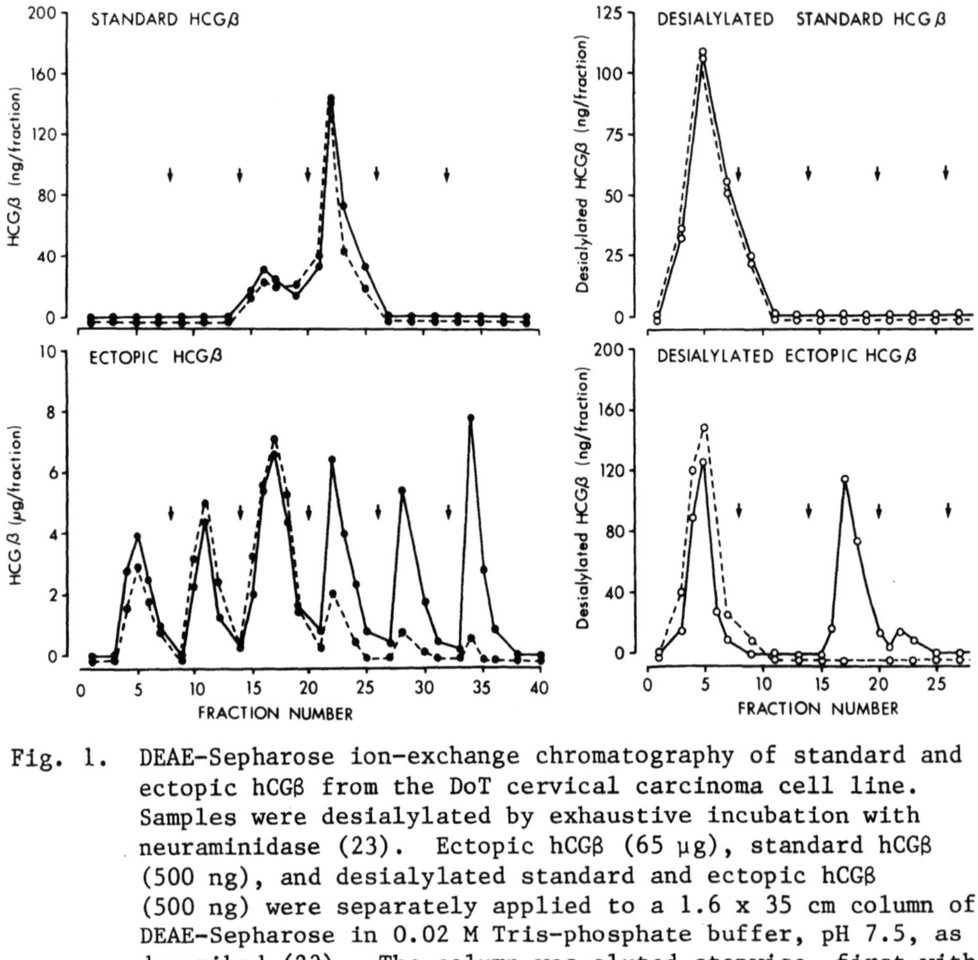

Fig. 1. DEAE-Sepharose ion-exchange chromatography of standard and ectopic hCGβ from the DoT cervical carcinoma cell line. Samples were desialylated by exhaustive incubation with neuraminidase (23). Ectopic hCGβ (65 μg), standard hCGβ (500 ng), and desialylated standard and ectopic hCGβ (500 ng) were separately applied to a 1.6 x 35 cm column of DEAE-Sepharose in 0.02 M Tris-phosphate buffer, pH 7.5, as described (23). The column was eluted stepwise, first with 0.04 M Tris-phosphate, pH 7.5, then with 0.06, 0.12, 0.18, and 1.0 M NaCl in 0.04 M Tris-phosphate, pH 7.5 (*vertical arrows*). *Dashed lines*, radioimmunoassay using CTP-directed antiserum H100; *solid lines*, radioimmunoassay using core-directed antiserum H1a.

By contrast, form II is recognized only by the core-directed antiserum, and not at all by the CTP-directed antiserum.

These and other observations, summarized in Table 5, suggest that ectopic hCGβ-II lacks the carboxy-terminal peptide found on both standard hCGβ and ectopic hCGβ-I. As described above, antisera directed against the internal (core) portion of hCGβ recognized all forms of hCGβ: ectopic hCGβ-I, ectopic hCGβ-II, and standard hCGβ. Ectopic hCGβ-II, unlike standard hCGβ and ectopic hCGβ-I, is not recognized by antisera to the CTP. Another observation comes from an experiment with thermolysin, a protease that cleaves the CTP from standard hCGβ. Incubation with thermolysin reduced the apparent size of both standard hCGβ and ectopic hCGβ-I on molecular exclusion chromatography, but did not alter the elution position of ectopic hCGβ-II. The final observation comes from a binding experiment with the peanut agglutinin, *Arachis hypogaea*, specific for terminal galactosyl residues in the *O*-linked oligosaccharides found only on the CTP of hCGβ. After desialylation to expose the galactosyl residues, both standard hCGβ and ectopic hCGβ-I bound to the lectin, whereas ectopic hCGβ-II failed to bind, as would be expected if it lacked the CTP. Paradoxically, ectopic hCGβ-II, the form which apparently lacks the CTP, eluted in gel filtration prior to the position of standard hCGβ and ectopic hCGβ-I, suggesting that ectopic hCGβ-II is larger and may contain additional peptide or carbohydrate elsewhere (24). This and other altered forms of hCG and its subunits are summarized in Table 6.

Table 5. Characteristics of hCGβ from Cervical Carcinoma Cells (DoT Cell Line)

Characteristic	Standard hCGβ	Ectopic hCGβ-I	Ectopic hCGβ-II
Recognition by core-directed antisera	+	+	+
Recognition by CTP-directed antisera	+	+	-
Size relative to standard hCGβ	Same	Same	Larger
After thermolysin	Smaller	Smaller	No change
Binding (asialo derivative) to *Arachis hypogaea* lectin	+	+	-

For details see ref. 24.
Abbreviation: CTP, carboxy-terminal peptide of hCGβ.

Table 6. Altered Forms of hCG

Altered form	Reference
Free α- or β-subunits	1
Hyperglycosylated α- or β-subunit	23, 25-27
Asialo-CTP fragment of hCGβ (choriocarcinoma urine)	28
Absence of sialic acid in urinary hCG from choriocarcinoma patients but not from normal pregnancy or hydatidiform mole patients	28, 29
hCGβ minus CTP (cervical carcinoma)	24
Multiple forms of pre-hCGβ	30
Multiple genes for hCGβ	88, 89

Abbreviation: CTP, carboxy-terminal peptide of hCGβ.
See text for further details.

Survey of Altered hCG Species (Table 6)

Circulating free α- and β-subunits, rather than or in addition to intact hormone, have been reported by many authors and are reviewed elsewhere (1). Forms of both subunits containing more than the normal complement of carbohydrate have been described (23, 25-27). Amr and colleagues (28) have discovered small fragments of hCGβ which contain the carboxy-terminal peptide but lack portions of the core peptide, in urine from choriocarcinoma patients but not in normal pregnancy urine. Since this modified peptide was not present in the serum of the choriocarcinoma patients, it is possible that the modification occurred in the kidney. Amr and co-workers (28) and Nishimura and colleagues (29) described the absence of sialic acid in urinary hCG from choriocarcinoma patients, but not from normal pregnancy or hydatidiform mole patients. The altered form of hCGβ which lacks the carboxy-terminal peptide was described above.

Recently, Godine and associates (30) reported two forms of pre-hCGβ translated from placental mRNA in a wheat germ cell-free incubation. In the laboratories of Boime and of Fiddes, hybridization experiments have identified multiple genes for hCGβ in the normal human genome (88, 89). These observations imply that there may be multiple forms of the β-subunit of hCG, originating from different genes, in the normal placenta.

Depending on the specificity of a given analytical procedure, an altered form of hCG may or may not lead to an aberrant result. Therefore, it is important that we as diagnosticians be aware of the existence of altered forms of hCG, and that we consider the possible influence of such forms on the specificity of our clinical detection procedures for hCG.

ABERRANT hCG RESULTS

Aberrant results in hCG determinations have been described for a number of factors in addition to modified forms of hCG (Table 7). Common among these is the presence of elevated levels of LH in the blood (31-37), despite claims of insignificant LH cross-reaction by the manufacturers and distributors of a number of commercial kits. In this regard, Vaitukaitis and associates (31, 32) have pointed out that the immunoreactivities of pituitary, urinary, and plasma hLH differ markedly. The presence of circulating antibodies or binding proteins for hCG (38-40) will influence the results of some hCG procedures but not others. Baulieu and associates (41) obtained evidence for anti-rabbit IgG antibodies in nine human sera. This artifact resulted in falsely elevated results in double antibody radioimmunoassays for hCG as well as for other hormones. High or low levels of immunoglobulin or other proteins can affect the results of assays that employ polyethylene glycol as precipitating agent (42-44). Procedures using this precipitating agent can also yield falsely high results when the serum contains above-normal lipid concentrations (45). Less well characterized "nonspecific" serum or plasma factors influence different types of hCG detection procedures in various ways (31, 33, 46, 47). The use of different hCG reference preparations by different kits and in different laboratories results in disparate results and considerable confusion when comparing results (34, 48, 49). Higgins (50) obtained false-positive hCG results, caused by carryover from preceding specimens containing high levels of hCG, when using a positive-displacement pipetting system.

Table 7. Causes of Aberrant hCG Radioimmunoassay Results

Factor in serum	Reference
Altered forms of hCG	Table 6
LH	31-37
Antibodies or specific binding proteins for hCG	38-40
Anti-rabbit gamma globulin	41
IgG (high or low)	42, 43
Low serum protein (nephrotic syndrome)	44
Hyperlipidemia	45
"Nonspecific" serum or plasma factors	31, 33, 46, 47
Different hCG reference preparations	34, 38, 49

See text for details

DISCORDANT hCG RESULTS

To test the hypothesis that some hCG detection procedures might be giving aberrant results, we selected a number of patients (Table 8) who had displayed persistent low-positive hCG results in

Table 8. Patients Studied

Patient	Condition
1	MTD[a] following mole
2	Spontaneous abortion
3	Chorioadenoma destruens
4	Chorioadenoma destruens
5	Undifferentiated carcinoma
6	Choriocarcinoma
7	Undifferentiated carcinoma
8	Decidualization with endometriosis; possible abortion
9	Spontaneous abortion
10	Hydatidiform mole

[a]Abbreviation: MTD, metastatic trophoblastic disease

one hCG procedure or another, and repeated the analysis in alternate detection procedures. Five of the patients were trophoblast disease patients who appeared to be approaching remission. Patients 2 and 9 had both had spontaneous abortions with no antecedent mole, although the diagnosis was not confirmed with pathology for Patient 9. Patients 5 and 7 were males with undifferentiated carcinomas, and Patient 8 was a 40 year-old with endometriosis and marked decidualization, who had undergone total hysterectomy with bilateral ovariectomy several weeks prior to serum analysis.

Serum specimens from these patients were analyzed for hCG by two or more of the ten procedures listed in Table 9. The first 6 procedures (A-F) were radioimmunoassays that detected either intact hCG or the free β-subunit of hCG. Of these 6, procedures A, D, and E were commercial kits, and were used as recommended by the suppliers. Procedures B, C, and F were double antibody radioimmunoassays using antisera raised against hCG (B) or hCGβ (assays C and F). In method B, the low hLH cross-reactivity was eliminated by

Table 9. hCG Detection Procedures Studied

Assay	Specificity	Sensitivity (mIU/ml hCG)	Antibody or kit	Standard
A	hCG/hCGβ	3	GammaDab (Clinical Assays)	1st IRP[a] hCG
B	hCG/hCGβ	5	H1a Anti-hCG[b] (1, 51)	2nd IS hCG
C	hCG/hCGβ	2	H2 Anti-hCGβ[c]	2nd IS hCG
D	hCG/hCGβ	0.5	Concep-7-β-hCG (Leeco Diagnostics)	1st IRP hCG
E	hCG/hCGβ	3	Beta-Tec (Wampole Lab)	2nd IS hCG
F	hCG/hCGβ	7	SB6 Anti-hCGβ (31)	2nd IS hCG
G	hCG (not hCGβ)	2.5-5	Tandem-R hCG (49) (Hybritech, Inc.)	2nd IS hCG
H	α-Subunit	0.4[d]	H7 Anti-hCGα (52)[e]	CR-115 hCGα
I	hCGβ (not hCG)	9[d]	IE5 Anti-hCGβ (53) (monoclonal)	CR-115 hCGβ
J	PEG test for autoantibodies	---	^{125}I-hCG + serum	Pos/neg

[a]Abbreviations: IRP, International Reference Preparation for hCG; IS, International Standard for hCG; IRMA, immunoradiometric assay; PEG, polyethylene glycol.
[b]Antiserum H1a was raised in rabbits against hCG (51); LH cross-reaction was reduced by immunosorption with hLH-Sepharose (1).
[c]Antiserum H2 was raised in rabbits against hCGβ.
[d]Expressed as ng/ml of subunit.
[e]Antiserum H7 was raised in rabbits against the large α-subunit secreted by choriocarcinoma cells in culture (52).

pretreatment of the antiserum with hLH-Sepharose (1). The double antibody radioimmunoassays (assays B, C, and F) were performed as previously described (1, 22, 23, 24, 47, 51). Procedure G was a commercial immunoradiometric assay that measures intact hCG but not free α- or β-subunits. Radioimmunoassay H, described by Elegbe *et al.* (52), detected predominantly free α-subunit, while radioimmunoassay I detected only free hCGβ but not intact hCG or free α-subunit (53). Procedure J was devised to detect polyethylene glycol-precipitable, circulating immunoglobulins for hCG.

Before considering the results on the select group of problem cases with persistent low-positive hCG titers, it should be emphasized that for most patients, particularly trophoblast disease patients, most detection procedures yielded concordant results. This is illustrated in Table 10 for Patient 1, who had developed metastatic trophoblastic disease following evacuation of a mole. In all but the last two procedures, the hCG titer decreased with time, although the date at which the result became negative varied by several weeks. That assay D had not yet yielded a negative result by the most recent date may have reflected the high sensitivity (0.5 mIU/ml) of the procedure. Assays I and J, which were negative on all occasions, detected free hCGβ and hCG autoantibodies, respectively.

Table 10. Concordant Results: Post-Molar Trophoblastic Disease (Patient 1)

Assay	Assay result (mIU or ng per ml)					
	8/3	8/10	8/17	8/31	9/8	9/23
A						
B	172	47	16	Neg	Neg	Neg
C						
D		32	16		2.7	1.3
E						
F	136	32	16	Neg	Neg	Neg
G			35		5	Neg
H	2	1.5	2.4	1.7	Neg	Neg
I			Neg		Neg	Neg
J	Neg		Neg		Neg	Neg

Table 11 depicts the hCG titers in a patient who had a spontaneous abortion. In general, there was again a trend with time, from high levels of hCG down into remission. Again, the date at which the result became negative varied by many weeks, depending on the procedure. As the procedures are arranged, the nearer to the top of the array, the longer the result remained positive. Assays A and B never failed to produce positive results; to rely solely on either of them would beg the diagnosis of occult trophoblastic disease. On the other hand, multiple analyses with procedures C-H, in concert with a lack of suspicious clinical symptoms, provides a more compelling argument for an hCG-negative status for this patient. The hCG levels are currently being monitored at monthly intervals for this patient.

Table 12 illustrates the results from several hCG assay procedures for a single serum date from each of 9 different patients. Underlined results appear to be inconsistent with the results from most of the other procedures and with the clinical status of the patient, although this status is currently still somewhat indefinite in some of the patients. The procedures toward the top of the array tend to yield positive results, while those at the bottom tend to

Table 11. hCG Titers in Patient 2 (Spontaneous Abortion)

Assay	Assay result (mIU or ng per ml)						
	2/12	3/1	3/15	4/5	7/6	8/16	9/13
A		40	12	6	4	6	31
B	300	24	12	13	7	15	16
C						Neg	Neg
D		13	3	1	Neg	Neg	0.5
E		25	8	Neg	Neg	Neg	
F			Neg				Neg
G		8.5	3	Neg		Neg	Neg
H	1.6	Neg	0.5	Neg	Neg	Neg	Neg
I		Neg	Neg	Neg		13	Neg
J			Neg			Neg	Neg

Table 12. Discordant Results: Ten hCG Procedures

Assay	Patient no. 1	3	4	5	6	7	8	9	10
A				Neg	34	20	57	34	
B	Neg	Neg	11	30	7	6	19	11	20
C				Neg	Neg		36	12	
D	1.3	4			3	7	6	3	13
E				17		28	Neg	Neg	
F	Neg	Neg	Neg	Neg	Neg	Neg	8	Neg	20
G	Neg	Neg	Neg	Neg	Neg	Neg	Neg	Neg	32
H	Neg			Neg	Neg		Neg	2	Neg
I	Neg	Neg	Neg	Neg	Neg	Neg	Neg	Neg	Neg
J	Neg	Neg		Neg	Neg	Pos		Neg	B/L[a]

[a]B/L, Borderline

give negative results. Note that Patient 7, a male with palpable undifferentiated carcinoma, was positive in 5 different procedures and negative in 3. Patient 8, who had undergone a total abdominal hysterectomy for endometriosis several weeks before, was positive in 5 procedures and negative in 4. Patient 9, who presumably had had a spontaneous abortion 8 months prior, was positive in 5 procedures and negative in 5 procedures. For these last two patients, comparable results were obtained for several other serum dates. Before it can be determined which procedures were really correct, we must await more definitive resolution of the clinical status of these patients, and biochemical information on the nature of the immunoreactive material. Even at this early time, however, it appears that none of the ten procedures has been completely reliable in predicting the clinical status by itself of all of these patients.

From this experience, it seems prudent to verify persistent stable low-positive hCG cases with alternate procedure(s), until the cause of the discordant results can be determined. To reduce or minimize aberrant results, the alternate procedure(s) should ideally employ a different technology than the first procedure. These findings justify a systematic evaluation of this phenomenon on a large series of patients, using several alternate procedures. In patients with discordant results in different assays, biochemical studies should be performed to elucidate the factor(s) -- such as modified molecular forms of hCG -- responsible for producing the aberrant result. This seems important in view of the ever-increasing number of highly sensitive hCG detection procedures (which differ in specificity) that are commercially available.

NEW HORIZONS IN CLINICAL DETECTION OF hCG

The last major topic to address in the realm of new hCG horizons deals with advances in technology for clinical detection of hCG (Table 13). Reports documenting the unbalanced secretion of the α and β subunits of hCG, first in nontrophoblastic tumor tissues and subsequently in placenta and trophoblastic tumors (1), have created interest in measuring the subunits clinically (54). In the management of gestational trophoblastic disease there appears to be added advantage in analyzing α-subunit levels as well as hCG levels (52,

Table 13. New Horizons in Clinical Detection of hCG

Technology	Reference
Free α and β subunit assays	52, 54-65
Monoclonal antibodies (single and mixed; for RIA and IRMA)	49, 53, 66-73
Two-site immunometric assays (enzyme-, radio-)	49, 68, 74
Enzyme immunoassay	73, 75-84
High-sensitivity RIA for urine concentrates	85-87
Adaptation of high technology for practical use in developing countries	First World Trophoblast Congress

See text for details.

54-58). Dawood and associates (55) observed that α-subunit levels increased while hCG and hCGβ decreased or disappeared in patients with choriocarcinoma in whom cerebral metastases eventually developed. Without monitoring α-subunit levels, therefore, the persistence of disease could be missed once the serum hCG level became normal, if a small focus of tumor cells produced only α-subunit. Ashitaka and co-workers (56, 59) found that the response of patients with choriocarcinoma or hydatidiform mole to therapy was more rapidly reflected by α-subunit levels than by hCG levels. This is undoubtedly a reflection of the shorter plasma half-life of α-subunit compared with the half-life of hCG. Quigley *et al.* (57, 58) suggested that routine analysis of α-subunit levels in patients successfully treated for trophoblastic disease may help identify patients who require additional or more intensive follow-up or additional chemotherapy. These investigators found that measurements of α-subunit were useful in detecting recurrences in patients with choriocarcinoma in remission, but only when pituitary gonadotropin secretion was first suppressed with oral contraceptives (58). The rationale for this is that the pituitary gonadotropins, which share the α-subunit with hCG, cross-react in the radioimmunoassay for α-subunit. Quigley *et al.* (58) suggested that consideration be given to the routine measurement of α-subunit in those patients being followed after treatment for gestational trophoblastic neoplasia once there is no detectable hCG (β-subunit radioimmunoassay) and recommended the use of routine pituitary gonadotropin-suppressive therapy in these patients.

Increased α-subunit levels have been reported in patients with other conditions: inevitable abortion, ectopic pregnancy, preeclampsia, or eclampsia (59, 60). Benveniste and co-workers (62) found abnormally elevated α-subunit levels, but normal hCG levels, in diabetic pregnancy and in third-trimester patients with fetal growth retardation. Patients with chronic renal failure have elevated serum levels of glycoprotein hormone α-subunit (63, 64), a consequence of defective clearance of the subunit by the kidney. Levels of α-subunit immunoreactivity are higher in postmenopausal women than in premenopausal women or males, probably reflecting cross-reaction from pituitary gonadotropins that circulate in higher concentrations in the postmenopausal women (1).

Elevated serum levels of α-subunit have been found in a variety of different nontrophoblastic malignancies including cancers of the gastrointestinal tract, lung, breast, and others (54). Serum gastrin and α-subunit appear to be useful tumor markers in management of patients with metastatic gastrinoma, and possibly in patients with breast cancer, as reviewed elsewhere (54). In a series that included 532 cancer patients, Blackman *et al.* (61) measured serum levels of α- and β-subunit of all four glycoprotein hormones. They found that both α-subunit and hCGβ, especially when measured in combination, were potentially useful as markers for certain malignancies. These workers emphasized, however, that the actual clinical utility of these markers remains to be established in prospective studies. There appears to be a relatively high incidence of free β-subunit secretion in males with hCG-positive nonseminomatous testicular germ-cell tumors (65; D. Sevier, M. B. Khazaeli, personal communications). Many laboratories have now developed radioimmunoassays designed to detect either free α-subunit or free hCGβ.

In the last few years, interest in producing monoclonal antibodies to hCG and its subunits has become intense (49, 53, 66-73). Monoclonal antibodies have a number of advantages. They are homogeneous; the reagent is a pure product rather than a mixture of thousands of different antibodies, as in conventional polyclonal antisera. They have high specificity, and the antibodies can be obtained in unlimited supply. Monoclonal antibodies are consistent from batch to batch in their immunologic properties, and can be purified in large quantities by normal chemical procedures; affinity purification is unnecessary since they are not contaminated with thousands of other antibodies. Monoclonal antibodies can be blended with other monoclonal antibodies to give mixtures with different properties than the individual constituent antibodies. Finally, contaminant antigens are not a problem with monoclonal antibody production, since the contaminants would be recognized by different spleen cells than the desired antigen. The undesirable spleen cells are eliminated during the hybridization, cloning, and selection steps. A number of useful applications of monoclonal antibodies are listed in Table 14.

Table 14. Uses of Monoclonal Antibodies

Immunoassays
Immunometric assays
Agglutination (precipitation)
Counterimmunoelectrophoresis
Nephelometry
Structure elucidation
Antigen topography
Antibody combining site
Hormone-receptor combining site
Immunoscintigraphy
Immunotherapy
Immunopurification
Antigens
Cells

Courtesy of Dr. E. D. Sevier, Hybritech, Inc.

A possible caveat of monoclonal antibodies is that they may be too specific to detect even slightly altered forms of hCG. For example, monoclonal antibody IE5 recognizes the free β-subunit of hCG, but neither the α-subunit nor the intact hCG molecule (53). As shown in Table 15, reduction of the disulfide bonds eliminates recognition by the antibody. More surprisingly, removal of amino acids from either the N-terminal or C-terminal portion of the β-subunit also eliminates recognition, as does splitting of the C-terminal peptide by thermolysin; neither the resulting core fragment nor the C-terminal peptide are recognized by the antibody.

Two-site immunometric assays (Table 13) are becoming more popular as clinical detection procedures for hCG (49, 68, 74). In contrast to immunoassays, where labeled and unlabeled ligand compete for a limited number of binding sites on the antibody and result in a response that is inversely proportional to ligand concentration,

Table 15. Specificity of Monoclonal Antibody IE5

Ligand	Recognition relative to hCGβ (%)
hCGβ	100
Intact hCG (CR-119)	<9
hCGα (CR-115)	<0.3
hCGβ in 8M urea	100
Desialylated, RCM[a] hCGβ	<3
LAP-digested hCGβ	<10
CPA Y-digested hCGβ	<7
hCGβ core peptide[b]	<4
Synthetic CTP (residues 131-145, no sugars)	<0.05

[a]Abbreviations: RCM, reduced and S-carboxymethylated; CTP, COOH-terminal peptide of hCGβ; CPA Y, carboxypeptidase Y; LAP, leucine aminopeptidase.
[b]Thermolysin cleavage product, minus residues 115-145.

immunometric assays give a proportional response. In immunometric assays there is excess antibody, so that all the ligand molecules bind to antibody. Shimizu *et al.* (49) described a two-site immunoradiometric assay that is specific for intact hCG but will not detect either free subunit. It uses two monoclonal antibodies, the first of which, specific for determinants on the α-subunit, is coupled (in excess) to a polystyrene bead. The second antibody is directed at determinants on the β-subunit. The second antibody, also added in excess, is labeled either with radioactivity (immunoradiometric assay) or with an enzyme (immunoenzymetric assay). The amount of label (after washing) that is measured is proportional to the amount of labeled second antibody that bound to the hCG, that has in turn combined with the anti-α on the bead.

Another refinement in hCG immunoassay technology (Table 13) is the use of enzymes, such as β-galactosidase, penicillinase, horse radish peroxidase, or alkaline phosphatase, as labels instead of ^{125}I-iodide (73, 75-82). The advantage of enzyme-linked assays include longer shelf-life of the labeled reagents, absence of radiation hazard and contamination, and colorimetric endpoint. Assay sensitivity can be enhanced with fluorogenic substrates (83, 84) or by concentration of hCG from urine with kaolin or Vitachange (85-87, Table 13). The concentrate is analyzed in RIAs using CTP-directed or other hCG-specific antisera. Such assays appear to be suitable for application in developing countries, including Africa.

SUMMARY

The advent of high technology in the field of hCG measurement has created a greater requirement for high expertise in the analysis and evaluation of hCG levels, particularly low-positive levels, and for the concomitant clinical management of the patient. This implies an imperative to treat trophoblastic disease patients in trophoblast disease referral centers.

ACKNOWLEDGEMENTS

This work was supported by PHS Grant Number 2 R01 CA23357 awarded by the National Cancer Institute, DHHS. The generous supplies of Gamma Dab and Tandem hCG kits by Clinical Assays, Inc., and Hybritech, Inc., respectively, are greatly appreciated.

REFERENCES

1. Hussa, R. O., Human chorionic gonadotropin, a clinical marker: review of its biosynthesis, The Ligand Review 3 (Suppl. 2): 1 (1981).

2. Livingston, V. W. C. and Livingston, A. M., Some cultured immunological and biochemical properties of *Progenitor cryptocides*, Trans. N. Y. Acad. Sci. 36:569 (1974).
3. Cohen, H. and Strampp, A., Bacterial synthesis of substance similar to human chorionic gonadotropin, Proc. Soc. Exp. Biol. Med. 152:408 (1976).
4. Acevedo, H. F., Slifkin, M., Pouchet, G. R., and Pardo, M., Immunohistochemical localization of a choriogonadotropin-like protein in bacteria isolated from cancer patients, Cancer 41: 1217 (1978).
5. Maruo, T., Cohen, H., Segal, S. J., and Koide, S. S., Production of choriogonadotropin-like factor by a microorganism, Proc. Natl. Acad. Sci. USA 76:6622 (1979).
6. Borkowski, A. and Marquardt, C., Human chorionic gonadotropin in the plasma of normal, nonpregnant subjects, New Engl. J. Med. 301:298 (1979).
7. Ayala, A. R., Nisula, B. C., Chen, H. C., Hodgen, G. D., and Ross, G. T., Highly sensitive radioimmunoassay for chorionic gonadotropin in human urine, J. Clin. Endocrinol. Metab. 47: 767 (1978).
8. Chen, H. C., Hodgen, G. D., Matsuura, S., Lin, L. J., Gross, E., Reichert, L. E., Jr., Birken, S., Canfield, R. E., and Ross, G. T., Evidence for a gonadotropin from nonpregnant subjects that has physical, immunological, and biological similarities to human chorionic gonadotropin, Proc. Natl. Acad. Sci. USA 73:2885 (1976).
9. Robertson, D. M., Suginami, H., Hernandez Montes, H., Puri, C. P., Choi, S. K., and Diczfalusy, E., Studies on a human chorionic gonadotrophin-like material present in nonpregnant subjects, Acta Endocrinol. 89:492 (1978).
10. Braunstein, G. D., Rasor, J., and Wade, M. E., Presence in normal human testes of a chorionic-gonadotropin-like substance distinct from human luteinizing hormone, New Engl. J. Med. 293:1339 (1975).
11. Braunstein, G. D., Kamdar, V., Rasor, J., Swaminathan, N., and Wade, M. E., Widespread distribution of a chorionic gonadotropin-like substance in normal human tissues, J. Clin. Endocrinol. Metab. 49:917 (1979).
12. Hartree, A. S., Shownkeen, R. C., Matsuura, S., and Chen, H. C., The constancy of immunoactive HCG content in pooled human pituitary glands, Endocrinology (Suppl.) 108:A283 (1981) (Abstract).
13. Odell, W. D., Glycopeptide hormones and neoplasms, New Engl. J. Med. 297:609 (1977).
14. Yoshimoto, Y., Wolfsen, A. R., and Odell, W. D., Human chorionic gonadotropin-like substance in nonendocrine tissues of normal subjects, Science 197:575 (1977).
15. Yoshimoto, Y., Wolfsen, A. R., and Odell, W. D., Glycosylation, a variable in the production of hCG by cancers, Amer. J. Med. 67:414 (1979).

16. Sporn, M. B. and Todaro, G. J., Autocrine secretion and malignant transformation of cells, New Engl. J. Med. 303: 878 (1980).
17. Pattillo, R. A. and Gey, G. O., The establishment of a cell line of human hormone-synthesizing trophoblastic cells *in vitro*, Cancer Res. 28:1231 (1968).
18. Pattillo, R. A., Ruckert, A., Hussa, R., Bernstein, R., and Delfs, E., The JAr cell line - continuous human multi-hormone production and controls, In Vitro 6:398 (1971)(Abstract).
19. Pattillo, R. A. and Ruckert, A. C. F., Establishment of a continuous line of human breast cancer cells in vitro, In Vitro 9:382 (1974)(Abstract).
20. Pattillo, R. A., Hussa, R. O., Story, M. T., Ruckert, A. C. F., Shalaby, M. R., and Mattingly, R. F., Tumor antigen and human chorionic gonadotropin in CaSki cells: a new epidermoid cervical cancer cell line, Science 196:1456 (1977).
21. Pattillo, R. A., Hussa, R. O., Ruckert, A. C. F., Story, M. T., and Mattingly, R. F., HCG-beta production by epidermoid carcinoma of the cervix, Endocrinology (Suppl.) 100:A179 (1977)(Abstract).
22. Story, M. T., Cole, L. A., and Hussa, R. O., A procedure using immobilized antibody for the isolation of the β-subunit of human chorionic gonadotropin from the culture fluid of a β-subunit-secreting nontrophoblastic cell line, J. Clin. Endocrinol. Metab. 53:1090 (1981).
23. Cole, L. A. and Hussa, R. O., Use of glycosidase digested human chorionic gonadotropin β-subunit to explain the partial binding of ectopic glycoprotein hormones to Con A, Endocrinology 109:2276 (1981).
24. Cole, L. A., Birken, S., Sutphen, S., Hussa, R. O., and Pattillo, R. A., Absence of the COOH-terminal peptide on ectopic human chorionic gonadotropin β-subunit (hCGβ), Endocrinology 110:2198 (1982).
25. Dean, D. J., Weintraub, B. D., and Rosen, S. W., De novo synthesis and secretion of heterogeneous forms of human chorionic gonadotropin and its free alpha subunit in the human choriocarcinoma clonal cell line, JEG-3, Endocrinology 106:849 (1980).
26. Fein, H. G., Rosen, S. W., and Weintraub, B. D., Increased glycosylation of serum human chorionic gonadotropin and subunits from eutopic and ectopic sources: comparison with placental and urinary forms, J. Clin. Endocrinol. Metab. 50:1111 (1980).
27. Morrow, J. S. and Rosen, S. W., Sodium butyrate and dibutyryl cyclic AMP differentially regulate glycosylation of ectopic alpha subunit (α) by Chang liver cells, Endocrinology (Suppl.) 110:A313 (1982)(Abstract).
28. Amr, S., Wehmann, R. E., Birken, S., Canfield, R. E., and Nisula, B. C., Characterization of a carboxyterminal peptide fragment of hCGβ excreted in the urine of a woman with

choriocarcinoma, Endocrinology (Suppl.) 110:A129 (1982) (Abstract).

29. Nishimura, R., Endo, Y., Tanabe, K., Ashitaka, Y., and Tojo, S., The biochemical properties of urinary human chorionic gonadotropin from the patients with trophoblastic disease, J. Endocrinol. Invest. 4:349 (1981).
30. Godine, J. E., Chin, W. W., and Habener, J. F., Detection of two precursors to each of the subunits of human chorionic gonadotropin translated from placental mRNA in the wheat germ cell-free system, Biochem. Biophys. Res. Commun. 104: 463 (1982).
31. Vaitukaitis, J. L., Braunstein, G. D., and Ross, G. T., A radioimmunoassay which specifically measures human chorionic gonadotropin in the presence of human luteinizing hormone, Amer. J. Obstet. Gynecol. 113:751 (1972).
32. Vaitukaitis, J. L., Practical considerations of specific hCG assays for clinical use, The Ligand Review 3 (Suppl. 2):45 (1981).
33. Knox, B. S., McKee, J. W., Hair, P. I., and France, J. T., Determination of beta-choriogonadotropin in human plasma; evaluation and comparison of five "kit" methods, Clin. Chem. 26:1890 (1980).
34. Boyko, W. L. and Barrett, B., Detection and quantitation of the β-subunit of human chorionic gonadotropin in serum by radioimmunoassay, Fertil. Steril. 33:141 (1980).
35. Javadpour, N. and Soares, T., False-positive and false-negative alpha-feto protein and human chorionic gonadotropin assays in testicular cancer: a double blind study, Cancer 48:2279 (1981).
36. Fowler, J. E., Platoff, G. E., Kubrock, C. A., and Stutzmann, R. E., Commercial radioimmunoassay for beta subunit of human chorionic gonadotropin: falsely positive determinations due to elevated serum luteinizing hormone, Cancer 49:136 (1982).
37. Ketchum, C., Maclaren, N., Jensen, J., Phillips, I., Weiner, R., and Kappy, M., False increases of β-subunit choriogonadotropin in commercial kit results because of cross-reactivity with lutropin, Clin. Chem. 28:1998 (1982).
38. Chan, D. W., Bill, M. J., and Rosenshein, N., Specific binding proteins for human chorionic gonadotrophin in a patient with trophoblastic disease, Amer. J. Clin. Pathol. 76:214 (1981).
39. Musch, K., Wolf, A. S., and Lauritzen, C., Antibodies to human chorionic gonadotropin in humans, Clin. Chim. Acta 113:95 (1981).
40. Nieschlag, E., Bernitz, S., and Topert, M., Antigenicity of human chorionic gonadotrophin preparations in men, Clin. Endocrinol. 16:483 (1982).
41. Baulieu, J. L., Lepape, J., Baulieu, F., and Besnard, J. C., Falsely elevated results of radioimmunoassays using double antibody method: arguments for a third anti-rabbit IgG

antibody present in certain human sera, Eur. J. Nucl. Med. 7:121 (1982).
42. Chen, I. W., Heminger, L., Maxon, H. R., and Tsay, J. Y., Nonspecific binding as a source of error in thyrotropin radioimmunoassay with polyethylene glycol as separating agent, Clin. Chem. 26:487 (1980).
43. Jawad, M. J. and Wilson, E. A., Effect of variations in globulin concentrations on serum radioimmunoassay results, as exemplified by choriogonadotropin, Clin. Chem. 27:1993 (1981).
44. Regester, R. F. and Painter, P., False-positive radioimmunoassay pregnancy test in nephrotic syndrome, J. Amer. Med. Assoc. 246:1337 (1981).
45. Fritz, T. J., Bunker, D. M., and Lawlor, J., Hyperlipidemia interference in radioimmunoassays, Clin. Chem. 28:2325 (1982).
46. McReady, J., Braunstein, G. D., Helm, D., and Wade, M. E., Modification of the choriogonadotropin beta-subunit radioimmunoassay for determination of urinary choriogonadotropin, Clin. Chem. 24:1958 (1978).
47. Rao, C. V. and Hussa, R. O., A simple way to determine nonspecific effects of plasma and serum components in radioreceptor assays and radioimmunoassays for human chorionic gonadotropin, Amer. J. Obstet. Gynecol. 142:153 (1982).
48. Bangham, D. R. and Storring, P. L., Standardisation of human chorionic gonadotropin, HCG subunits, and pregnancy tests, Lancet 1:390 (1982).
49. Shimizu, S. Y., Present, W. A., Sevier, E. D., Wang, R., and Saunders, R. L., Choriogonadotropin measured by use of monoclonal antibodies in a two-site immunoradiometric assay, Clin. Chem. 28:546 (1982).
50. Higgins, T., Source of error in β-choriogonadotropin determinations, Clin. Chem.28:1822 (1982).
51. Hussa, R. O. and Mattingly, R. F., Semiquantitative use of Biocept-G radioreceptorassay, Obstet. Gynecol. 54:199 (1979).
52. Elegbe, R. A., Hussa, R. O., Pattillo, R. A., Damole, I. O., Hoffmann, R. G., and Finlayson, W., Glycoprotein hormone alpha subunit and human chorionic gonadotropin in normal pregnancy and gestational trophoblastic disease (GTD), Abstracts of the First World Congress on Trophoblast Neoplasms, Oct. 25-27, 1982, Nairobi.
53. Khazaeli, M. B., England, B. G., Dieterle, R. C., Nordblom, G. D., Kabza, G. A., and Beierwaltes, W. H., Development and characterization of a monoclonal antibody which distinguishes the β-subunit of human chorionic gonadotropin (βhCG) in the presence of hCG, Endocrinology 109:1290 (1981).
54. Hussa, R. O., Clinical utility of hCG and α-subunit measurements, Obstet. Gynecol. 60:1 (1982).
55. Dawood, M. Y., Saxena, B. B., and Landesman, R., Human chorionic gonadotropin and its subunits in hydatidiform mole and choriocarcinoma, Obstet. Gynecol. 50:172 (1977).
56. Nishimura, R., Ashitaka, Y., and Tojo, S., The clinical

evaluation of the simultaneous measurements of human chorionic gonadotropin (hCG) and its alpha-subunit in sera of patients with trophoblastic diseases, Endocrinol. Jap. 26:575 (1979).
57. Quigley, M. M., Tyrey, L., and Hammond, C. B., α-Subunit in sera of choriocarcinoma patients in remission, J. Clin. Endocrinol. Metab. 50:98 (1980).
58. Quigley, M. M., Tyrey, L., and Hammond, C. B., Utility of assay of alpha subunit of human chorionic gonadotropin in management of gestational, trophoblastic malignancies, Amer. J. Obstet. Gynecol. 138:545 (1980).
59. Ashitaka, Y., Nishimura, R., Takemori, M., and Tojo, S., Production and secretion of HCG and HCG subunits by trophoblastic tissue, in: "Chorionic Gonadotropin," S. J. Segal, ed., Plenum Press, New York (1980), p. 147.
60. Gaspard, U. J., Hustin, J., Reuter, A. M., Lambotte, R., and Franchimont, P., Immunofluorescent localization of placental lactogen, chorionic gonadotrophin and its alpha and beta subunits in organ cultures of human placenta, Placenta 1:135 (1980).
61. Blackman, M. R., Weintraub, B. D., Rosen, S. W., Kourides, I. A., Steinwascher, K., and Gail, M. H., Human placental and pituitary glycoprotein hormones and their subunits as tumor markers: a quantitative assessment, J. Natl. Cancer Inst. 65:81 (1980).
62. Benveniste, R., Barnea, E., Ulep, E., and Scommegna, A., Measurement of choriogonadotropin (hCG) alpha-subunit in normal and pathological pregnancy, Endocrinology (Suppl.) 108:A283 (1981)(Abstract).
63. Hagen, C., Gilby, E. D., McNeilly, A. S., Olgaard, K., Bondy, P. K., and Rees, L. H., Comparison of circulating glycoprotein hormones and their subunits in patients with oat cell carcinoma of the lung and uraemic patients on chronic dialysis, Acta Endocrinol. 83:26 (1976).
64. Blackman, M. R., Weintraub, B. D., Kourides, I. A., Solano, J. T., Santner, T., and Rosen, S. W., Discordant elevation of the common α-subunit of the glycoprotein hormones compared to β-subunits in serum of uremic patients, J. Clin. Endocrinol. Metab. 53:39 (1981).
65. Mann, K., Haidl, P., Hammerl, B., and Karl, H. J., Incidence of hCG subunits in patients with HCG-positive nonseminomatous testicular germ cell tumors, Acta Endocrinol. (Suppl.) 96: 80 (1981).
66. Kennett, R. H., McKearn, T. J., and Bechtol, K. B., eds., "Monoclonal Antibodies," Plenum Press, New York (1980).
67. Gupta, S. K. and Talwar, G. P., Development of hybridomas secreting anti-human chorionic gonadotropin antibodies, Indian J. Exp. Biol. 18:1361 (1980).
68. Sevier, E. D., David, G. S., Martinis, J., Desmond, W. J., Bartholomew, R. M., and Wang, R., Monoclonal antibodies in clinical immunology, Clin. Chem. 27:11 (1981).

69. Moyle, W. R., Ehrlich, P. H., and Canfield, R. E., Use of monoclonal antibodies to subunits of human chorionic gonadotro- to examine the orientation of the hormone in its complex with receptor, Proc. Natl. Acad. Sci. 79:2245 (1982).
70. Wada, H. G., Danisch, R. J., Baxter, S. R., Federici, M. M., Fraser, R. C., Brownmiller, L. J., and Lankford, J. C., Enzyme immunoassay of the glycoprotein tropic hormones - choriogonadotropin, lutropin, thyrotropin - with solid-phase monoclonal antibody for the α-subunit and enzyme-coupled monoclonal antibody specific for the β-subunit, Clin. Chem. 28:1862 (1982).
71. Nakamura, R. M. and Maggio, E. T., Biomolecular advances. 2. Monoclonal antibodies - methods of production and applications, The Ligand Review 3:6 (1981).
72. Stenman, U. H., Tanner, P., Ranta, T., Schroder, J., and Seppala, M., Monoclonal antibodies to chorionic gonadotropin: use in a rapid radioimmunoassay for gynecological emergencies, Obstet. Gynecol. 59:375 (1982).
73. Nakamura, R. M., Dito, W. R., and Tucker, E. S., eds., "Immunoassays. Clinical Laboratory Techniques for the 1980s," Alan R. Liss, Inc., New York (1980).
74. Hales, C. N. and Woodhead, J. S., Labeled antibodies and their use in the immunoradiometric assay, Meth. Enzymol. 70:334 (1980).
75. Yorde, D. E., Sasse, E. A., Wang, T. Y., Hussa, R. O., and Garancis, J. C., Competitive enzyme-linked immunoassay with use of soluble enzyme/antibody immune complexes for labeling. I. Measurement of human choriogonadotropin, Clin. Chem. 22: 1372 (1976).
76. Schuurs, A. H. W. M. and van Weemen, B. K., Enzyme-immunoassay, Clin. Chim. Acta 81:1 (1977).
77. Nakamura, R. M., Dito, W. R., and Tucker, E. S., eds., "Immunoassays in the Clinical Laboratory," Alan R. Liss, Inc., New York (1979).
78. Bos, E., Bosch, A., and Schuurs, A., Enzyme immunoassay. A colorful test, The Ligand Review 3:35 (1981).
79. Joshi, U. M., Roy, R., Sheth, A. R., and Shah, H. P., A simple and sensitive color test for the detection of human chorionic gonadotropin, Obstet. Gynecol. 57:252 (1981).
80. Sekiya, T., Furuhashi, Y., Goto, S., Kaseki, S., Tomoda, Y., and Kato, K., Specific enzyme immunoassay for human chorionic gonadotrophin, Acta Endocrinol. 97:562 (1981).
81. Wisdom, G. B., Recent progress in the development of enzyme immunoassays, The Ligand Review 3:44 (1981).
82. Mehta, H. C. and MacDonald, D. J., A sensitive enzyme immunoassay specific for human chorionic gonadotrophin, Clin. Chim. Acta 121:245 (1982).
83. Estes, G. B., Virella, G., Quantitative immunofluorescence using the FIAX fluoroimmunoassay system, The Ligand Review 3:26 (1981).
84. Maggio, E. T. and Nakamura, R. M., Biomolecular advances. 3.

85. Ayala, A. R., Nisula, B. C., Chen, H. C., Hodgen, G. D., and Ross, G. T., Highly sensitive radioimmunoassay for chorionic gonadotropin in human urine, J. Clin. Endocrinol. Metab. 47: 767 (1978).
86. Wehmann, R. E., Harman, S. M., Birken, S., Canfield, R. E., and Nisula, B. C., Convenient radioimmunoassay for urinary human choriogonadotropin without interference by human lutropin, Clin. Chem. 27:1997 (1981).
87. Shimizu, T., Matsuura, S., Oh, S., Ohashi, M., Ashitaka, Y., and Tojo, S., Efficient extraction and radioimmunoassay of chorionic gonadotropin in human urine, Endocrinology (Suppl.) 110:A310 (1982)(Abstract).
88. Boorstein, W. R., Vamvakopoulos, N. C., and Fiddes, J. C., Human chorionic gonadotropin β-subunit is encoded by at least eight genes arranged in tandem and inverted pairs, Nature 300: 419 (1982).
89. Policastro, P., Ovitt, C. E., Hoshina, M., Fukuoka, H., Boothby, M. R., and Boime, I., The β subunit of human chorionic gonadotropin is encoded by multiple genes, J. Biol. Chem. 258:11492 (1983).

THE CARBOHYDRATE ON HUMAN CHORIONIC GONADOTROPIN PRODUCED BY CANCER CELLS

Laurence A. Cole and Robert O. Hussa

Department of Pharmacology
University of Michigan
Ann Arbor, Michigan 48109, USA
and
Department of Gynecology & Obstetrics
Medical College of Wisconsin
Milwaukee, Wisconsin 53226, USA

INTRODUCTION

Standard hCG and its subunits in pregnancy urine and serum contain *N*-linked biantennary oligosaccharides (1), through which they bind the lectin Con A (2). However, as recently shown, that produced by nontrophoblastic malignancies and *in vitro* by choriocarcinoma cells only partially binds this lectin (Table 1). On this basis, it has been suggested that cancer cell hCG subunits have an alternative oligosaccharide structure (3, 4), or a reduced carbohydrate content or are sugar-free (4). The DoT and CaSki cell lines were established from the tumors of two patients with epidermoid carcinoma of the cervix. Immunoreactive hCG/hCGβ was detected in the serum of both patients and in the spent medium from the corresponding cell lines (5, 6). The hCGβ from DoT and CaSki cell lines only partially binds Con A. To study this phenomenon, the hCGβ produced by DoT cells was compared with standard hCGβ in terms of its oligosaccharide structure. Methods are described whereby the oligosaccharides on trace amounts of ectopic glycoprotein can be compared to those of glycoprotein with known oligosaccharide structure. Methods, developed with mg quantities of standard hCGβ, were applied to trace amounts of ectopic hCGβ from DoT culture fluids.

MATERIALS AND METHODS

Purified hCGβ (Batch CR-123) was kindly provided by the Hormone

Table 1. Binding to Con A-Sepharose of hCG Produced by Normal Placenta and Neoplastic Tissues

hCG preparation	Percent bound	Reference
Standard hCG[a]	100	7
Standard hCGβ[b]	98	8
Pregnancy serum hCG	100	4
Placenta hCG	92.5 ± 0.9[c]	4
Nontrophoblastic cancer		
Tissue hCG	31 ± 9.1	4
Serum hCG	55 ± 12	4
Cervical cancer hCGβ (*in vitro*)	60	9
Choriocarcinoma hCGβ (*in vitro*)	58	Peters, Cole, and Ruddon[d]
Glycopeptides from choriocarcinoma hCG (*in vitro*)	52	Peters, Cole, and Ruddon
Glycopeptides from choriocarcinoma hCGα (*in vitro*)	44	Peters, Cole, and Ruddon
Cervical carcinoma hCGα (*in vitro*)	85	3

[a]Purified from pregnancy urine.
[b]Purified from pregnancy urine hCG.
[c]Standard error of the mean.
[d]Unpublished observations.

Distribution Program, NIAMDD, and antiserum H100 was a gift from Dr. H-C Chen, NICHHD. Con A-Sepharose and DEAE-Sepharose were purchased from Pharmacia Fine Chemicals, Inc. (Piscataway, NJ), and Bio-Gel P100 and P10 from Bio-Rad Laboratories (Richmond, CA). NaB^3H_4 and ^3H-glucose were obtained from New England Nuclear Corp. (Boston, MA). Azocoll was purchased from Calbiochem-Behring Corp.

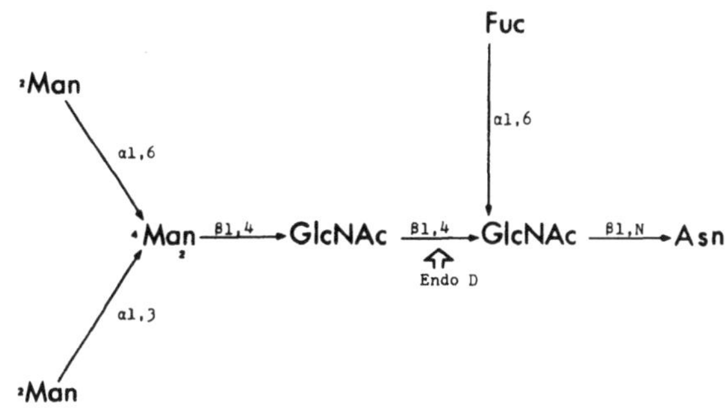

Fig. 1. Con A binding site and endo D cleavage site on *N*-linked oligosaccharides. The Con A binding determinant on "complex" *N*-linked oligosaccharides, such as those on standard hCGβ (1), is Manα1-6(Manα1-3)Manβ1-4GlcNAc (2). Con A binding is blocked by residues linked to C-2 and C-4 on the βMan component of this determinant or to C-4 and C-6 on the αMan component. However, residues linked to C-2 on the αMan components do not block Con A binding. Endo D specifically cleaves the *di-N*-acetylchitobiose component of this structure (12). However, the enzyme fails to cleave this structure when additional residues are linked to C-2 on the αMan components. Abbreviations: Man, mannosyl; GlcNAc, *N*-acetylglucosaminyl; Fuc, fucosyl; Asn, asparaginyl; Endo D, endo-β-*N*-acetylglucosaminidase D.

(La Jolla, CA), and *Ricinus communis*-120 lectin and *Arachis hypogaea* agglutinin, both linked to agarose, from E-Y Laboratories (San Mateo, CA). Highly purified endo-β-*N*-acetylglucosaminidase D (endo D) came from Miles Biochemicals (Elkart, IN). This enzyme specifically cleaves the *di-N*-acetylchitobiose component of exoglycosidase digested "complex" *N*-linked oligosaccharides (Fig. 1). Affinity-purified neuraminidase from *Clostridium perfringens* (Type X) was purchased from Sigma Chemical Co. (St. Louis, MO), as were crude preparations of β-galactosidase and β-*N*-acetylglucosaminidase from *Aspergillus niger*, and all other reagents.

Enzymes

The specificity of each glycosidase preparation was determined using the *para*-nitrophenyl (PNP) substrates PNP-β-galactose, PNP-β-*N*-acetylglucosamine, PNP-α-mannose, PNP-β-mannose, PNP-α-*N*-acetylgalactosamine, and PNP-*N*-acetylneuraminyl lactose (10, 11). Proteolytic activity was determined using the substrate Azocoll, an insoluble collagen-dye complex that is chromogenic upon incubation with proteases (9). Contaminant glycosidase or protease activity was not detected in the neuraminidase preparation. Minimal β-*N*-acetylglucosaminidase activity was detected in the endo D preparation. The crude β-*N*-acetylglucosaminidase preparation contained significant β-galactosidase and α-*N*-acetylgalactosaminidase activities, and the crude β-galactosidase preparation contained significant protease activity as well as multiple contaminant glycosidase activities.

The crude β-galactosidase and β-*N*-acetylglucosaminidase preparations were purified by ion-exchange chromatography according to the method of Bahl and Agrawal (13). The purification procedures significantly improved the specific activities of both enzymes, and diminished contaminant protease and glycosidase activities in the β-galactosidase preparation. The purification procedures failed to diminish the α-*N*-acetylgalactosaminidase activity in the β-*N*-acetylglucosaminidase preparation; therefore, α-*N*-acetylgalactosaminyl residues in the terminal position may also be substrates for this enzyme.

Glycosidase Digestion

Samples were incubated with glycosidases at 37° for 24 hr. Following each glycosidase digestion, the products were separated on 0.9 x 15 cm Bio-Gel P10 columns, and lyophilized. Digestions were performed as follows: i) neuraminidase, enzyme (3 additions of 1 unit) in 0.1 M sodium acetate, pH 5 (1 ml); ii) β-galactosidase or β-*N*-acetylglucosaminidase (3 additions of 0.8 unit) in 0.1 M sodium citrate, pH 4 (0.5 ml); iii) endo D, enzyme (single addition of 0.1 unit) in 0.1 M Tris acetate, pH 6.5 (450 μl). A drop of toluene was added to all reaction mixtures to inhibit bacterial growth.

Reduction and S-Carboxymethylation

Neuraminidase-digested samples were dissolved in 0.5 M Tris-HCl, pH 8.5 (1 ml), containing 8 M urea and 0.1 M EDTA, then mixed with 0.3 M dithiothreitol (1.3 ml). The mixtures were incubated for 30 min at 37° under nitrogen, then an additional 30 min in the dark after the addition of 2 M iodoacetic acid (2 ml). Reduced and S-carboxymethylated samples were desalted on 1.6 x 25 cm Bio-Gel P10 columns, then lyophilized.

Gel Filtration

Samples were analyzed by gel filtration on a Bio-Gel P100, -400 mesh column, as described previously (8). The column was calibrated with ovalbumin (Stokes radius 28 Å), carbonic anhydrase (23.5 Å), soybean trypsin inhibitor (22 Å), myoglobin (20 Å), and cytochrome c (16 Å). Blue dextran 2000 was used to mark the void volume.

Sugar Analyses

After each glycosidase digestion, ^{3}H-glucose was added for determination of recovery, and the products were analyzed after separation on Bio-Gel P10 columns. Neuraminic acid was quantitated by the thiobarbituric acid method (14). Galactose was measured by a specific enzyme assay (15, 16). Total *N*-acetylhexosamines were determined by the Elson-Morgan reaction, as modified by Reissig (17). *N*-acetylglucosamine was quantitated as glucosamine, the product of acid deacetylation (6 N HCl, 80°, 2 hr). The glucosamine was measured by a compound enzyme assay (15). The differential mannose content of the endo D substrate and protein product were used as a measure of $(Man)_3$GlcNAc release by this enzyme. The mannose content was determined after acid hydrolysis (6 N HCl, 110°, 4 hr) and cation exchange (18) by a compound enzyme assay (15).

Lectin Affinity Chromatography

Con A binds the determinant Manα1-6(Manα1-3)Manβ1-4GlcNAc on *N*-linked oligosaccharides (Fig. 1). Samples were applied to 1 x 4 cm columns of Con A-Sepharose equilibrated with phosphate-buffered saline (PBS, 0.15 M NaCl, 50 mM Na_2HPO_4, 15 mM NaN_3) containing 1 mM $MgCl_2$ and $CaCl_2$. Following sample application, the columns were washed with 7 ml buffer. Because the elution of samples from Con A may be retarded or incomplete (19), the percent bound was determined from the equation:

$$\text{Percent bound} = \frac{\text{Total - Unbound - NSB}}{\text{Total - NSB}}$$

where NSB is the portion nonspecifically bound.

The NSB was determined using Con A columns equilibrated with buffer containing the specific inhibitor, α-methylglucopyranoside.

Ricinus communis-120 lectin specifically binds *N*- and *O*-linked oligosaccharides on glycoproteins with nonreducing terminal β-galactosyl residues (20, 21). Samples (1 ml) were applied to 1 x 4 cm columns of *Ricinus communis*-120 lectin linked to agarose. The columns were then washed with 7 ml PBS. As was observed, the elution of samples from *Ricinus communis*-120 was retarded or incomplete. For this reason, the percent bound was also determined as in the case of Con A binding (above). The NSB was determined using *Ricinus communis*-120 columns equilibrated with buffer containing lactose, a specific inhibitor of binding.

Arachis hypogaea agglutinin binds *O*-linked oligosaccharides on glycoproteins with nonreducing terminal Galβ1-3GalNAc (21, 22). Samples (1 ml) were applied to 1 x 4 cm columns of *Arachis hypogaea* agglutinin linked to agarose. The columns were washed with 7 ml PBS. Bound proteins were eluted with PBS containing 0.2 M lactose (8 ml). The columns were washed with 21 ml PBS before reuse. Using this procedure, 95 to 100% recovery of samples was achieved.

Radioimmunoassay (RIA)

Assays were performed for hCGβ and its derivatives according to the double antibody procedure, as previously described (23). The assays employed ^{125}I-hCG as tracer, prepared by the lactoperoxidase method (24), and the carboxy-terminal peptide (CTP)-directed antiserum, H100 (final dilution 1:5000), or the core-directed antiserum, H1a (final dilution 1:50,000), as first antibody. The data obtained in the RIAs were analyzed by the logit-log method of Rodbard and associates (25) using a program arranged for the Texas Instruments T159/PC100C calculator.

Reductive Methylation

Tritiated hCGβ was prepared by reductive methylation, according to the method of Tack *et al.* (26). The hCGβ (750 μg in 250 μl of borate buffer, 0.2 M, pH 8) was mixed at 4° with formaldehyde (12.5 μl, 0.2 M), then cooled on ice in a sealed vial containing NaB^3H_4 (10 μl, 1 Ci/ml in 10 mM NaOH) for 10 min. The mixture was removed from the vial with a syringe, and separated on a 0.9 x 15 cm Bio-Gel P10 column. The specific activity of the ^{3}H-hCGβ was 1.7 μCi/nmol by RIA with antiserum H1a or H100. Amino acid analysis demonstrated modification of 50% of lysyl residues by reductive methylation.

Cell Culture

The DoT and CaSki lines of epidermoid carcinoma of the cervix cells in culture ectopically secrete hCGβ and hCG (9). Cells were routinely cultured in serum-containing medium as previously described (9).

Purification of Ectopic hCGβ

Antibody produced against the β-subunit of hCG was linked to Sepharose 4B and used to isolate ectopic hCGβ from DoT spent culture fluids (27). Briefly, fluids were dialyzed, then concentrated by lyophilization. Samples were taken up in PBS and processed as follows: i) by adsorption to anti-hCGβ linked to Sepharose 4B; ii) by elution with 3 M guanidine HCl, pH 3.0; iii) by desalting of the eluate on Sephadex G25; iv) by repeating steps (i), (ii), and (iii). From 16 liters of DoT spent fluids, 50.9 μg purified ectopic hCGβ was isolated, representing a 207,000-fold purification. The purified preparation contained less than 1% hCG. Gel filtration, ion-exchange chromatography, and RIA using various antisera were all used to compare the physical and immunologic properties of ectopic hCGβ in spent culture fluids with that purified as described. In all cases, the properties of purified ectopic hCGβ were not distinguished from those for that in spent culture fluids.

RESULTS

Glycosidase Digestion of Intact hCGβ

In an effort to examine the oligosaccharides on nanogram amounts of purified ectopic hCGβ, a glycosidase digestion procedure was developed for intact glycoproteins (Fig. 2). Figure 3 shows the structure of the oligosaccharides on standard hCGβ as determined by Kessler and associates (28). In validation studies, the glycosidase digestion procedure was first applied to 12 mg standard hCGβ, a quantity which allowed quantification of the released sugars (Table 2). The results are consistent with the presence of 11 NeuAc, 8 β-Gal, 4 β-GlcNAc (antennary), 3 to 4 α-GalNAc, and 6 Man residues per molecule. Since these results are in good agreement with the carbohydrate composition of standard hCGβ as determined by Kessler *et al.* (1, 28) using glycopeptides, and by Endo and coworkers (29) using isolated oligosaccharides, it is concluded that the glycosidase digestion procedure for intact hCGβ is valid.

An assay was required capable of measuring picomole amounts of hCGβ following the various stages of the glycosidase digestion procedure (Fig. 2). These conditions were met by the RIA using the CTP antiserum, H100, since this antibody did not distinguish

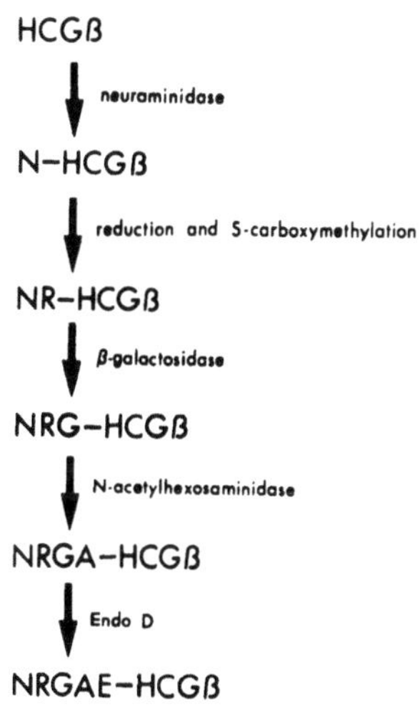

Fig. 2. Summary of glycosidase digestion procedure. Abbreviations: N-hCGβ, neuraminidase-digested hCGβ; NR-hCGβ, reduced and S-carboxymethylated N-hCGβ; NRG-hCGβ, β-galactosidase-digested NR-hCGβ; NRGA-hCGβ, β-*N*-acetylhexosaminidase-digested NRG-hCGβ; NRGAE-hCGβ, endo D-digested NRGA-hCGβ. The modifications were performed as described in MATERIALS AND METHODS.

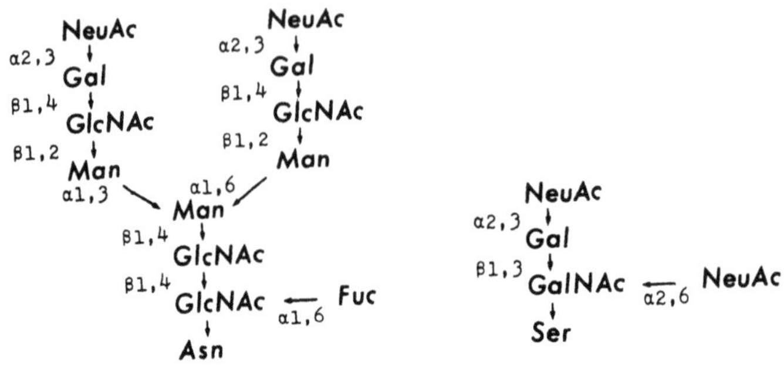

Fig. 3. Structure of the oligosaccharides attached to standard hCGβ. Two branched-chain oligosaccharides (left) are attached to the β-subunit by *N*-asparagine linkage at residues 13 and 30 (1), and 4 tetrasaccharides (right) are attached via *O*-serine linkage to the CTP at residues 121, 127, 132, and 138 (28). Abbreviations: NeuAc, *N*-acetyl-neuraminyl; Gal, galactosyl; GlcNAc, *N*-acetylglucosaminyl; Man, mannosyl; Fuc, fucosyl; Asn, asparaginyl; GalNAc, *N*-acetylgalactosaminyl; Ser, seryl.

standard hCGβ from reduced and S-carboxymethylated hCGβ, nor from reduced and carboxymethylated hCGβ digested with glycosidases (Fig. 4). In contrast, the more sensitive RIA using the core-directed antiserum H1a, failed to recognize reduced and S-carboxymethylated hCGβ derivatives (Fig. 5).

The derivatives generated by the glycosidase digestion of standard hCGβ were analyzed by gel filtration (Fig. 6) and the Stokes radius determined (Fig. 7). Neuraminidase digestion reduced the molecular size of standard hCGβ, from a Stokes radius of 28Å to a Stokes radius of 24 Å. Reduction and S-carboxymethylation in denaturing conditions increased the Stokes radius, consistent with increased molecular linearity. Glycosidase digestion of this hCGβ derivative (NR-hCGβ) reduced the Stokes radius from 28 Å to 20 Å.

To ascertain whether the glycosidase digestion procedure was applicable to trace quantities of glycoprotein, the method was applied to 30 μg ^{3}H-hCGβ. In order to mimic the substrate concentrations used in the initial study, ^{3}H-hCGβ was supplemented with 30 mg bovine fetuin, another glycoprotein (30). The similarity of the gel filtration elution volumes of ^{3}H-hCGβ derivatives (Fig. 8) and standard hCGβ derivatives in the initial study (Fig. 6), validated the glycosidase digestion procedure for microgram amounts of glycoprotein. It is noteworthy that the glycosidase digestion procedure did not significantly alter the specific activity of ^{3}H-hCGβ (Table 3).

Table 2. Glycosidase Digestion[a] of Standard hCGβ

Substrate and treatment	^{3}H-Glucose recovery (%)	Sugar product: sugar	μmoles[d]	specific activity[c]
hCGβ (0.50 μmole)				
↓ NEURAMINIDASE	94	NeuAc	5.5	11.0
N-hCGβ (0.44 μmole)				
↓ RCM[b]				
NR-hCGβ (0.32 μmole)				
↓ β-GALACTOSIDASE	97	Gal	2.5	7.8
NRG-hCGβ (0.26 μmole)				
↓ β-*N*-ACETYL-GLUCOSAMINIDASE	99	GlcNAc	1.1	4.2
		GalNAc	0.89	3.4
NRGA-hCGβ (0.14 μmole)				
↓ ENDO D	60	Man[e]	0.83	5.9
NRGAE-hCGβ				

[a]Incubations were performed as described in MATERIALS AND METHODS. Following glycosidase digestion, ^{3}H-glucose was added to each reaction mixture to determine recovery, and the products were analyzed after separation on Bio-Gel P10 columns.
[b]Reduction and S-carboxymethylation.
[c]Moles of sugar released per mole hCGβ.
[d]Corrected for recovery.
[e]Determined from the differential Man content of NRGA-hCGβ (6.4 mole Man per mole NRGA-hCGβ) and NRGAE-hCGβ (0.48 mole/mole).
Other abbreviations are defined in Figs. 1-3.

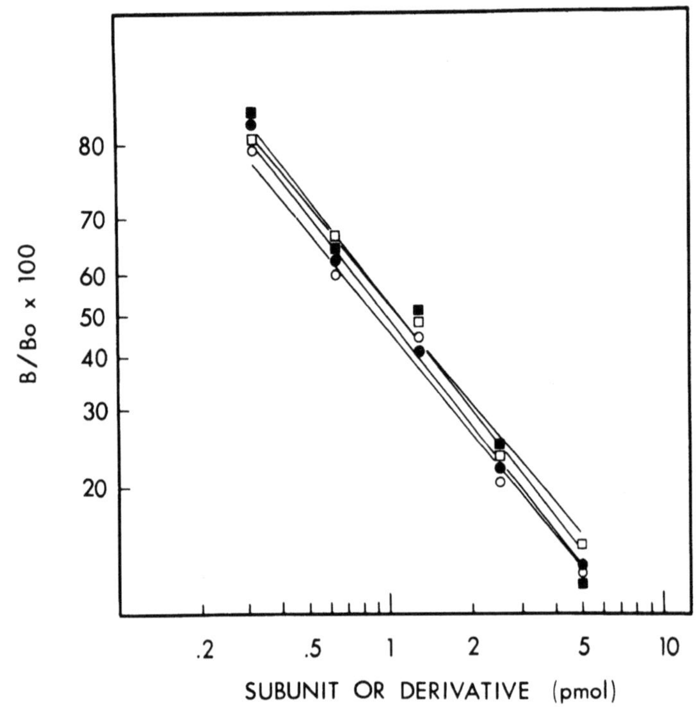

Fig. 4. Competition studies using antiserum H100 and ^{125}I-hCG tracer. The competitors used are: *solid circles*, hCGβ; *open circles*, neuraminidase-digested hCGβ (N-hCGβ); *solid squares*, reduced and S-carboxymethylated N-hCGβ (NR-hCGβ); *open squares*, endo/exoglycosidase-digested NR-hCGβ (NRGAE-hCGβ). The dosage of competitor is given on the abscissa in picomoles per tube. The corresponding percent counts bound is calculated as the B/Bo x 100, where B is the counts bound for a specific dose and Bo for zero dose (both corrected for nonspecific binding).

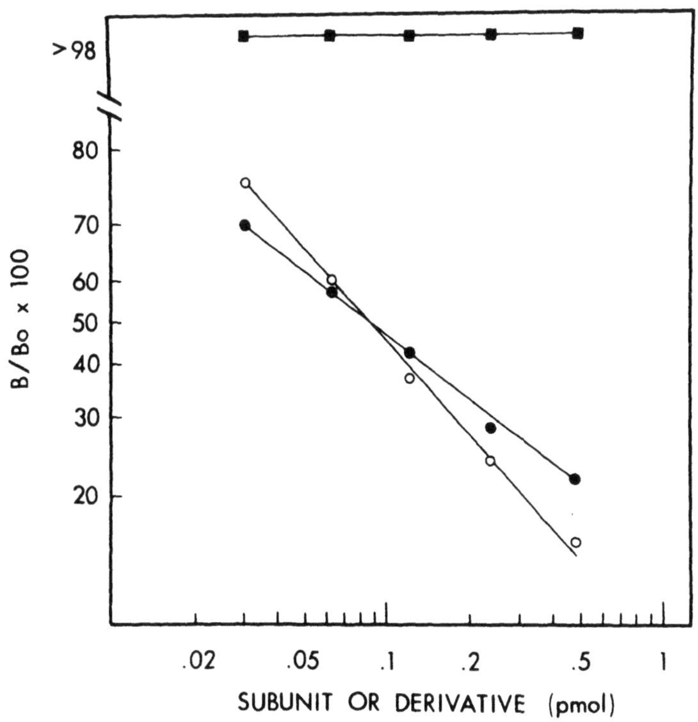

Fig. 5. Competition studies using antiserum H1a and ^{125}I-hCG tracer. The competitors used are: *solid circles*, hCGβ; *open circles*, neuraminidase-digested hCGβ (N-hCGβ); *solid squares*, reduced and S-carboxymethylated N-hCGβ (NR-hCGβ). The dosage of competitor is given on the abscissa in picomoles per tube. The corresponding percent counts bound is calculated as the B/Bo x 100, where B is the counts bound for a specific dose and Bo for zero dose (both corrected for nonspecific binding).

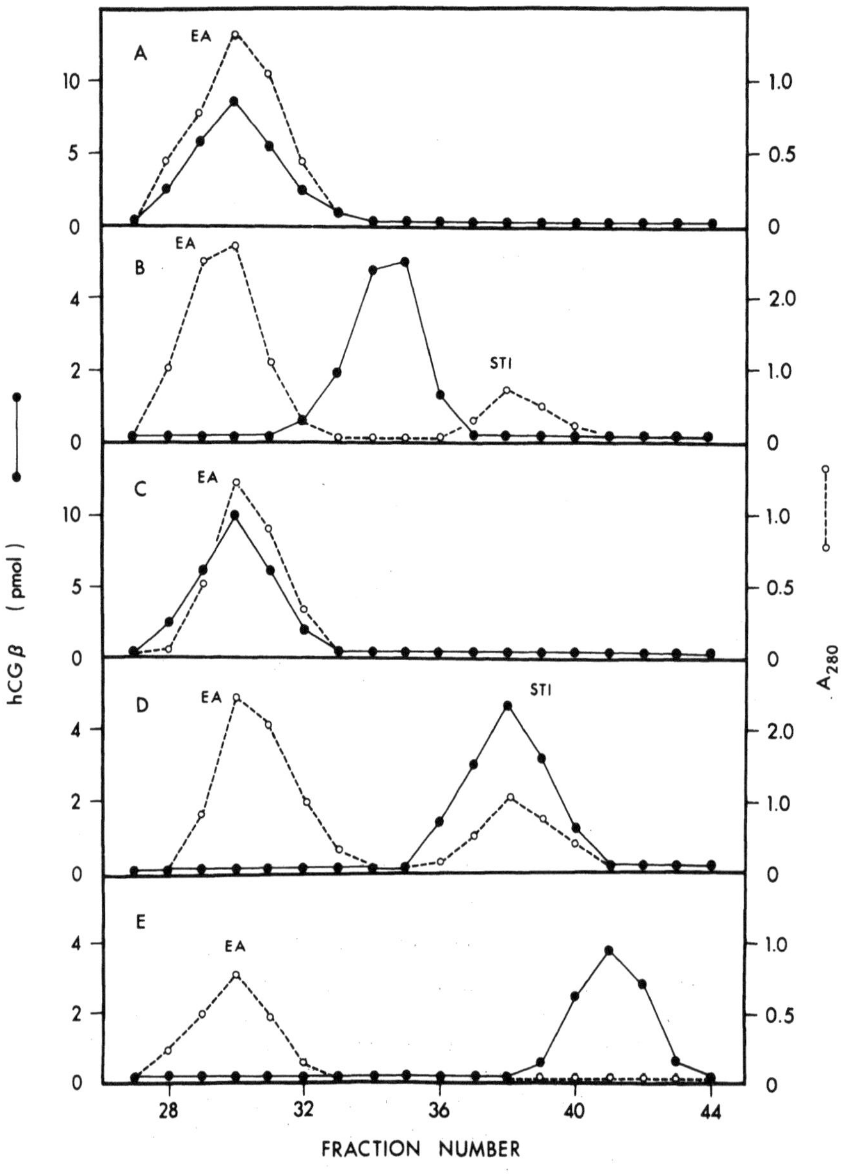

Fig. 6. Bio-Gel P100 gel filtration of hCGβ and glycosidase-digested derivatives. *Panel A*, hCGβ; *panel B*, neuraminidase-digested hCGβ (N-hCGβ); *panel C*, reduced and S-carboxymethylated N-hCGβ (NR-hCGβ); *panel D*, β-galactosidase- and β-*N*-acetylglucosaminidase-digested NR-hCGβ (NRGA-hCGβ); *panel E*, endo D-digested NRGA-hCGβ (NRGAE-hCGβ). Eluates were monitored for hCGβ and derivatives by RIA with antiserum H100, and for protein by absorbance at 280 nm. See Fig. 2 for glycosidase digestion scheme. Abbreviations: EA, ovalbumin; STI, soybean trypsin inhibitor.

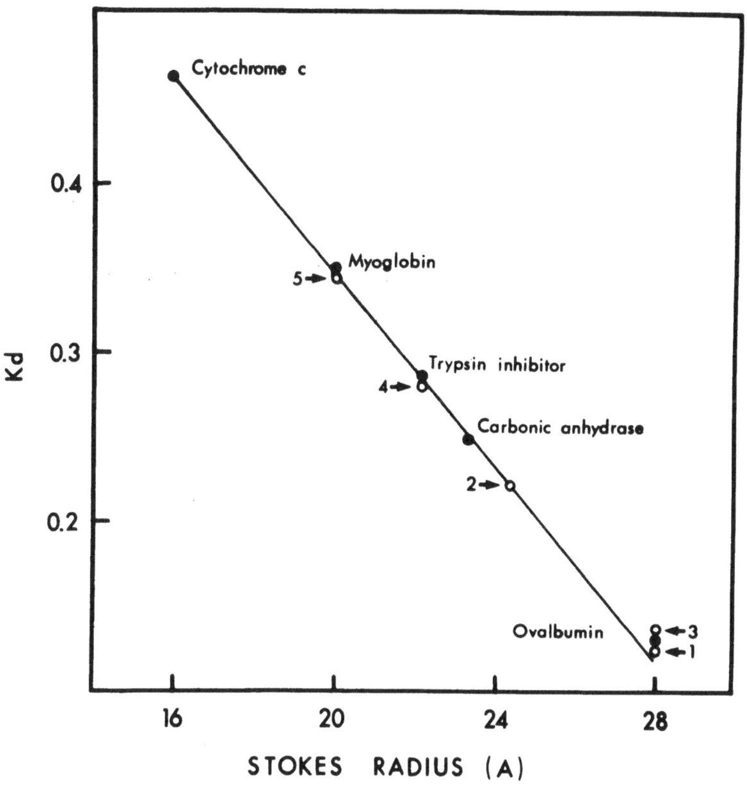

Fig. 7. Stokes radius of hCGβ and derivatives. The gel filtration distribution coefficient, Kd, was calculated from the relationship, Kd = (Ve - Vo)/(Vt - Vo), where Ve (elution volume) is the volume corresponding to the elution peak of the protein, Vo (void volume) is the volume corresponding to the peak of Blue dextran 2000, and Vt is the total volume of the Bio-Gel P100 column. *Arrow 1*, hCGβ; *arrow 2*, N-hCGβ; *arrow 3*, NR-hCGβ; *arrow 4*, NRGA-hCGβ; *arrow 5*, NRGAE-hCGβ. Abbreviations are as described in Figs. 2 and 6.

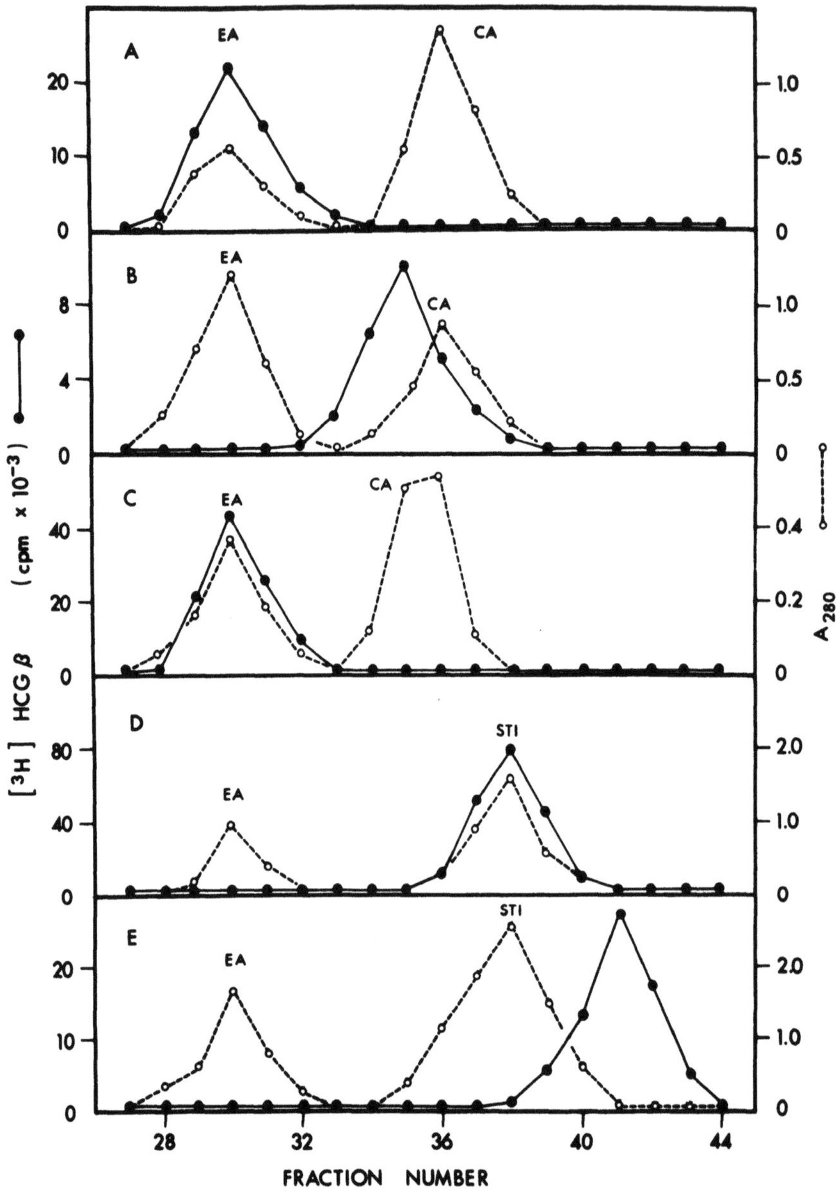

Fig. 8. Bio-Gel P100 gel filtration of ^{3}H-hCGβ and glycosidase-digested derivatives, prepared from ^{3}H-hCGβ by the procedure summarized in Fig. 2. *A*, ^{3}H-hCGβ; *B*, N-^{3}H-hCGβ; *C*, NR-^{3}H-hCGβ; *D*, NRGA-^{3}H-hCGβ; *E*, NRGAE-^{3}H-hCGβ. Eluates were monitored for ^{3}H-hCGβ and derivatives by liquid scintillation spectrometry, and for protein by absorbance at 280 nm. Abbreviations: EA, ovalbumin; CA, carbonic anhydrase; STI, soybean trypsin inhibitor.

Table 3. Specific Activity of ^{3}H-hCGβ Derivatives[a]

Sample and treatment	Specific activity[b] (dpm/pmole)
^{3}H-hCGβ	3423
↓ NEURAMINIDASE	
N-^{3}H-hCGβ	3954
↓ REDUCTION AND S-CARBOXYMETHYLATION	
NR-^{3}H-hCGβ	4111
↓ β-GALACTOSIDASE	
NRG-^{3}H-hCGβ	
↓ β-*N*-ACETYLGLUCOSAMINIDASE	
NRGA-^{3}H-hCGβ	
↓ ENDO D	
NRGAE-^{3}H-hCGβ	3488

[a]Derivatives were analyzed by RIA using antiserum H100, and by liquid scintillation spectrometry (counting efficiency, 26%).

[b]Specific activity = $\frac{ED_{50}\ ^{3}\text{H-hCG}\beta\ \text{(in dpm)}}{ED_{50}\ \text{hCG}\beta\ \text{(in picomoles)}}$, where

ED_{50} is the concentration of antigen necessary to inhibit binding of tracer to antibody by 50%.

Finally, the procedure (Fig. 2) was applied to 30 μg purified ectopic hCGβ, supplemented with 30 mg fetuin and ^{3}H-hCGβ as internal standard. The completeness of the procedure was indicated by the similarity of the gel filtration elution volumes of the internal standard (Fig. 9) and similarly-treated standard hCGβ in the initial study (Fig. 6).

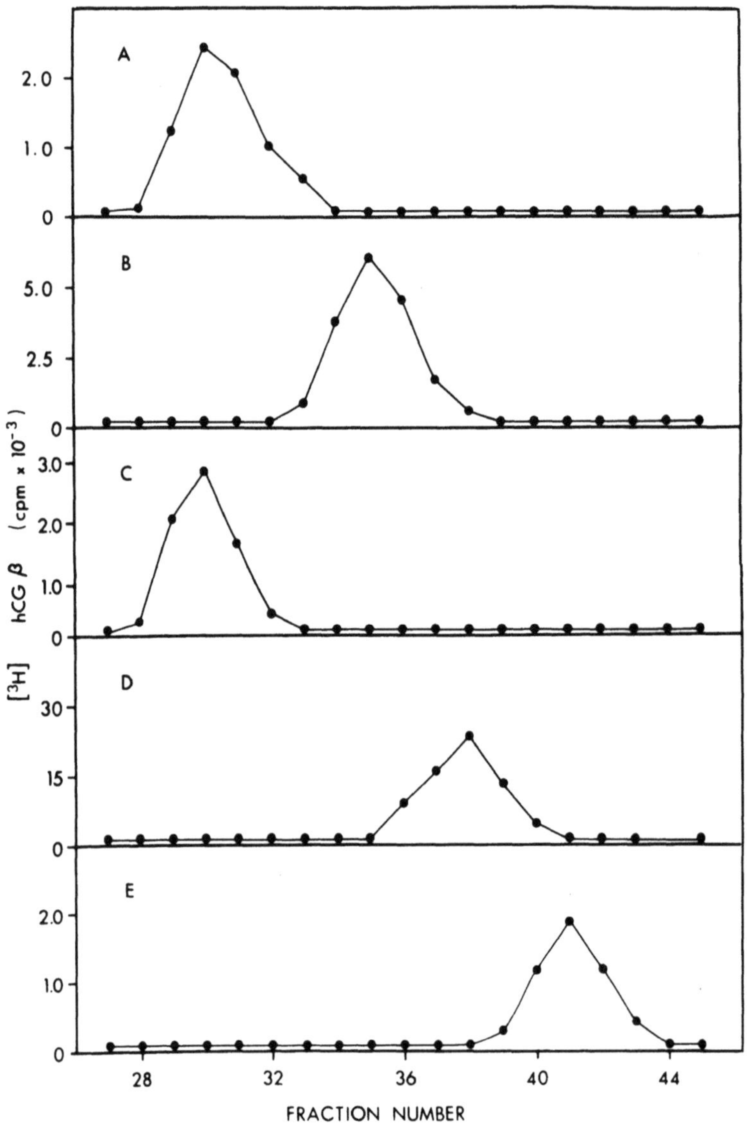

Fig. 9. Bio-Gel P100 gel filtration of ^{3}H-hCGβ internal standard. The glycosidase digestion procedure (Fig. 2) was applied to purified ectopic hCGβ supplemented with fetuin and with ^{3}H-hCGβ as internal standard. *A*, ^{3}H-hCGβ; *B*, N-^{3}H-hCGβ; *C*, NR-^{3}H-hCGβ; *D*, NRGA-^{3}H-hCGβ; *E*, NRGAE-^{3}H-hCGβ. The ^{3}H-hCGβ internal standard and derivatives in eluates were quantitated by liquid scintillation spectrometry.

Table 4. Binding of hCGβ Derivatives to Con A-Sepharose[a]

Sample and treatment	% Bound
hCGβ	98
↓ NEURAMINIDASE	
N-hCGβ	
↓ REDUCTION AND S-CARBOXYMETHYLATION	
NR-hCGβ	
↓ β-GALACTOSIDASE	
NRG-hCGβ	
↓ β-*N*-ACETYLGLUCOSAMINIDASE	
NRGA-hCGβ	98[b]
↓ ENDO D	
NRGAE-hCGβ	3[c]

[a]Samples (1 nmole) were applied to Con A-Sepharose columns in 400 μl PBS. Columns were washed, and unbound samples were eluted with PBS containing 1 mM $MgCl_2$ and $CaCl_2$. Fractions were analyzed by RIA using antiserum H100.

[b]Mannose content 6.4 mole per mole hCGβ.

[c]Mannose content 0.45 mole per mole hCGβ.

Lectin Affinity Chromatography

Con A-Sepharose chromatography was used to confirm the completeness of the glycosidase digestion of intact hCGβ. Con A binds *N*-linked oligosaccharides containing the structure, Manα1-6(Manα1-3)Manβ1-4GlcNAc (Fig. 1). Since this structure is cleaved by endo D (12, 31), and since nonreducing terminal αMan is essential for endo D activity (12, 32), Con A binding can be used

Table 5. Binding of ^{3}H-hCGβ and Derivatives to Con A-Sepharose[a]

Sample and treatment	% Bound
^{3}H-hCGβ	
↓ NEURAMINIDASE	
N-^{3}H-hCGβ	
↓ REDUCTION AND S-CARBOXYMETHYLATION	
NR-^{3}H-hCGβ	97
↓ ENDO D	
NRE-^{3}H-hCGβ	92
↓ β-GALACTOSIDASE (from NR-^{3}H-hCGβ)	
NRG-^{3}H-hCGβ	94
↓ β-*N*-ACETYLGLUCOSAMINIDASE	
NRGA-^{3}H-hCGβ	96
↓ ENDO D	
NRGAE -^{3}H-hCGβ	3

[a]Samples were applied to Con A-Sepharose columns in 50 μl PBS. Columns were washed, and unbound samples were eluted with PBS containing 1 mM $MgCl_2$ and $CaCl_2$. Fractions were analyzed by liquid scintillation spectrometry.

to follow endo D digestion and confirm the prior cleavage of peripheral sugars (αNeuAc, βGal, and βGlcNAc) on "complex" oligosaccharides. Endo D digestion of exoglycosidase-digested standard hCGβ (NRGA-hCGβ) decreased the mannose content by 93% and decreased Con A binding from 98% down to 3% (Tables 2 and 4). Likewise, endo D digestion of exoglycosidase-digested ^{3}H-hCGβ (NRGA-^{3}H-hCGβ) lowered Con A binding from 96% down to 3% (Table 5). In a control experiment, endo D treatment failed to alter the Con A binding

Table 6. Binding of Ectopic hCGβ and Derivatives to Con A-Sepharose[a]

Sample and treatment	% Bound
Ectopic hCGβ	60
↓ NEURAMINIDASE	
N-Ectopic hCGβ	61
↓ REDUCTION AND S-CARBOXYMETHYLATION	
NR-Ectopic hCGβ	60
↓ ENDO D	
NRE-Ectopic hCGβ	61
↓ β-GALACTOSIDASE (from NR-Ectopic hCGβ)	
NRG-Ectopic hCGβ	63
↓ β-*N*-ACETYLGLUCOSAMINIDASE	
NRGA-Ectopic hCGβ	96
↓ ENDO D	
NRGAE-Ectopic hCGβ	2

[a]Samples (20 pmoles) were applied to Con A-Sepharose columns in 100 μl PBS. Columns were washed, and unbound samples were eluted with PBS containing 1 mM $MgCl_2$ and $CaCl_2$. Fractions were analyzed in the RIA using antiserum H100.

properties of NR-^{3}H-hCGβ, which still contained Gal and GalNAc residues peripheral to Man (Table 5). These results confirmed the completeness of the glycosidase digestion of ^{3}H-hCGβ.

Table 6 shows the ability of ectopic hCGβ and its derivatives to bind to Con A-Sepharose. Ectopic hCGβ, ectopic hCGβ treated with neuraminidase (N-ectopic hCGβ), and reduced and S-carboxymethylated then digested with β-galactosidase (NRG-ectopic hCGβ) bound only

Table 7. Binding of Ectopic hCGβ to Immobilized Lectins[a]

Sample	Treatment	Percent Bound		
		Con A	RC[b]	AH[c]
Standard hCGβ	None	94	36	5
	Neuraminidase		97	93
Ectopic hCGβ	None	57	60	7
	Neuraminidase		88	89

[a]Samples (5 pmoles) were applied to columns of Con A-Sepharose, *Ricinus communis*-120 lectin linked to agarose, and *Arachis hypogaea* agglutinin linked to agarose. Con A columns were washed, and unbound samples were eluted with PBS containing 1 mM $MgCl_2$ and $CaCl_2$. *Ricinus communis*-120 and *Arachis hypogaea* columns were washed with PBS. Samples were eluted from *Arachis hypogaea* columns with PBS containing 0.2 M lactose. Fractions were analyzed by RIA with antiserum H100.

[b]*Ricinus communis*-120 lectin.

[c]*Arachis hypogaea* agglutinin.

partially to Con A. However, following digestion with β-*N*-acetylglucosaminidase (NRGA-ectopic hCGβ), 96% was bound by Con A. Like standard hCGβ (Table 4), Con A binding of NRGA-ectopic hCGβ was ablated by digestion with endo D (NRGAE-ectopic hCGβ), confirming the completeness of the glycosidase digestion of ectopic hCGβ.

Ricinus communis-120 lectin binds neuraminic acid-free oligosaccharides on glycoproteins with nonreducing terminal βGal residues (20, 21). As shown in Table 7, 36% of standard hCGβ and 60% of ectopic hCGβ bind this lectin. Following neuraminidase digestion, greater than 85% of standard and ectopic hCGβ bind *Ricinus communis*-120. *Arachis hypogaea* agglutinin binds *O*-linked oligosaccharides on glycoproteins with nonreducing terminal structure Galβ1-3GalNAc (21, 22). As shown in Table 7, ectopic hCGβ, like standard hCGβ, binds this lectin, but only after neuraminidase digestion.

DISCUSSION

The techniques traditionally used to examine the oligosaccharides on glycoproteins have involved proteolysis and glycosidase digestion of the resulting glycopeptides (1, 33). Protease

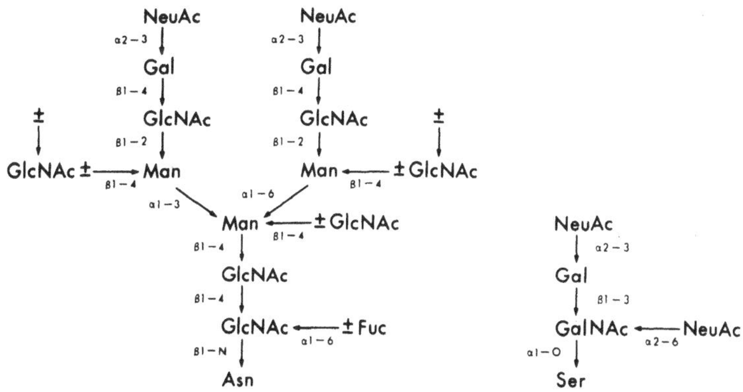

Fig. 10. Possible structures of the *N*-linked and *O*-linked oligosaccharides attached to ectopic hCGβ. The linkages assumed are those of standard hCGβ. Three possible attachment sites of Con A-blocking βGlcNAc residues are shown. These sites and their linkages are those found on other Con A-nonbinding oligosaccharides (30, 34-41).

treatment was required primarily to avoid steric hindrance in subsequent glycosidase action. These experiments demonstrate an alternative method for reducing the steric hindrance, while maintaining intact, although denatured, polypeptide. Using an RIA that recognizes denatured glycoprotein, or using a labeled molecule, this method permits the complete glycosidase digestion of trace amounts of intact glycoprotein. Since carbohydrate disproportionately affects the molecular size of proteins, gel filtration can be used to follow the procedure, and to compare the products of the glycosidase digestion of modified glycoprotein with those of similarly treated normal glycoprotein of known oligosaccharide structure.

Possible structures for the *N*- and *O*-linked oligosaccharides on ectopic hCGβ are presented in Fig. 10. These structures were formulated on the basis of several observations:

1. *Arachis hypogaea* agglutinin specifically binds glycoproteins containing the nonreducing terminal sequence, Galβ1-3GalNAc (21). This is the sequence of the *O*-linked oligosaccharides on neuraminidase-digested standard hCGβ (Fig. 3), which binds to *Arachis hypogaea* agglutinin. With respect to this lectin, the binding properties of neuraminidase-digested ectopic hCGβ are analogous to those of similarly treated standard hCGβ (Table 7). It is inferred that *O*-linked oligosaccharides containing the sequence Galβ1-3GalNAc are attached to ectopic hCGβ (Fig. 10). Neuraminidase digestion is a prerequisite for binding of standard hCGβ or ectopic hCGβ to *Arachis hypogaea* agglutinin (Table 7).

This shows that the lectin determinant on ectopic hCGβ, like that on standard hCGβ, is blocked by bound neuraminic acid. The indicated positions and linkages of neuraminic acid (Fig. 10) are those reported on the *O*-linked oligosaccharides of standard hCGβ (Fig. 3).

2. Endo D cleaves the Con A-binding determinant on *N*-linked oligosaccharides (Fig. 1). Several investigators have used Con A binding, and diminution of Con A binding with endo D treatment, to identify the endo D substrate, Manα1-3(Manα1-6)Manβ1-4GlcNAcβ1-4-GlcNAc, on *N*-linked oligosaccharides (12, 32). In "complex" oligosaccharides, such as those on standard hCGβ (Fig. 3), βGlcNAc, *N*-acetyllactosamine, or sialyl-*N*-acetyllactosamine are bound to the endo D substrate (1, 33). Some laboratories have identified "complex" oligosaccharides on glycopeptides by demonstrating that neuraminidase, β-galactosidase, and β-*N*-acetylglucosaminidase treatments are a prerequisite for endo D cleavage (32, 34). As shown in Table 6, Con A binding of NR-ectopic hCGβ is ablated only by treatment with endo D following β-galactosidase and β-*N*-acetylglucosaminidase digesiton. This clearly indicates that ectopic hCGβ contains "complex" *N*-linked oligosaccharides like those on standard hCGβ.

3. Ectopic hCGβ only binds partially to Con A (Table 6). This is also the case after treatment with neuraminidase, reduction and S-carboxymethylation, and treatment with β-galactosidase. However, 96% of the ectopic hCGβ binds to Con A after treatment with β-*N*-acetylglucosaminidase. This clearly suggests that the Con A-binding determinant on a portion of the *N*-linked oligosaccharides is blocked by an attached residue removed by β-*N*-acetylglucosaminidase. Several investigators (33-36) have noted such a residue, GlcNAc, which when linked β1-4 to a core mannosyl residue on *N*-linked oligosaccharides (Fig. 1), blocks Con A binding. Oligosaccharides containing this residue linked to the core βMan have been reported on IgG (35), IgA (37), ovalbumin (36, 38), and glycophorin A (34); and to the core αMan (triantennary oligosaccharides) on α_1-acid glycoprotein (39), ceruloplasmin (40), α_1-protease inhibitor (41), and fetuin (30). In many instances, oligosaccharides containing or not containing the Con A-blocking βGlcNAc may occupy the same site on a heterogeneous population of molecules (30, 37, 40, 41). This can result in partial Con A binding (2), as applies with ectopic hCGβ (Table 6). If ectopic hCGβ, like standard hCGβ, contains two *N*-linked oligosaccharides, it is likely that the Con A binding determinant on both of them is blocked to prevent lectin binding.

4. *Ricinus communis*-120 lectin binds glycoproteins with non-reducing terminal βGal residues (20, 21), such as neuraminidase-digested standard hCGβ (Fig. 3). As shown in Table 7, neuraminidase-digested ectopic hCGβ (88%) binds to this lectin. It is inferred that *N*- and/or *O*-linked oligosaccharides on ectopic hCGβ contain βGal residues.

Using the methods described, it is not possible to determine the number of *N*- and *O*-linked oligosaccharides on ectopic hCGβ. On standard hCGβ there are two NeuAc residues on each *N*- and *O*-linked oligosaccharide, so that the number of NeuAc residues is proportional to the number of oligosaccharides. Ectopic hCGβ and desialylated ectopic hCGβ are of similar molecular size to the standard preparations (gel filtration and RIA with anti-CTP antisera, data not presented). This suggests that ectopic hCGβ is sialylated to a similar extent as standard hCGβ, so the number of oligosaccharides on ectopic hCGβ could be similar to the number on standard hCGβ. There is a Fuc attached to the *N*-linked oligosaccharides of standard hCGβ (Fig. 3). Using the methods described, it was not possible to determine if this residue is also found on the *N*-linked oligosaccharides of ectopic hCGβ. Recently, a second form of ectopic hCGβ was identified (22). This form lacks the characteristic hCGβ carboxy-terminal peptide, and as such is unrecognized by the RIA used in this study. Like the ectopic hCGβ described herein, and that produced by other cancers, this molecule only partially binds to Con A, and binds to *Ricinus communis*-120 following neuraminidase digestion.

Intact hCG and free hCG subunits, which only partially bind to Con A, are found in cancer tissues, cancer sera, and the medium of cultured trophoblastic and nontrophoblastic cancer cells (Table 1). Our studies with DoT cancer of the cervix cells clearly indicate that the partial binding could be the consequence of the linkage of extra βGlcNAc residues.

ACKNOWLEDGEMENTS

The authors acknowledge Dr. Roland A. Pattillo, Medical College of Wisconsin, for providing DoT cultures, and Drs. Barry Peters and Richard Cummings for their expert advice. This investigation was supported by PHS Grant Number 2 R01 CA23357-03A3, awarded by the National Cancer Institute, Department of Health and Human Services, National Institutes of Health.

REFERENCES

1. Kessler, M. J., Reddy, M. S., Shah, R. H., and Bahl, O. P., Structures of *N*-glycosidic carbohydrate units of human chorionic gonadotropin, J. Biol. Chem. 254:7901 (1979).
2. Baenziger, J. U. and Fiete, D., Structural determinants of concanavalin A specificity for oligosaccharides, J. Biol. Chem. 254:2400 (1979).
3. Cox, G. S., Glycosylation of the chorionic gonadotropin alpha subunit synthesized by HeLa cells, Cancer Res. 41:3087 (1981).
4. Yoshimoto, Y., Wolfsen, A., and Odell, W. D., Glycosylation, a

variable in the production of hCG by cancers, Amer. J. Med. 67:414 (1979).

5. Pattillo, R. A., Hussa, R. O., Story, M. T., Ruckert, A. C. F., Shalaby, M. R., and Mattingly, R. F., Tumor antigen and human chorionic gonadotropin in CaSki cells: a new epidermoid cervical cancer cell line, Science 196:1456 (1977).
6. Hussa, R. O., Pattillo, R. A., Ruckert, A. C. F., and Scheuermann, K. W., Effects of butyrate and dibutyryl cyclic AMP on hCG-secreting trophoblastic and non-trophoblastic cells, J. Clin. Endocrinol. Metab. 46:69 (1978).
7. Braunstein, G. D., Kamdar, V., Rasor, J., Swaminathan, N., and Wade, M. E., Widespread distribution of chorionic gonadotropin-like substance in normal human tissues, J. Clin. Endocrinol. Metab. 49:917 (1979).
8. Cole, L. A. and Hussa, R. O., Use of glycosidase digested human chorionic gonadotropin β-subunit to explain the partial binding of ectopic glycoprotein hormones to Con A, Endocrinology 109: 2276 (1981).
9. Cole, L. A., Hussa, R. O., and Rao, C. V., Discordant synthesis and secretion of human chorionic gonadotropin and subunits by cervical carcinoma cells, Cancer Res. 41:1615 (1981).
10. Cassidy, J., Jourdian, G. W., and Roseman, S., Sialidase from *Clostridium perfringens*, Methods Enzymol. 8:680 (1966).
11. Li, Y. and Li, S., Studies on the glycosidases in Jack bean meal, J. Biol. Chem. 243:3994 (1968).
12. Tarentino, A. and Maley, R., A comparison of the substrate specificities of endo-β-*N*-acetylglucosaminidases from *Streptomyces griseus* and *Diplococcus pneumonae*, Biochem. Biophys. Res. Commun. 253:455 (1975).
13. Bahl, O. P. and Agrawal, K. M. L., Glycosidases of *Aspergillus niger*, J. Biol. Chem. 244:2970 (1969).
14. Warren, L., The thiobarbituric acid assay of sialic acids, J. Biol. Chem. 234:1971 (1959).
15. Schachter, J., Enzymic microassays for D-mannose, D-glucose, D-galactose, L-fucose, and D-glucosamine, Methods Enzymol. 41:3 (1975).
16. Wallensfell, K. and Kurz, G., β-D-Galactose dehydrogenase from *Pseudomonas saccharophilia*, Methods Enzymol. 4:112 (1964).
17. Ressig, J. L., Stominger, J. L., and Leloir, L. E., A modified colorimetric method for the estimation of *N*-acetylamino sugars, J. Biol. Chem. 217:959 (1955).
18. Davidson, E. A., Analysis of sugars found on mucopolysaccharides, Methods Enzymol. 8:52 (1966).
19. Narasimhan, S., Wilson, J. R., Martin, E., and Schachter, H., Structural basis for four distinct elution profiles on concanavalin A-Sepharose affinity chromatography of glycopeptides, Can. J. Biochem. 57:83 (1979).
20. Baenziger, J. U. and Fiete, D., Structural determinants of *Ricinus communis* agglutinin and toxin specificity for oligosaccharides, J. Biol. Chem. 254:7975 (1979).

21. Goldstein, I. J. and Hayes, C. E., Lectins: carbohydrate binding proteins, Adv. Carbohydrate Chem. Biochem. 35:127 (1978).
22. Cole, L. A., Birken, S., Sutphen, S., Hussa, R. O., and Pattillo, R. A., Absence of the COOH-terminal peptide on ectopic human chorionic gonadotropin β-subunit (hCGβ), Endocrinology 110:2198 (1982).
23. Hussa, R. O., Immunologic and physical characterization of hCG and its subunits in cultures of human malignant trophoblast, J. Clin. Endocrinol. Metab. 44:1154 (1977).
24. Miyachi, Y., Vaitukaitis, J. L., Nieschlag, E., and Lipsett, M. B., Enzymatic radioiodination of gonadotropins, J. Clin. Endocrinol. Metab. 34:23 (1972).
25. Rodbard, D., Statistical quality control and routine data processing for radioimmunoassays and immunoradiometric assays, Clin. Chem. 20:1255 (1974).
26. Tack, B. F., Dean, J., Eilat, D., Lorenz, P. E., and Schechter, A. N., Tritium labeling of proteins to high specific activity by reductive methylation, J. Biol. Chem. 255:8842 (1980).
27. Story, M. T., Cole, L. A., and Hussa, R. O., A procedure using immobilized antibody for the isolation of the β-subunit of human chorionic gonadotropin from the culture fluid of a β-subunit-secreting nontrophoblastic cell line, J. Clin. Endocrinol. Metab. 53:1090 (1981).
28. Kessler, M. J., Mise, T., Ghai, R. D., and Bahl, O. P., Structure and location of the *O*-glycosidic carbohydrate units of human chorionic gonadotropin, J. Biol. Chem. 254:7909 (1979).
29. Endo, Y., Yamashita, K., Tachibana, Y., Tojo, S., and Kobata, A., Structure of the asparagine-linked sugar chains of human chorionic gonadotropin, J. Biochem. 85:669 (1979).
30. Baenziger, J. U. and Fiete, D., Structure of the complex oligosaccharides of fetuin, J. Biol. Chem. 254:789 (1979).
31. Muramatsu, T., Endo-β-*N*-acetylglucosaminidase D from *Diplococcus pneumoniae*, Methods Enzymol. 50:555 (1978).
32. Atkinson, P. H. and Hakimi, J., Alterations in glycoproteins of the cell surface, in: "The Biochemistry of Glycoproteins and Proteoglycans," W. J. Lennarz, ed., Plenum Press, New York (1980), p. 191.
33. Kornfeld, R. and Kornfeld, S., Structure of glycoproteins and their oligosaccharide units, in: "The Biochemistry of Glycoproteins and Proteoglycans," W. J. Lennarz, ed., Plenum Press, New York (1980), p. 1.
34. Irimura, T., Tsuji, T., Tagami, S., Yamamoto, K., and Osawa, T., Structure of a complex-type sugar chain of human glycophorin A., Biochemistry 20:560 (1981).
35. Harpaz, N. and Schachter, H., Control of glycoprotein synthesis, J. Biol. Chem. 255:4894 (1980).
36. Narasimhan, S., Harpaz, N., Longmore, G., Carver, J. P., Grey, A. A., and Schachter, H., Control of glycoprotein synthesis,

J. Biol. Chem. 255:4876 (1980).
37. Baenziger, J. U. and Kornfeld, S., Structure of the carbohydrate units of IgA immunoglobulin, J. Biol. Chem. 249: 7260 (1974).
38. Yamashita, K., Tachibana, Y., and Kobata, A., The structure of the galactose-containing sugar chains of ovalbumin, J. Biol. Chem. 253:3862 (1978).
39. Fournet, B., Montrevil, J., Strecker, G., Dorland, L., Haverkamp, J., Vliegenthart, J., Binette, P., and Schmid, K., Determination of the structures of 16 asialo-carbohydrate units derived from human plasma α_1-acid glycoprotein by 360 MHz 1H NMR spectroscopy and permethylation analysis, Biochemistry 17:5206 (1978).
40. Yamashita, K., Liang, C-J., Funakoshi, S., and Kobata, A., Structural studies of asparagine-linked sugar chains of human ceruloplasmin, J. Biol. Chem. 256:1283 (1981).
41. Mega, T., Lujan, E., and Yoshida, A., Studies on the oligosaccharide chains of human α_1-protease inhibitor, J. Biol. Chem. 255:4057 (1980).

PARADOXICAL EFFECT OF ANTIBODIES AGAINST CHORIONIC GONADOTROPIN ON BeWo CHORIOCARCINOMA CELLS IN VITRO AND IN VIVO: EVIDENCE FOR HETEROGENEITY OF CELL TYPES

S. K. Gupta and G. P. Talwar

Department of Biochemistry
All India Institute of Medical Sciences and
National Institute of Immunology
New Delhi-110 029
India

INTRODUCTION

Human chorionic gonadotropin (hCG), a major hormone of early pregnancy, is also secreted by a variety of trophoblastic and nontrophoblastic tumors (1-3). Anti-hCG immunization has been proposed as an approach for control of fertility (4-6). The impact of anti-hCG immunization on tumors making hCG is a matter of concern. The antibodies could have an enhancing effect as noticed for some tumors (7), or could exercise a cytotoxic action on cancer cells secreting this hormone, especially in view of the report on localization of hCG on the surface of tumor cells (8).

Previous studies on the action of antibodies on viability of tumor cells are conflicting. Antibodies raised in rabbits against partially purified intact hCG were shown to produce extensive ultrastructural damage in both normal and malignant trophoblast cells in primary culture (9-11). Nisula and Kohler (12), however, failed to observe a cytotoxic effect of anti-hCG antibodies on BeWo choriocarcinoma cells *in vitro*, even though a reduction in the tumor size was recorded in hamsters bearing choriocarcinoma cells in the cheek pouch of animals treated with anti-hCG antibodies. Knecht (13) reported an unrestricted growth of choriocarcinoma cells in hamsters actively immunized with β-subunit of hCG linked to tetanus toxoid.

This study was undertaken to investigate the reasons for the disparity of results on the action of anti-hCG antibodies on choriocarcinoma cells. Data reported in this communication suggest the presence in the BeWo choriocarcinoma cell line of more than one subpopulation of cells with differing characteristics, and thereby differential sensitivity to anti-hCG antibodies.

MATERIALS AND METHODS

Choriocarcinoma Cells and Maintenance *In Vitro*

The BeWo cell line of human choriocarcinoma was obtained from Dr. K. D. Bagshawe, Department of Medical Oncology, Charing Cross Hospital, London. The cells were grown in RPMI-1640 medium (Flow Laboratories, U. K.) supplemented with 10% fetal calf serum (FCS), 10 mM Hepes buffer, penicillin (100 units/ml), and streptomycin (100 µg/ml), in plastic culture flasks (25 or 75 cm^2 growth area) or 35 mm petri dishes (Falcon Plastic Co., Oxnard, California) at 37° C in a humidified atmosphere of 5% CO_2 and 95% air. Confluent cultures growing in monolayer were dispersed by adding 2 to 5 ml of RPMI-1640 medium containing 0.1% trypsin and 0.02% EDTA. The culture vessel was incubated at 37° C, the cells were detached in 5 to 10 min. The cells were collected with help of Pasteur pipette, mixed with an equal volume of growth medium (RPMI-1640 medium supplemented with 10% FCS), and centrifuged for 10 min at 800 x g. The cell pellet was washed once more with the growth medium, and cells were counted in a hemocytometer and inoculated in fresh flasks at a density of 0.2 to 0.3 x 10^6 cells in 5 ml of growth medium per 25 cm^2 flask.

Anti-hCG Antibodies

Sera of rhesus monkeys (*Macaca mulatta*) or baboons (*Papio cynocephalis*) immunized with Pr-β-hCG-TT as described elsewhere (14, 15) were used as source of anti-β-hCG antibodies. Blood was collected from the animals previously screened for high titers of anti-hCG antibodies. Sera were separated, stored at -20° C and decomplemented before use in the cytotoxicity assay.

Complement

Freshly-bled guinea pig serum was used as source of complement. Animals were screened for complement titers using the standard procedure of sheep red blood cells-hemolysin; only sera from animals with high complement titers were used in the study.

Cytotoxicity Assay

Twenty-four hr after subculture, the BeWo cells growing in monolayer were washed once with medium, and incubated with fresh growth medium containing various dilutions of anti-β-hCG antibodies plus complement. Nonimmune monkey or baboon sera were used as controls.

At 24 and 48 hr after addition of antibodies and complement, the cells were examined under inverted microscope for morphologic changes. Viability of the cells detached from the surface of the culture vessel, floating in the medium was checked by trypan blue dye exclusion and by their ability to grow in fresh culture flasks. The residual adhering cells were stained with Leishman's stain and photographed.

In addition to morphologic criteria, the cytotoxic effect of anti-β-hCG antibodies was investigated by incorporation of ^{3}H-thymidine (s.a. 6.7 Ci/mmole, Amersham International, Ltd., Amersham, U. K.) and ^{3}H-leucine (s.a. 51 Ci/mmole, New England Nuclear Corp., Boston, Massachusetts). After 48 hr of antibody treatment, cultures were pulsed for 24 hr with ^{3}H-thymidine or ^{3}H-leucine (1 μCi/ml) in medium. Cells were detached by freeze-thaw, and the suspension was collected by repeated aspiration with an 18G needle attached to a syringe. The suspension was filtered on Whatman No. 1 disc and washed twice with 4 or 5 ml cold isotonic saline, cold 5% trichloroacetic acid (TCA), and 2 ml absolute methanol. The disc was removed from the filtration assembly, dried at 37° C for an hour, and transferred to scintillation vials containing 7 ml scintillation mixture (4 g PPO and 0.5 g POPOP in 1 liter of sulfur-free toluene). The radioactivity was measured in a Packard Beta Counter with counting efficiency of 50% for tritium.

For studies of ^{3}H-leucine incorporation, the detached cell suspension was centrifuged at 1500 x g for 15 min, the supernatant was discarded, and the pellet was washed twice with ice-cold 5% TCA. The pellet was dissolved in 100 μl Soluene-350 (Packard Instrument Co., Illinois) by incubation overnight at 37° C. The solubilized pellet was transferred to a counting vial along with scintillation mixture, and kept overnight before counting.

Transplantation of Choriocarcinoma Cells in Hamster Cheek Pouch

Hamsters of either sex (6 week) were purchased from Ciba Geigy Research Center, Bombay, India. The animals were maintained in the Institute animal house facility and fed *ad libitum*. BeWo choriocarcinoma cells (approximately 5 million per 0.05 ml medium) were harvested from culture flasks and transplanted into hamsters according to a previously described method (16). Five mg of hydrocortisone (Allenburys, Glaxo Laboratories, India) was injected subcutaneously with a repeat dose after 3 days. After 5 days, animals were checked daily for tumor growth. Appearance of a tumor mass as a very small nodule having firm consistency and dark purplish hue was taken as evidence of growth of the tumor and the end of the lag phase. At the end of the lag phase, anti-β-hCG antibodies were injected daily at the indicated doses for a period of nine days. Changes in tumor volume were noted daily by measuring the diameter of tumor nodule in three different perpendicular directions. Tumor volume was calculated according to the method of Friedell and associates (17).

Estimation of hCG

A specific double-antibody radioimmunoassay was used to estimate hCG in the culture fluid or serum. Rabbit anti-β-hCG serum (SB6), kindly made available by the National Institutes of Health, Bethesda, Maryland, was used as the first antibody. Purified hCG (10,000 IU/mg), calibrated against the Second International Reference Preparation of hCG for radioimmunoassay, was used as tracer after radioiodination and also as standard. Iodination of hCG with sodium ^{125}I was by the chloramine T method adopted by Vaitukaitis and coworkers (18). Labeled hormone was separated from unreacted $^{125}I^-$ by gel filtration using Sephadex G-75. The radioimmunoassay contained 100 μl of the test sample or hCG standard, 100 μl of ^{125}I-hCG (10,000 to 12,000 cpm), 100 μl antiserum at a dilution which bound 30-40% of the ^{125}I-hCG in the absence of cold hCG, and assay buffer (0.1 M phosphate buffer, pH 7.4, containing 0.15 M NaCl, 0.01% merthiolate, 0.5% bovine serum albumin, and 0.015 M EDTA) to give a final volume of 700 μl. Test samples, hCG standards, and antiserum were diluted in assay buffer, whereas ^{125}I-hCG was diluted in assay buffer supplemented with 0.5% normal (nonimmune) rabbit serum. Tubes were mixed on a vortex mixer and incubated for 18 to 20 hr at 4° C. After incubation, 100 μl donkey anti-rabbit gamma globulin (1:40 initial dilution, supplied through World Health Organization Quality Control Program) was added to precipitate antigen bound to antibody. The tubes were vortex mixed, incubated for 16 to 18 hr at 4° C, and centrifuged at 2000 x g for 30 min at 4° C. The supernatant fluid was discarded and the pellet was counted in a Packard Autogamma Counter. The dose-response curve was plotted as logit B/Bo *vs* logarithmic dose. A straight line was fitted using the least squares linear regression method. The sensitivity of the assay was 6.25 mIU/ml at 95% confidence limit.

Localization of hCG

BeWo choriocarcinoma cells, growing as monolayer, either in a 30mm petri dish (Falcon Plastic Co., Oxnard, California) or on a cover slip inside a Leighton tube, were fixed for 1 hr with periodate-lysine-paraformaldehyde buffered solution (0.01 M periodate, 0.075 M lysine, 2% paraformaldehyde, and 0.037 M phosphate buffer) as described by Mclean and Nakane (19). The fixed cells were washed twice with 50 mM phosphate-buffered saline, pH 7.4 (PBS), containing 4% sucrose. Cells were then covered with appropriate dilutions of monospecific anti-β-hCG serum and incubated for 16 hr at 4° C on a rocking platform. Cells were subsequently washed with several changes of PBS-sucrose over a period of 2 hr, and treated with Protein A linked to horseradish peroxidase (HRPO, Sigma Type VI) at 1:50 dilution in PBS-sucrose for 60 min at 37° C. Cells were washed extensively with several changes of PBS-sucrose, and then incubated for 20 min in the dark with a solution of 3',3'-diaminobenzidine tetrahydrochloride (DAB, 2 mg/10 ml) with 0.015 ml 30% H_2O_2. Cells were washed with PBS-sucrose, mounted in 5% glycerol, and examined by light microscopy for evidence of specific immunostaining. The following controls were run concurrently: 1) cells incubated with nonimmune serum, 2) cells incubated with Protein A-HRPO conjugate only, and 3) cells reacted with DAB.

For immunoenzymatic quantitation of anti-hCG-reacting antigens, DAB was omitted as substrate for peroxidase. Instead, cells were incubated with 2 ml of 0.05 M phosphate buffer, pH 7.3, containing 1×10^{-3} M H_2O_2, 0.01 M phenol, and 1.4×10^{-3} M 4-aminophenazone for 15 to 20 min at 37° C for color development. The reaction was terminated by decanting off the buffered substrate reagent in separate tubes. Absorbance of the reaction product was measured at 515 nm in a Pye-Unicam Spectrophotometer SP8-100.

RESULTS

Cytotoxic Effect of Anti-β-hCG Antibodies *In Vitro*

Fig. 1 shows the morphology of the cells as viewed after 48 hr from addition of the monkey anti-Pr-β-hCG-TT serum to the culture. It is evident that in cultures in which anti-β-hCG antibodies were added, the cells have a rounded morphology, with vacuolated cytoplasm and pyknosis (Fig. 1a). Many cells were detached from the surface of the culture flask. In parallel experiments, BeWo cells cultured in the presence of nonimmune monkey serum grew normally without observable cytopathic changes (Fig. 1b).

In order to exert a cytotoxic effect, anti-β-hCG antibodies required the presence of complement, since no inhibition of ^{3}H-thymidine uptake was seen in cultures in which de-complemented immune serum was added without guinea pig serum as source of complement, as compared to those treated with nonimmune serum (Table 1).

Cytotoxic Effect of Anti-β-hCG Antibodies *In Vivo*

In view of the widespread cytotoxic effect ofthe anti-β-hCG antibodies on the BeWo choriocarcinoma cells *in vitro*, *in vivo* experiments were undertaken to reassess the effect of anti-Pr-β-hCG-TT antibodies on growth of the tumor in the hamster cheek pouch. Progressively increasing amounts of antibodies were administered daily for a period of nine days after the end of the lag phase. The data in Fig. 2 show the regressive effect of the antibodies at the initial stages on the growth of the tumor, although this effect was statistically insignificant. As time progressed, the tumor size was similar in control animals and in animals administered antibody.

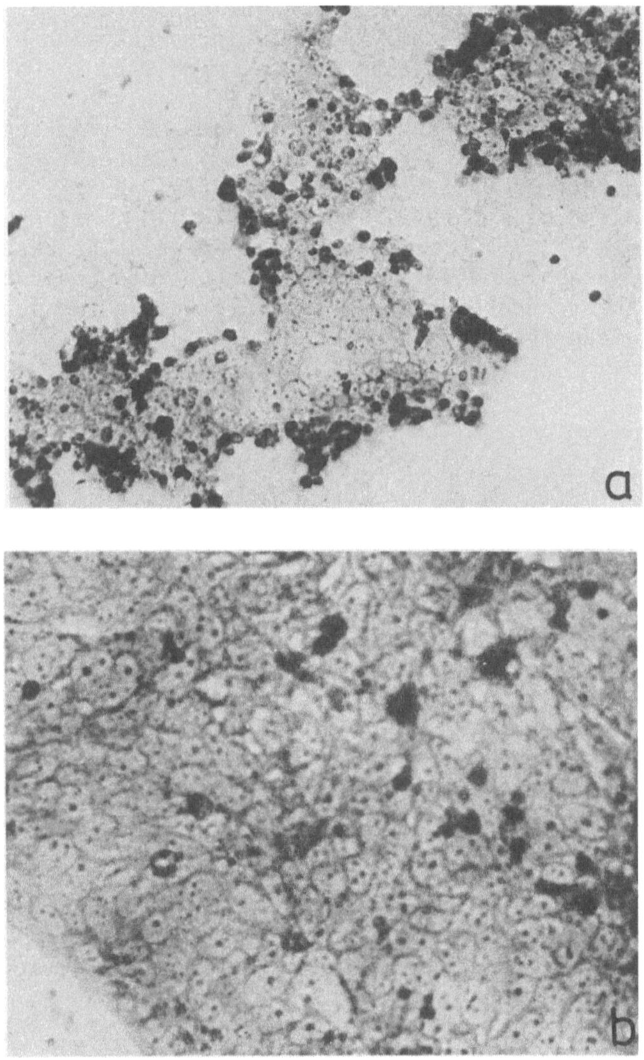

Fig. 1. Effect of anti-Pr-β-hCG-TT antibodies on the growth of BeWo choriocarcinoma cells. *a*, Photomicrograph of BeWo cells in the presence of 10% anti-β-hCG serum plus 5% guinea pig serum (x280); *b*, photomicrograph of BeWo cells in the presence of 10% normal monkey serum plus 5% guinea pig serum (x280).

Table 1. Effect of Monkey Anti-Pr-β-hCG-TT Serum on Incorporation of ^{3}H-Thymidine into BeWo Choriocarcinoma Cells

Set	Treatment	Incorporation[a] (cpm/flask)	Inhibition (%)
I	10% NMS[b] + 5% GPS	7,759	
	10% Anti-Pr-β-hCG-TT	7,695	0.82
	5% GPS + Anti-Pr-β-hCG-TT		
	1%	4,876	37.2
	5%	2,571	66.9
	10%	1,137	85.3
II	10% NMS + 5% GPS	26,100	
	20% Anti-Pr-β-hCG-TT	26,850	0
	5% GPS + Anti-Pr-β-hCG-TT		
	5%	20,800	20.1
	20%	11,200	57.2

[a]Mean of duplicate determinations.
[b]Abbreviations: NMS, normal monkey serum; GPS, guinea pig serum.

Antibody-Sensitive and -Resistant Subpopulations

While the antibodies caused appreciable damage to cells *in vitro* as visualized morphologically, they were ineffective *in vivo* in ultimate analysis. To understand this paradox, further studies were undertaken on the effect of antibodies on BeWo choriocarcinoma cells in culture.

The antibodies did not kill all cells despite the addition of saturating amounts of antibodies and complement. The cytotoxic effect of antibodies on only a fraction of the choriocarcinoma cells was revealed by studies on the incorporation of ^{3}H-thymidine (Tables 1 and 2) and ^{3}H-leucine (Table 3) by these cells. Dose-dependent inhibition of ^{3}H-thymidine incorporation occurred with the antibodies, until a plateau effect was reached at 10% final concentration of antiserum (Table 1). Prolongation of the time of action of the antibodies did not induce a total kill. The ability of the BeWo cells to resist cytotoxic effect was verified by (a) the continued viability as measured by trypan blue exclusion, and (b) the capability of the cells to grow after subculture.

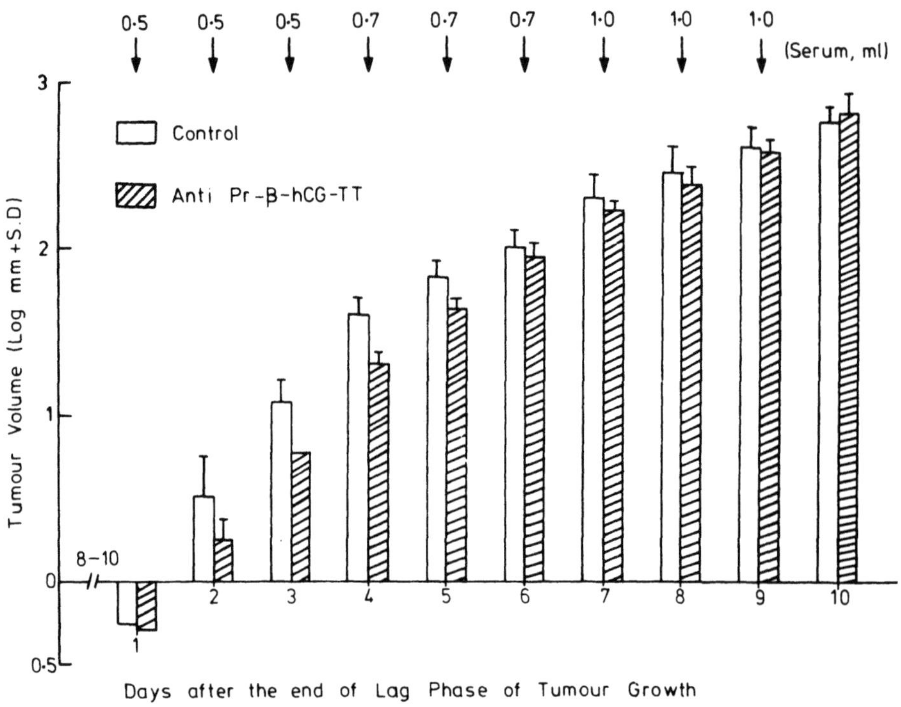

Fig. 2. Effect of passive administration of anti-Pr-β-hCG-TT antibodies on the tumor volume of human choriocarcinoma transplanted in the hamster cheek pouch. Each bar represents the mean and SEM of 5 animals.

The microheterogeneity of cell population was further evident by experiments on immunoenzymatic localization of hCG. This probe detected hCG on the surface lining of some but not all cells (Fig. 3). Assuming that the hCG-bearing cells were vulnerable to immune attack by anti-hCG antibodies plus complement, continuous culture of cells in the presence of antibodies and complement should select out the resistant category of the cells. As a consequence, culture of BeWo choriocarcinoma cells was carried out for 7 days in the presence of anti-β-hCG antibodies and complement. The culture medium, containing fresh antibodies and complement, was changed at 48-hour intervals. The residual cells were washed several times with RPMI-1640 medium and transferred to fresh growth medium devoid of antibodies. The hCG secreted by these cells (the BeWo-R subpopulation) was determined by radioimmunoassay, as was the hCG produced by the parent cell line without treatment with antibody. The results in Table 4 indicate the absence of hCG secretion by BeWo cells resistant to antibody, in contrast to the parent cells not treated with antibody and which produced hCG. The resistant cell population also failed to bind anti-hCG antibodies

Table 2. Effect of Increasing Concentration of Complement on Anti-Pr-β-hCG-TT Antibody-Mediated Inhibition of ^{3}H-Thymidine Incorporation in BeWo Choriocarcinoma Cells

Set	Treatment	Incorporation (cpm/flask)[a]	Inhibition (%)
I	10% GPS[b]	46,617	
	10% GPS + 10% Anti-Pr-β-hCG-TT	17,901	61.1
II	15% GPS	82,795	
	15% GPS + 10% Anti-Pr-β-hCG-TT	36,714	55.7

[a]Mean of duplicate determinations.
[b]Abbreviation: GPS, guinea pig serum.

Table 3. Effect of Baboon Anti-Pr-β-hCG-TT Serum on ^{3}H-Leucine Incorporation in BeWo Cells

Treatment	Incorporation (cpm/flask)[a]	Inhibition (%)
Control (10% normal baboon serum + 5% guinea pig serum)	2,953	
10% Anti-Pr-β-hCG-TT + 5% guinea pig serum	1,308	55.7

[a]Mean of duplicate determinations.

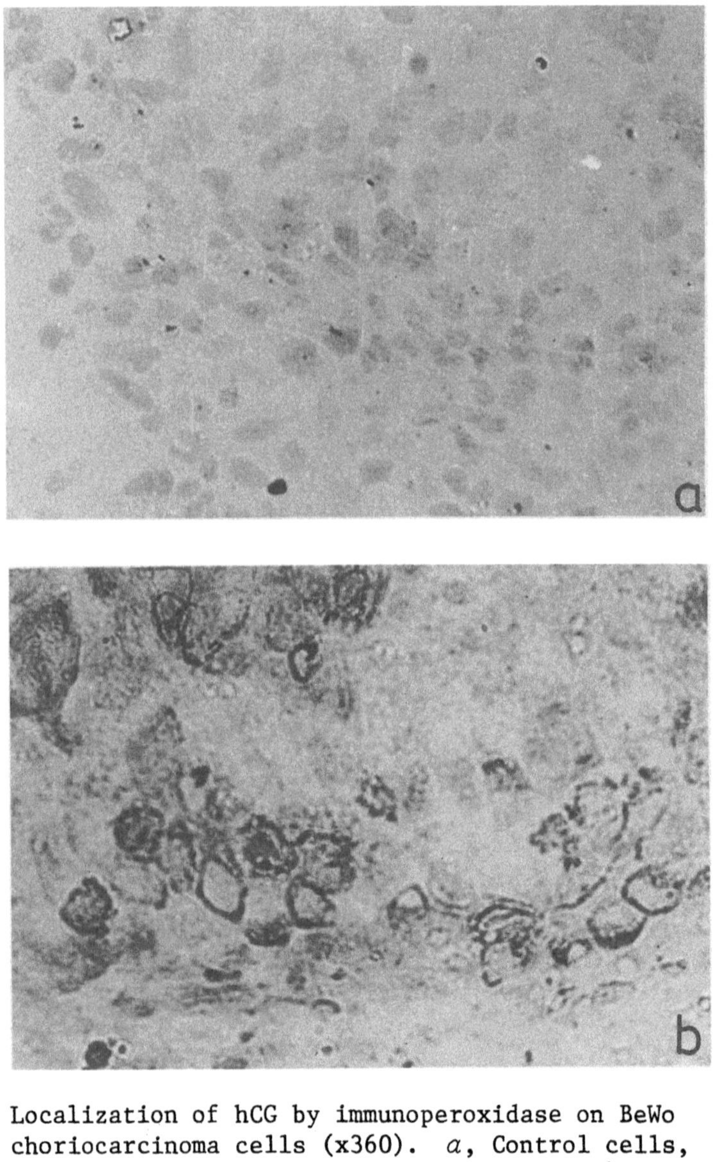

Fig. 3. Localization of hCG by immunoperoxidase on BeWo choriocarcinoma cells (x360). *a*, Control cells, incubated with nonimmunized monkey serum; *b*, experimental cells, incubated with monkey anti-β-hCG.

Table 4. Quantitation by Radioimmunoassay of hCG Secreted by Parent BeWo Cells and BeWo Cells Resistant to Anti-hCG

BeWo cell type	hCG (mIU/mg cellular protein)
Parent	28.9 $\pm$ 2.8[a]
Resistant	<6.25

[a]Mean $\pm$ SEM.

Table 5. Immunoenzymatic Quantitation of Antigens Reactive to Anti-hCG on Parent and Anti-hCG-Resistant BeWo Cells

BeWo cell type	Treatment	Absorbance at 515 nm/mg protein
Parent	Nonimmune serum	189
	Anti-β-hCG	262
Resistant	Nonimmune serum	171
	Anti-β-hCG	172

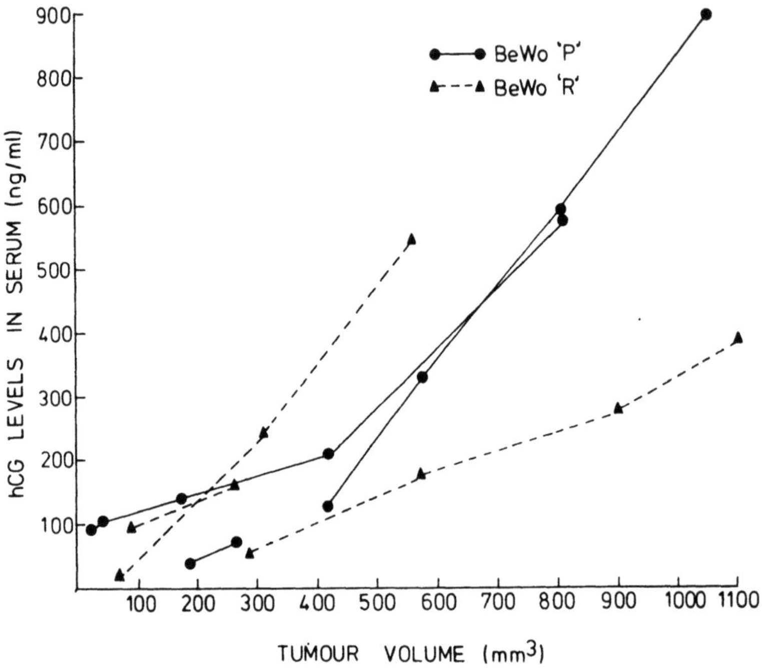

Fig. 4. Comparison of the tumor volume and the amount of hCG secreted by parent BeWo choriocarcinoma cells (BeWo 'P') and BeWo cells resistant to antibody (BeWo 'R') maintained in the hamster cheek pouch. After the end of the lag phase, blood was collected on alternate days for estimation of hCG from tumor-bearing animals. At the time of collection of blood, tumor volume and hCG level were determined and are plotted for 3 different animals in each category.

as determined by quantitative immunoenzymatic assay (Table 5).

To determine whether the block in production and secretion of hCG by the resistant subpopulation of the BeWo cell line was a stable or a transient property, the cells were reimplanted in the hamster cheek pouch. Serum hCG and tumor volume were determined for these animals. Fig. 4 gives the results for three hamsters implanted with resistant BeWo cells (BeWo 'R'), and for three hamsters implanted with parent BeWo cells (BeWo 'P'). No significant difference was observed in the hCG secretion pattern in the two cases.

DISCUSSION

Our results demonstrate complement-dependent cytotoxic action of anti-Pr-β-hCG-TT antibodies on the BeWo choriocarcinoma cell line maintained in tissue culture. This cytotoxicity was manifested morphologically as well as by incorporation of radioactive thymidine and leucine. The effect was partial in that no concentration of antibodies in conjunction with excess complement killed all of the BeWo cells. These observations indicate the presence of two subpopulations of cells, one sensitive to the action of the antibody and the other resistant. The resistant cells, obtainable on continuous culture of cells in the presence of antibodies, did not show the presence of hCG on the surface of cells as visualized by immunoenzymatic technique. Parental cells, on the other hand, consisted of a mixed population of cells, with some of the cells carrying immunoreactive hCG on the cell surface. Another major difference in cells before treatment with antibodies and those selected out by treatment with antibodies was the significant loss in the amount of hCG secreted into the medium. Parent cultures produced 28.9 $\pm$ 2.8 mIU hCG per mg cellular protein, whereas the antibody-resistant cells secreted no detectable hCG into the medium (<6.25 mIU hCG/ml) after 4 days of culture. The loss of ability of BeWo cells to secrete hCG after years in continuous culture has been reported by Pattillo and associates (20). These workers also noted the presence of anti-β-hCG-reactive material on only a fraction of the BeWo cells (21).

The production of hCG by BeWo cells may be regulated at several points: 1) the expression of the genome to make the peptide subunits; 2) the transport and secretion of the synthesized hormone, a process accompanied by glycosylation, and 3) the uptake of hCG by binding proteins on the surface of the cell. This trait could also be a reflection of the passage of the hormone from the intracellular to the extracellular compartment, with transient presence of hCG on the membrane. The morphological data do not permit distinction between this phenomenon and an active receptor type of binding. The above postulates are supported by various observations. The ability of trophoblast to make hCG varies considerably in early and late pregnancy placenta (22). Secondly, the messenger RNA activity for α- and β-subunits of hCG in polysomes is much reduced in term placenta (23). Also, many somatic cells make hCG but at very low levels (24, 25). Malignant transformation enhances the ability of the cells to make this hormone (1-3). In choriocarcinoma, blocks at some of these points can be removed by treatment with dibutyryl adenosine 3', 5'-monophosphate (26). A cell quiescent for the synthesis of hCG *in vitro* can regain the ability to synthesize and secrete hCG *in vivo*. Such modulations provide explanation for lack of hCG secreted by the resistant subpopulation of BeWo cells *in vitro* in the present study, and regain of this ability upon reimplantation into the hamster cheek pouch.

Experiments on the effect of antibodies on the growth of the tumor in the hamster cheek pouch indicate an inhibitory effect of the anti-Pr-β-hCG-TT antibodies at the initial stages. However, with time no difference was evident in the tumor size in either control or antibody-treated animals. One interpretation of this result could be the suppression by antibodies of the sensitive subpopulation of cells in the initial stages. As time progressed, the resistant cells would dominate. Another factor contributing to the escape of tumor from the possible noxious effect of antibodies is the access that antibody has to cells containing hCG on the cell surface. This could be quite different *in vivo* as compared to that obtainable *in vitro*. Choriocarcinoma grown *in vivo* contains extensive areas of necrosis with lack of blood supply which would not be susceptible to immunologic attack by antibodies. Nisula and Kohler (12) reported inhibition of tumor growth after passive administration of whole hCG antiserum to the BeWo choriocarcinoma-bearing hamsters. Anti-tumor activity of anti-hCG antibodies was based on a single time point after tumor inoculation, rather than over an entire time spectrum of tumor growth. Whether the passive use of anti-hCG antibodies significantly reduced tumor weight at other time points was not recorded. However, tumors treated with antibodies did not differ from control tumors on histological examination. The observation of Knecht (13) on the lack of effect of active immunization with Pr-β-hCG-TT on the growth of human choriocarcinoma in the hamster cheek pouch is in conformity with our findings.

Heterogeneity of cell type and the susceptibility *in vitro* of only those cells which have the target antigen disposed on the surface, suggest that a polyvalent approach consisting of antibodies directed against more than one cell surface marker expressed on choriocarcinoma may be required to kill all the tumor cells.

ACKNOWLEDGEMENT

This work was supported by research grants from International Development Research Centre of Canada, Family Planning Foundation of India, and Rockefeller Foundation. We thank Lady Tata Memorial Trust for fellowship support to S. K. G. Shri. K.K. Sarin and Pardeep Roy rendered valuable technical assistance. Gurpreet Singh is acknowledged for useful discussion and preparation of the manuscript.

SUMMARY

Antisera raised in monkey or baboon against purified β-subunit of human chorionic gonadotropin (β-hCG) coupled to tetanus toxoid exert complement-dependent cytotoxic effects on BeWo choriocarcinoma cells maintained in tissue culture. The cytotoxic effect is manifested morphologically as well as by incorporation of radioactive thymidine and leucine. However, in the presence of saturating amounts of anti-β-hCG antibodies and complement, antibodies failed to kill all of the BeWo choriocarcinoma cells. Evidence is presented to suggest that the partial and not complete cytotoxic effect of antibodies may be due to the heterogeneity of cell types, one sensitive to immune attack by anti-β-hCG antibodies, the other resistant. Immunoenzymatic localization of hCG revealed its presence on the cell surface of only a fraction of BeWo cells. The antibody-resistant BeWo cell population had no demonstrable hCG on the cell surface. Resistant cells did not secrete hCG into the medium when cultured for up to 4 days. However, the resistant cell population, upon transplantation to the hamster cheek pouch, regained the ability to secrete hCG. Heterogeneity of cell types may explain the refractoriness of the BeWo cells transplanted to the hamster cheek pouch to an inhibitory effect of antibodies at later stages of tumor growth.

REFERENCES

1. Braunstein, G. D., Vaitukaitis, J. L., Carbone, P. P., and Ross, G. T., Ectopic production of human chorionic gonadotropin by neoplasms, Ann. Intern. Med. 78:39 (1973).
2. Gailani, S., Chu, T. N., Nussbaum, A., Ostrander, M., and Christoff, N., HCG in non-trophoblastic neoplasms, Cancer 38:1684 (1976).
3. Dawood, M. Y., Saxena, B. B., and Landesman, R., Human chorionic gonadotropin and its subunits in hydatidiform mole and choriocarcinoma, Obstet. Gynecol. 50:172 (1977).
4. Talwar, G. P., Sharma, N. C., Dubey, S. K., Salahuddin, M., Das, C., Ramakrishnan, S., Kumar, S., and Hingorani, V., Isoimmunization against human chorionic gonadotropin with conjugates of processed β-subunit of the hormone and tetanus toxoid, Proc. Natl. Acad. Sci. USA 73:218 (1976).
5. Hearn, J. P., Short, R. V., and Lunn, S. R., The effect of immunizing marmoset monkeys against the β-subunit of hCG, in: "Physiological Effects of Immunity Against Hormones," R. G. Edwards and M. H. Johnson, eds., Cambridge University Press, Cambridge (1975) p. 239.
6. Stevens, V. C., Perspectives of development of a fertility control vaccine from hormonal antigens of the trophoblast, in: "Development of Vaccines for Fertility Regulation," Scriptor, Copenhagen (1976), p. 93.
7. Hellstrom, K. I. and Hellstrom, I., Lymphocyte-mediated cytotoxicity and blocking serum activity to tumor antigens, in: "Advances in Immunology," Vol. 18, F. J. Dixon and H. G. Kunel, eds., Academic Press, New York (1974), p. 209.
8. Naughton, M. A., Merrill, D. A., McManus, L. M., Fink, L. M., Berman, E., White, M. J., and Martinez-Hernandez, A., Localization of the β chain of human chorionic gonadotropin on

human tumor cells and placental cells, Cancer Res. 35:1887 (1975).
9. Morisada, M., Yamaguchi, H., and Iizuka, R., Toxic action of anti-hCG antibody to human trophoblast, Int. J. Fertility 17: 65 (1972).
10. Currie, G. A., Immunological studies of trophoblast in vitro, J. Obstet. Gynaecol. Brit. Commonwealth 74:841 (1967).
11. Morisada, M., Yamaguchi, H., and Iizuka, R., Immunobiological function of the syncytiotrophoblast: A new theory, Amer. J. Obstet. Gynecol. 125:3 (1976).
12. Nisula, B. C. and Kohler, P. O., Effect of antiserum to human chorionic gonadotropin on growth and function of choriocarcinoma *in vivo* and *in vitro*, Cancer Res. 34:512 (1974).
13. Knecht, M., The lack of an effect of active immunization with the β-subunit of chorionic gonadotropin coupled to tetanus toxoid on the growth of human choriocarcinoma maintained in the hamster cheek pouch, Endocrinology 106:150 (1980).
14. Talwar, G. P., Dubey, S. K., Salahuddin, M., and Shastri, N., Kinetics of antibody response in animals injected with processed beta-hCG conjugated to tetanus toxoid (Pr-β-hCG-TT), Contraception 13:153 (1976).
15. Talwar, G. P., Ramakrishnan, S., Das, C., Dubey, S. K., Salahuddin, M., Shastri, N., Tandon, A., and Singh, O., Anti-hCG immunization, in: "Recent Advances in Reproduction and Regulation of Fertility," G. P. Talwar, Ed., Elsevier/North Holland Biomedical Press, Amsterdam (1979), p. 453.
16. Hertz, R., Serial passage of choriocarcinoma of women in the hamster cheek pouch, in: "Choriocarcinoma," J. F. Holland and M. M. Hreshchyshyn, eds., Springer-Verlag, Berlin, Vol. 3, UICC Monograph Series (1967), p. 26.
17. Friedell, G. H., Sherman, J. D., and Sommers, S. C., Growth curves of human cancer transplants during experimental chemotherapy, Cancer 14:1117 (1961).
18. Vaitukaitis, J. L., Braunstein, G. D., and Ross, G. T., A radioimmunoassay which specifically measures human chorionic gonadotropin in the presence of human luteinizing hormone, Amer. J. Obstet. Gynecol. 113:751 (1972).
19. McLean, L. W. and Nakane, P. K., Periodate-lysine-paraformaldehyde fixative, a new fixative for immunoelectron microscopy, J. Histochem. Cytochem. 22:1077 (1974).
20. Pattillo, R. A., Hussa, R. O., Ruckert, A. C. F., Kurtz, J. W., Cade, J. M., and Rinke, M. L., hCG in BeWo trophoblastic cells after 12 years in continuous culture: retention of intact hCG secretion in mechanically versus enzyme-dispersed cells, Endocrinology 105:967 (1979).
21. Yorde, D. E., Hussa, R. O., Garancis, J. C., and Pattillo, R. A., Immunocytochemical localization of human choriogonadotropin in human malignant trophoblast. Model for human choriogonadotropin secretion, Lab. Invest. 40:391 (1979).

22. Vaitukaitis, J. L., Changing placental concentrations of hCG and its subunits during gestation, J. Clin. Endocrinol. Metab. 38:755 (1974).
23. Boothby, M., McQueen, S. D., McWilliams, D., Zernik, M., and Boime, I., Human chorionic gonadotropin α and β subunit mRNAs: Translatable levels during pregnancy and molecular cloning of DNA sequences complementary to hCG, in: "Chorionic Gonadotropin," S. J. Segal, Ed., Plenum Press, New York (1980), p. 253.
24. Braunstein, G. D., Rasor, J., and Wade, M. E., Presence in normal human testes of a CG-like substance distinct from hLH, New Engl. J. Med. 293:1339 (1975).
25. Yoshimoto, Y., Wolfsen, A. R., and Odell, W. D., Human chorionic gonadotropin-like substance in non-endocrine tissues of normal subjects, Science 197:575 (1977).
26. Hussa, R. O., Latent ability to produce hCG in response to dibutyryl adenosine 3',5'-monophosphate in the BeWo-NBC trophoblastic cell line, J. Clin. Endocrinol. Metab. 50: 5 (1980).

THE SURFACE CHARGE OF CELLS PRODUCING hCG

Lawrence L. Hause, Norio Tosaka, and R. A. Pattillo

Department of Pathology
Medical College of Wisconsin
8700 W. Wisconsin Avenue
Milwaukee, Wisconsin 53226, USA

INTRODUCTION

The cell surface is the interface between the cell and its environment. The surface acts to regulate cell function through antigens, receptors, cell-cell interaction, and other factors. One important and measurable property of the cell surface is charge. Surface charge results from the accumulation of exposed charge groups at the external surface of the cell membrane, and is peripheral to the region of transmembrane ion separation which defines transmembrane potential. The surface of normal human cells is negatively charged due to the presence of acidic oligosaccharide groups at the terminal regions of membrane glycoproteins (1).

Cell Surface Charge

Surface charge functions primarily as an averaging property which modulates cell interaction or biochemical activity. It is often complementary to more specific properties such as antigenicity. Cell surface charge is an important parameter in the function and characterization of cells (1-4). Surface charge has been used to study the cell membrane (5, 6), identify cell subpopulations (7, 8), identify cell disorders (9, 10), study malignancy (11-13), and separate cells (14).

A single sugar group, *N*-acetylneuraminic acid, is responsible for 75 to 94 percent of the surface charge of human red blood cells (1, 2). This observation was made by treating cells with the enzyme, neuraminidase, which specifically cleaves the neuraminic acid groups from surface glycoproteins. As a result, the cell surface charge is reduced significantly (1). Neuraminidase incubation destroys cell receptors to *Vibrio cholerae*, which produces this enzyme (15). About 2.4 x 10^7 charge groups were associated with the surface charge of normal human red blood cells (16). Hence, a significant number of negative charge groups contribute to membrane negativity and define averaging properties. A typical function of the surface charge of red cells and lymphocytes is to help suspend cells in the blood stream due to the electrostatic separation of similar charges.

Surface Charge Measurement

The surface charge of cells has been recognized since 1902 (17). The early work with cell surface charge concerned apparatus and charge fundamentals; applications have been most numerous since 1965 (3). Several physical principles have been used to detect cell surface charges. By far, the most extensive measurements of cell surface charge have used cell electrophoresis. Electrophoresis of cells typically consists of the microscopic measurement of cell movement under defined electric fields, a technique termed, microelectrophoresis. An extension of this technique, in which fields are applied across a moving layer of electrolyte with suspended cells, is called free-flow electrophoresis. Free-flow electrophoresis has been used to separate cells based on surface charge (14). Two recent techniques have been applied to help automate the measurement of surface charge which is labor intensive under most microelectrophoretic methods. These are laser doppler spectroscopy and flow cytology. The doppler interaction of laser light with moving cells (much like microwaves detect the speed of cars) has been used to measure the cell surface charges of lymphocyte populations (8). Finally, recent advances in flow cytology have been used with charge-specific dyes to identify surface charges in a manner which correlates well with cell electrophoresis (18). Each of the above methods requires the suspension of cells before measurement, an experimental approach that can present problems for cells in tissue or in culture. Microelectrode penetration has been used to measure membrane potentials of cultured cells without suspension (19). Future studies of surface charge can be expected to use automated procedures for more rapid measurements of surface charge in large cell populations.

Malignant Cell Surface Charge

An increased surface charge level was found for various types of cancer (13). It was hypothesized that increased charge and subsequent loss of contact inhibition were characteristic of malignancy (20). However, further studies found that increased surface charge was not always associated with malignancy (21). Thus, it appears that increased surface charge is characteristic of certain cancers and not others.

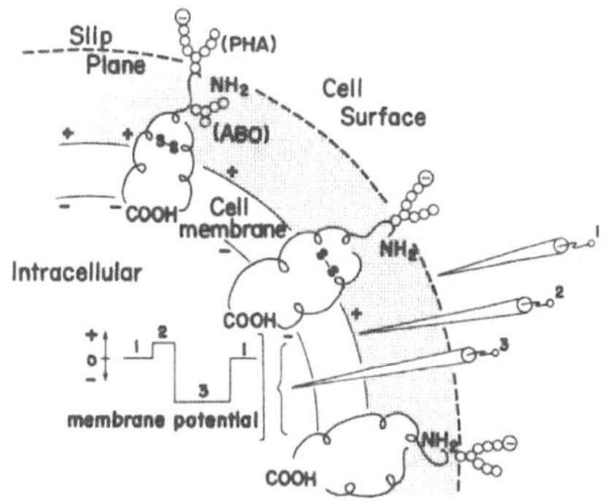

Fig. 1. Schematic diagram of the cell surface, representing glycoprotein units with attached polysaccharides. The conventional intracellular terminal COOH of glycoprotein is depicted, as well as representative disulfide bonds which regulate glycoprotein structure and surface charge exposure. The negative surface results from negative terminal polysaccharides. Cell electrophoresis measures the net surface charge exposed at the slip plane (*dotted line*). Microelectrode penetration can detect surface charge, as depicted in the membrane potential tracing.

The electrophysiology of malignant trophoblasts in culture (BeWo cell) was studied through microelectrode penetration (19). This technique did not require the suspension of cells before measurement, so that cell perturbation was minimized. It was found that as the electrode penetrated the cell membrane, it measured the typical transmembrane potential and also detected a prepotential prior to membrane penetration. Positive prepotentials have also been recorded for granulocytes (22). The prepotential appears positive relative to the peripheral surface charge as the electrode tip enters the relatively thick surface coat. During penetration the electrode measures a zero reference potential *1*) in the extracellular electrolyte, a positive potential *2*) referenced to the peripheral surface charge as the tip dimples the membrane and *3*), finally, the classical negative transmembrane potential after membrane penetration (Fig. 1). The magnitude of the prepotential was found to be dependent upon pH within the range of 6.6 to 8.0 where cells remain viable. Optimal prepotentials were recorded at high pH (pH = 8). The electrophoretic mobility of red blood cells was not variable in this pH range (1, 2). However, red blood cell mobility was increased by the reduction (breaking) of disulfide bonds in surface glycoproteins (Fig. 1), and these red blood cells were found to be more susceptible to lysis by complement (10). Consequently, cell surface charge is dependent on charged groups as well as configuration of the cell surface and/or surface

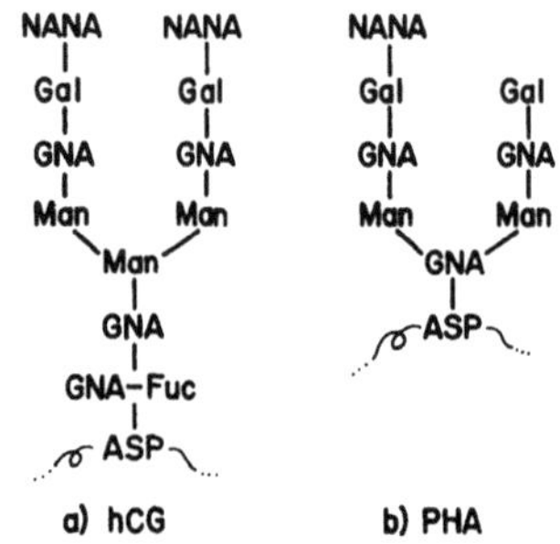

Fig. 2. Structures of oligosaccharides of hCG (24) and PHA receptor (25). Saccharide groups are: NANA, *N*-acetyl-neuraminic acid; GAL, galactose; GNA, *N*-acetylglucosamine; MAN, mannose; FUC, fucose. Oligosaccharides are attached to protein at asparagine (ASP) residues in both cases. Negative charge results from NANA groups, which are acidic at physiologic pH.

glycoproteins. This can affect charge measurement or cell function and warrants further investigation in cells such as BeWo.

The BeWo cell line was one of the first cell culture lines found to produce human chorionic gonadotropin (hCG) in culture (23). This hormone is a glycoprotein with *N*-glycosidic oligosaccharide units which terminate with negatively charged NANA groups (Fig. 2) (24). Very similar saccharide structures with terminal acid NANA groups have been described for hCG (24), PHA receptors (25), and cell surface charge (Fig. 1)(1, 2). Each of these glycoproteins can be expected to contribute to the surface charge of cells. This is especially true for hCG, which has been localized on the membrane of trophoblasts (26). As a result, the surface charge of several cell lines known to produce hCG components were studied with cell electrophoresis. The objective of these measurements was to compare hCG production and surface charge among these cell lines.

MATERIALS AND METHODS

Cell Culture and Suspension

Three cell lines known to produce various components of hCG were studied for cell surface charges after culture. These cell lines included: BeWo cells, derived from metastatic choriocarcinoma and which produce free α-subunit and intact hCG (23, 24); ElCo cells, derived from human epidermoid carcinoma of the breast and which produce the large α-subunit of hCG (24); and DoT cells, derived from human epidermoid carcinoma of the cervix and which produce primarily free β-subunit of hCG (27). All cells were cultured at 37° in media consisting of 40% Gey's balanced salt solution, 50% Waymouth MB 752/1 medium, and 10% newborn calf serum. Media were obtained from Grand Island Biological Company, New York. Cells were cultured for 3 or 7 days, with cell confluency after 3 days and multi-layered cell growth after 7 days.

Electrophoretic mobility was measured on cells which were suspended after culture. Cells were not suspended with enzymatic treatment such as trypsin, since trypsin cleaves glycoproteins and lowers the surface charge of human cells by 50 to 60% (5). Initial attempts to extract cells with collagenase (5 mg/ml)(ICN Nutritional Biochemical Company, Cleveland, Ohio) produced suspensions of a very low concentration. Further studies using a hypodermic needle were found to be quite effective in producing single cells, with sufficient recovery for measurement (28). Optimal suspensions were produced by drawing and expelling the cultured cells five times with the syringe and a 22-gauge stainless steel needle. This produced an acceptable suspension of 10^4 cells per ml for electrophoretic measurements from a 10 ml culture flask.

Measurement of Electrophoretic Mobility

After suspension, culture cells were washed in normal saline by centrifugation. Cells were suspended in 0.145 M saline at pH 7.4. Electrophoretic mobility was measured using dark field optics under constant current (5 mA) at 25° C as previously described (29). Human red blood cells were used as controls for each measurement. Measurements were analyzed from the mobility data for 15 cells for each experiment. The mean mobility and standard error of the mean were used to characterize the mobility of each respective group for comparative purposes.

The electrophoretic mobility measurements of 3 and 7 day cultures of BeWo, ElCo, and DoT cells are summarized in Table 1. All measurements were recorded on cells suspended in normal saline (0.145 M) and were followed by the measurement of human red blood cells as controls. The mean mobility ($\bar{m}$), which is the average of 15 cell readings, standard error of the mean (SEM), and number of preparations (N) are given for each cell group. Comparison of the mean mobility between cell groups based on the t-test show significant differences ($P<0.05$) according to cell type and culture period. Most cell types showed significant mobility differences, except for 3 and 7 day BeWo cells. Washing the cells in saline or Earle's balanced salt solution had little effect on the mobility.

Surface Charge Characteristics of hCG Producing Cells

The net surface charge of 3 and 7 day cultures of BeWo, ElCo, and DoT cells can be rated according to their mobility, and classified according to significance levels reported in Table 1.

Table 1. Comparative Electrophoretic Mobility of Human Cell Types

	BeWo 3 day	BeWo 7 day	ElCo 3 day	ElCo 7 day	DoT 7 day	Red blood cells
BeWo 3 day	$\bar{m} = 0.91$					
BeWo 7 day	N.S.	$\bar{m} = 0.89$				
ElCo 3 day	$P < 0.001$	$P < 0.001$	$\bar{m} = 1.25$			
ElCo 7 day	$P < 0.05$	$P < 0.001$	$P < 0.001$	$\bar{m} = 1.06$		
DoT 7 day	$P < 0.001$	$P < 0.001$	$P < 0.001$	$P < 0.02$	$\bar{m} = 1.14$	
Red blood cells	$P < 0.001$	$P < 0.001$	$P < 0.001$	N.S.	$P = 0.001$	$\bar{m} = 1.08$
	$\bar{m} = 0.91$ SEM=.002 N = 11	$\bar{m} = 0.89$ SEM=.004 N = 13	$\bar{m} = 1.25$ SEM=.007 N = 7	$\bar{m} = 1.06$ SEM=.007 N = 12	$\bar{m} = 1.14$ SEM=.001 N = 11	$\bar{m} = 1.08$ SEM=.014 (control)

Mobilities are significantly different when $P < 0.05$.
Abbreviations: N.S., not significant; $\bar{m}$, mean mobility;
SEM, standard error of the mean; N, number of preparations.

Rating produces four classes which differ significantly in mobility (Table 2). Mobility differences reflect variable surface charge or surface structure. In Table 2, charge levels of 3 and 7 day BeWo cultures are similar and significantly less than 7 day ElCo cultures. ElCo cultures, in turn, have a mobility similar to that of human red blood cells. The highest mobility for 3 day ElCo cells is 40 percent greater than that of 7 day BeWo cells.

The electrophoretic mobility of a cell is defined by the exposed surface charge at the slip plane (Fig. 1). This net charge is strongly affected by surface structure as well as by total charge. For example, microvilli commonly present on BeWo cells (26) may expose only a portion of surface charge to the slip plane for

Table 2. Relative Surface Charge According to Cell Type

Cell type	<	BeWo - 3 day BeWo - 7 day	<	ElCo - 7 day Red blood cells	<	DoT - 7 day	<	ElCo - 3 day
Mobility		0.91 0.89	<	1.06 1.08	<	1.14	<	1.25
hCG group		α and intact		α		β		α

electrophoresis while facilitating charge detection by increasing the apparent thickness of the surface coat for microelectrode penetration. In this manner, BeWo cells may show a very distinct prepotential by microelectrode penetration while demonstrating a relatively low electrophoretic mobility. Secondly, the oxidation or reduction of surface glycoproteins can result in the resultant contraction of extension of the protein structure so that the exposed surface charge is altered (Fig. 1). Disulfide bonds were considered important in the charge of red cells (10) and may contribute to pH dependence of prepotentials in BeWo cells. Charge groups and surface structure contribute to the measure of surface charge of cells and are likely to contribute to cell function.

The mobility levels of 7 day cultures show a relation to the hCG subgroups found for the cell types (Table 2). DoT cells produce primarily hCGβ and show the greatest 7 day mobility. Negatively charged neuraminic acid groups are most numerous in the hCG β-subunit (24). ElCo cells have a significantly lower mobility than DoT cells, and they produce hCGα which has a lower neuraminic acid content. BeWo cells, which produce intact and hCGα, show the lowest mobility level of the three 7 day cultures.

In exception to the 7 day strata, 3 day ElCo cells, which produce primarily α-subunit, have the highest mobility level of the hCG-producing cell lines (Table 2). The culture period may contribute to this difference, in that 3 day ElCo cultures yield about 3×10^6 cells while 7 day cultures yield about 12×10^6 cells per culture tube. The exposed hCG, and thereby the charge, may vary per cell. However, this is probably not the case for 3 and 7 day BeWo cultures which show similar mobility. Alternatively, differences in mobility may reflect the process of cell suspension, since ElCo cells suspend more readily than BeWo cells. Hence, the cause of these differences is not clearly defined. Further studies of hCG content, surface structure, and surface charge are required in order to resolve this question. For example, a bivariant measure of charge and hCG would be feasible with separate dyes in automated cytology.

Glycoproteins define the majority of surface charge on human cells (1, 2). A remarkable similarity can be observed in the structure of polysaccharides on the glycoproteins of hCG and PHA receptor (Fig. 2). Terminal sugar chains are nearly identical, differing only in the number of terminal neuraminic acid groups which carry negative charge. PHA contains one neuraminic acid group per oligosaccharide, as do most polysaccharides which define cell surface charge. In contrast, hCG contains two neuraminic acid groups per oligosaccharide. The relatively high negativity of hCG, coupled with the cell surface localization of hCG (26), would suggest its relation to cell surface charge, as was reported herein.

The oligosaccharide chains of both hCG and PHA receptor contain α-mannose linkages which act as a strong binding site for PHA (25). Therefore, a relationship between the two glycoproteins is suggested, but to date has not been defined. Antigen sites have also been identified for cell glycoproteins and hCG (3, 24). A common thread among the characteristics of cell surface charge and receptors is the surface glycoprotein.

As a consequence of surface glycoprotein, highly charged cells may circumvent contact inhibition and avoid immune rejection. These characteristics are common to normal human pregnancy and malignancy. Trophoblasts produce hCG during pregnancy. They show an increased surface charge and avoid immune rejection, characteristics that are often observed for malignant cells as well. Such similarities may be coincidental, but more probably result from an association between cell surface and glycoproteins such as hCG.

REFERENCES

1. Tenforde, T., Microelectrophoretic studies on the surface chemistry of erythrocytes, Adv. Biol. Med. Physics 13:43 (1971).
2. Seaman, G. V. F., Electrokinetic behavior of red cells, in: "The Red Cell," Vol. II, D. Surgenor, ed., Academic Press, New York (1975), p. 1135.
3. Pretlow, T. G. and Pretlow, T. P., International Review of Cytology 61:85 (1979).
4. Ambrose, E. J., ed., "Cell Electrophoresis," Churchill Ltd., London (1965).
5. Vassar, P. S., Hards, J. M., and Seaman, G. V. F., Surface properties of human lymphocytes, Biochim. Biophys. Acta 291: 107 (1973).

6. Seaman, G. V. F. and Uhlenbruck, G., The surface structure of erythrocytes from some animal sources, Arch. Biochem. Biophys. 100:493 (1963).
7. Chollet, P. H., Chassagne, C., Thierry, C., Sauvezie, B., Serrou, B., and Plagne, R., Isolation and electrophoretic mobility of three lymphoid populations in normal human blood, Eur. J. Cancer 13:333 (1977).
8. Kapken, J. H. and Uzgiris, Identification of T and B cell subpopulations in human peripheral blood: electrophoretic mobility distributions associated with surface marker characteristics, J. Immunol. 117:115 (1976).
9. Wiig, J. N., Electrophoresis of lymphoid cells. A study of Bruton type of agammaglobulinaemia, thymic dysplasia, chronic lymphatic leukaemia and of normal human thymocytes, Clin. Exptl. Immunol. 19:159 (1975).
10. Hause, L. L., Koethe, S. M., Rothwell, D. J., and Straumfjord, Jr., Relations between surface charge and *in vitro* lysis of red blood cells in paroxysmal nocturnal hemoglobinuria, Scand. J. Haematol. 16:241 (1978).
11. Field, E. J., Caspary, E. A., and Smith, K. S., Macrophage electrophoretic mobility (MEM) test in cancer: a critical evaluation, Brit. J. Cancer 28:208 (1973).
12. Hoffmann, W., Werner, W., Steiner, R., and Kaufmann, R., Cell electrophoresis for diagnostic purposes. I. Diagnostic value of the electrophoretic mobility test (EMT) for the detection of gynaecological malignancies, Brit. J. Cancer 43:
13. Ruhenstroth-Bauer, G., *in*: "Cell Electrophoresis," E. J. Ambrose, ed., Churchill, London, (1965), p. 66.
14. Zeller, K. and Hannig, K., Free-flow electrophoretic separation of lymphocytes. Evidence for specific organ distributions of lymphoid cells, Hoppe-Seyler's Z. Physiol. Chem. Bd. 352: 1162 (1971).
15. Gottschalk, A., Neuraminidase: the specific enzyme of influenza virus and *Vibrio cholerae*, Biochim. Biophys. Acta 23:645 (1957).
16. Eylar, E. H., Madoff, M. A., Brody, O. V., and Oncley, J. L., The contribution of sialic acid to the surface charge of the erythrocyte, J. Biol. Chem. 237:1992 (1962).
17. Lillie, R. S., On differences in the direction of the electrical connection of certain free cells and nuclei, Amer. J. Physiol. viii:273 (1902).
18. Valet, G., Bamberger, S., Hofmann, H., Schindler, R., and Ruhenstroth-Bauer, G., Flow cytometry as a new method for the measurement of electrophoretic mobility of erythrocytes using membrane charge staining by fluoresceinated polycations, J. Histochem. Cytochem. 27:342 (1979).
19. Hause, L. L., Pattillo, R. A., Sances, A., Jr., and Mattingly, R. F., Cell surface coatings and membrane potentials of malignant and nonmalignant cells, Science 169:601 (1970).

20. Currie, G. A. and Bagshawe, K. D., The masking of antigens on trophoblast and cancer cells, Lancet i:708 (1967).
21. Vassar, P. S., The electric charge density of human tumor cell surfaces, Lab. Invest. 12:1072 (1963).
22. Beckmann, A., Jenssen, H. L., Kalkoff, W., and Redmann, K., Transmembrane potential of white cells is found along with some surface potential, Separatum Experientia 26:186 (1970).
23. Pattillo, R. A. and Gey, G. O., The establishment of a cell line of human hormone-synthesizing trophoblastic cells in vitro, Cancer Res. 28:1231 (1968).
24. Hussa, R. O., Pattillo, R. A., Ruckert, A. C. F., and Scheuermann, K. W., Effects of butyrate and dibutyryl cyclic AMP on hCG-secreting trophoblastic and non-trophoblastic cells, J. Clin. Endocrinol. Metab. 46:69 (1978).
25. Kornfeld, R. and Kornfeld, S., The structure of a phytohemagglutinin receptor site from human erythrocytes, J. Biol. Chem. 245:2536 (1970).
26. Yorde, D. E., Hussa, R. O., Garancis, J. C., and Pattillo, R. A., Immunocytochemical localization of human choriogonadotropin in human malignant trophoblast, Lab. Invest. 40:391 (1979).
27. Cole, L. A., Birken, S., Sutphen, S., Hussa, R. O., and Pattillo, R. A., Absence of the COOH-terminal peptide on ectopic human chorionic gonadotropin β-subunit (hCGβ), Endocrinology 110:2198 (1982).
28. Mead, J. S., Horan, P. K., and Wheeless, L. L., Syringing as a method of cell dispersal, Acta Cytologica 22:86 (1978).
29. Hause, L. L., Rothwell, D. J., and Straumfjord, Jr., J. V., Measurement of cellular surface charge, Proc. 27th Ann. Conf. Engineer. Biol., Chevy Chase, Maryland (1974), p. 404.

THE ROLE OF TROPHOBLAST DIFFERENTIATION IN THE CONTROL OF THE hCG AND hPL GENES

Makoto Hoshina, Robert Hussa, Roland Pattillo,
H. Marvin Camel, and Irving Boime

Departments of Pharmacology and Obstetrics and Gynecology
Washington University School of Medicine
660 South Euclid Avenue
St. Louis, Missouri 63110
and
Department of Gynecology and Obstetrics
Medical College of Wisconsin
8700 W. Wisconsin Avenue
Milwaukee, Wisconsin USA 53226

INTRODUCTION

One of the unique features of the human placenta is its continued differentiation during gestation. Progeny of mitotically active mononucleated cytotrophoblasts fuse to form the mitotically inactive syncytiotrophoblast (1-3). During the differentiation, two major peptide hormones are produced, human chorionic gonadotropin (hCG) and human placental lactogen (hPL). Their temporal appearance in maternal serum during pregnancy is different: hCG peaks in the first trimester, while hPL reaches maximal levels at term. Therefore, the factors controlling their expression are not identical (4-7).

Gestational abnormalities of trophoblast development occur and are called hydatidiform mole, invasive mole, and choriocarcinoma (8-12). Hydatidiform mole is a relatively benign disease of the chorionic epithelium, which metastasizes and is invasive in only a small percentage of cases. Invasive mole invades the uterine muscle, but retains the same morphological features of hydatidiform mole. Choriocarcinoma is a malignant counterpart, which metastasizes early in its course. The risk of choriocarcinoma after molar pregnancy is 2000 to 4000 times higher than after normal pregnancy (8-12). One of the criteria for diagnosing these gestational trophoblastic tumors is the abnormally high serum level of hCG during the course of the disease. In contrast, serum hPL is very low or undetectable (13-17). Therefore, it appears that the aberrant expression of these hormonal genes in these tumors corresponds in some way with alterations in the pathway of placental differentiation. We previously demonstrated that in normal placenta the cytological distribution of hCGα and hPL mRNAs are different (20). This implies that expression of hCG and hPL is linked to and/or regulated by the pattern of placental differentiation. The availability of the trophoblastic tumor tissue permits us to test this hypothesis, since these neoplasms are in different stages of trophoblast differentiation. Here we report studies of the cytological distribution of the hCGα, hCGβ, and hPL mRNAs in normal placenta, choriocarcinoma, and hydatidiform mole tissue using the *in situ* hybridization technique. The attractive feature of this method is that it allows detection of specific mRNAs in individual cells. Using this technique, we assessed whether hCGα, hCGβ, and hPL mRNAs are transcribed in tissue components which are similar to their normal placental counterparts, and whether their expression is dependent on particular stages of trophoblast differentiation.

MATERIALS AND METHODS

Preparation of Double-Stranded Complementary DNA Probes

Isolation and purification of pBR322 clones bearing cDNAs complementary to hCGα, hCGβ, and hPL mRNAs were performed as previously described (18, 19). The following treatments were used as probes in this study: (a) a 440 base-pair *Pst*I restriction fragment which contains the complete 5'-noncoding sequence and all but the last eight amino acids of the coding region of the hCGα subunit; (b) a *Pst*I fragment of 540 base pairs that contains the information corresponding to the codons for amino acid 60 to the end of the peptide, and the contiguous 3'-noncoding region of hPL; (c) an *Hha*I fragment of 416 base pairs containing 20 base pairs of pBR322 flanking sequences, 90 base pairs of 5'-untranslated sequence, and remaining sequences corresponding to the translated region of hCGβ (21).

Preparation of ^{3}H-cDNA

The fragments were nick-translated in a 10 μl reaction mixture containing 200 ng of fragment, 700 pmol each of ^{3}H-dCTP, ^{3}H-dTTP, ^{3}H-dGTP, and ^{3}H-dATP (New England Nuclear Corp.), 25 pg of DNAse I, and 5 units of DNA polymerase I. The reaction mixtures were incubated overnight at 15 °C. The specific activity of the radioactive cDNA probe was 7.0-8.7 x 10^7 cpm per μg, and the size of the fragments was 60-80 base pairs under nondenaturing conditions. Salmon sperm DNA (denatured in NaOH and neutralized with HCl) was added to the labeled fragments and they were separated from unincorporated nucleotides by gel filtration on Sephadex G50-80. The material excluded from the Sephadex column was precipitated with ethanol. The precipitates were pelleted in an Eppendorf centrifuge and dissolved in water to a final concentration of 4 ng/μl.

Tissue Preparation and Slide Glass Treatment

The tissues were obtained either from hysterectomies or vacuum curettage, and immediately frozen in liquid nitrogen. *In situ* hybridization was performed using techniques described previously (20) except for the following modifications. After overnight hybridization, the slides were rinsed for 2 hours in 1X standard saline-citrate buffer containing 0.1% sodium dodecyl sulfate, and for 1 hour in 0.1X standard saline-citrate buffer. Microscope slides were pretreated with autoclaved gelatin instead of bovine serum albumin to avoid possible RNAse activity in the albumin.

Autoradiography

The slides were dipped in nuclear track emulsion (Kodak NTB-2) diluted with water (1:1) and prewarmed to 45 °C (20). They were dried in an upright position and exposed in a light-proof box for 1 week at 4 °C. The slides were developed with Kodak D-19 developer for 3 min at 20 °C, rinsed in cold water, fixed with Kodafix for 5 min at room temperature, and stained with hematoxylin-eosin.

RESULTS

Human placental villi (villous surface) are covered by the syncytiotrophoblast (syncytium, ST), which overlies a layer of cytotrophoblasts (Langhans cell, CT) and interstitial tissue (Fig. 1).

Messenger RNAs for hCGα, hCGβ, and hPL are abundant in first-trimester tissue (7). The distribution of these mRNAs in the trophoblast of first-trimester placenta was examined. Sections of 7- to 12-week placentae were hybridized to nick-translated probes corresponding to hPL and hCGα mRNAs. The distribution of grains is shown in bright and dark fields (Fig. 1). For both probes, most of the signal was seen in the syncytial (ST) regions, although in the case of hCGα significant signal was also seen in cytotrophoblasts (Fig. 1, C and D).

Fig. 2 shows the distribution of hCGβ mRNA in normal first-trimester placenta. Most of the signal was seen on the syncytial regions, although some was observed on a few cytotrophoblasts beneath the syncytium. Thus, like the hCGα mRNA, the hCGβ mRNA is not localized exclusively to syncytial trophoblast.

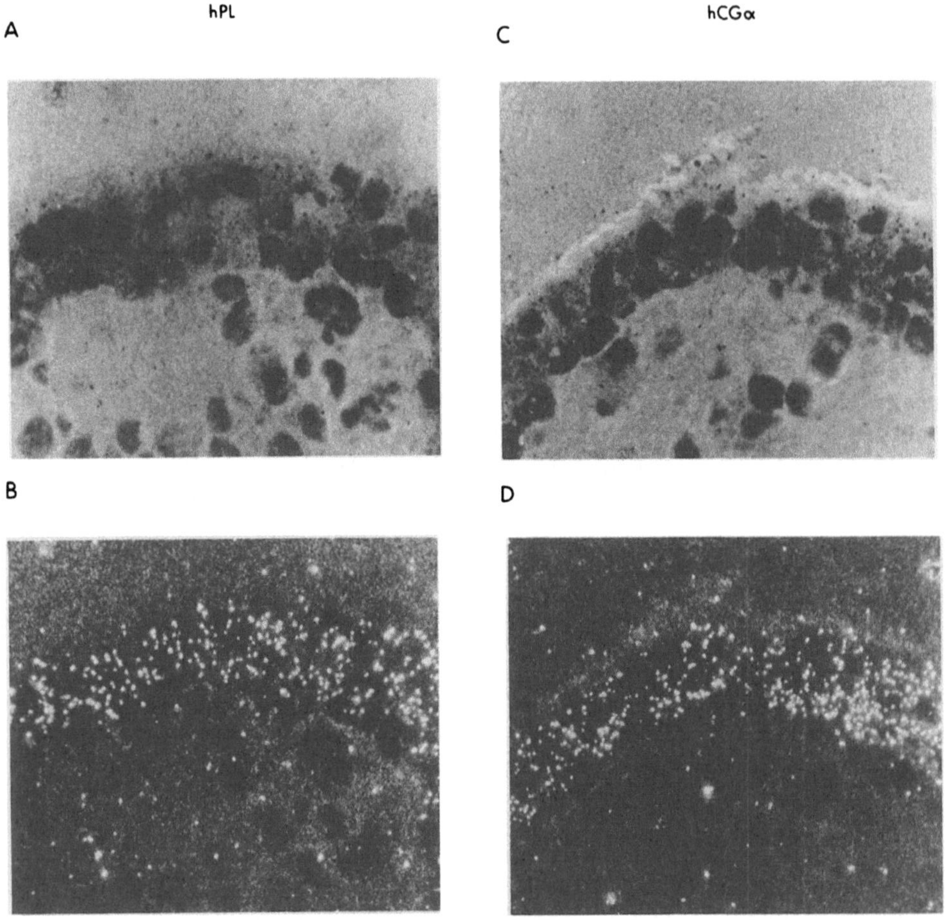

Fig. 1. Distribution of hPL (A, B) and hCGα (C, D) mRNAs in first-trimester placental sections viewed under high magnification (X260). Panels *B* and *D* are dark-field micrographs of the bright-field panels *A* and *C*. Note that in panels *C* and *D* the grains are closer to the core region of the villus, *i.e.*, they may overlie cytotrophoblasts.

Based on this result and our earlier studies (20), we proposed that the expression of hCG and hPL is linked to the differentiation of trophoblasts. Specifically, we suggested that the transcription of hCG subunit genes is activated during cytotrophoblast/syncytium conversion but before fusion into syncytium. In contrast, hPL mRNA synthesis is initiated later in differentiation, very likely concurrent with or after the stage of syncytiotrophoblast formation, and persists through the third trimester.

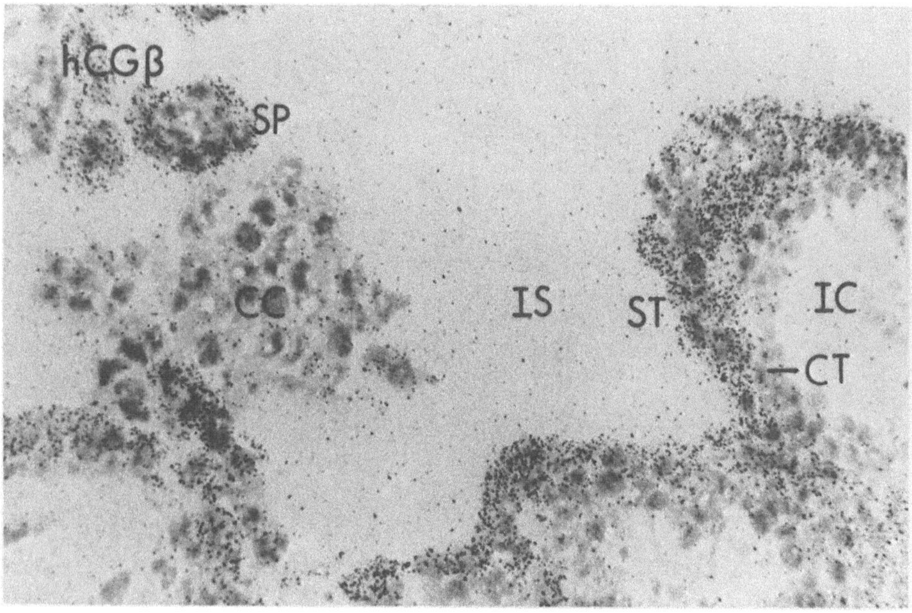

Fig. 2. Photomicrograph of an autoradiograph of first-trimester (8 week) placental tissue (5 μm cryostat sections) hybridized with 3.5×10^5 cpm of hCGβ probe (1 week exposure, hematoxylin-eosin stain). Silver grains are observed primarily over syncytiotrophoblast (*ST*) and syncytial sprout (*SP*) regions, and some are present over the cytotrophoblasts of villous surface (*CT*). Weak signals are seen over the cell column (*CC*) which consists of undifferentiated cells. *IS* and *IC* denote intervillous space and interstitial cells (villous stroma), respectively (X170).

Because choriocarcinoma contains trophoblasts that are not fully differentiated, we wanted to examine the distribution of hCGα, hCGβ, and hPL mRNAs in sections derived from choriocarcinoma tissue. Our hematoxylin-eosin stained sections of this tissue showed no villi, which is the typical histological pattern of this neoplasm. There were clusters of mononucleated cytotrophoblastic cells interspersed with foci of multinucleated cells reminiscent of syncytiotrophoblasts. Occasionally, some enlarged mononucleated cells were present. After hybridization of choriocarcinoma sections with nick-translated probes for hCGα and hCGβ, abundant grains were seen in syncytial cells (ST, Figs. 3A and 3B). Few grains were seen in the cytotrophoblastic cells (CT). In contrast to these findings, no signal above the background was seen when sections were hybridized to hPL cDNA probe with comparable specific activity to the hCG probes (Fig. 3C).

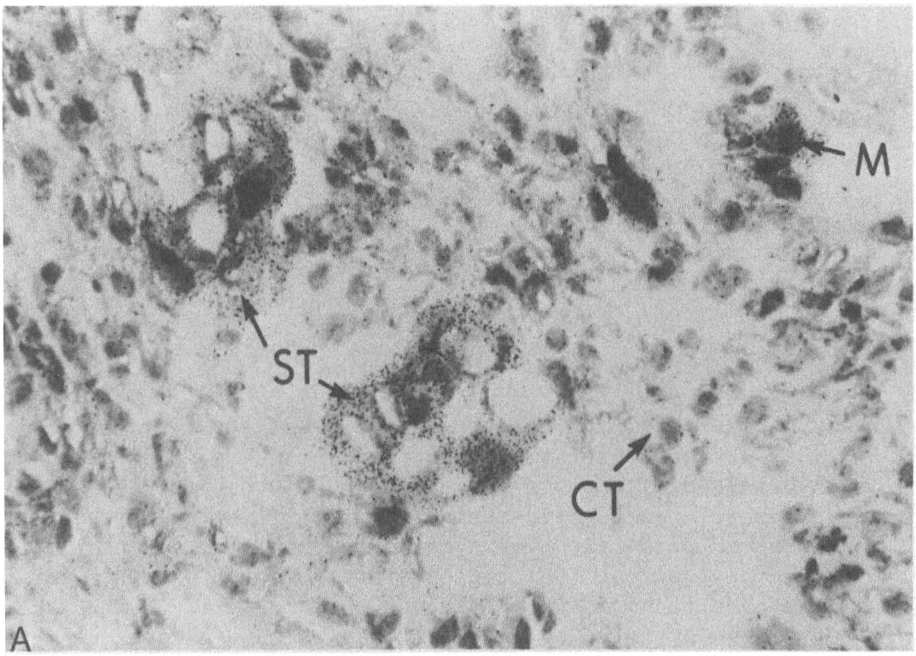

Fig. 3. *In situ* hybridization of sections of choriocarcinoma with hCGα (A), hCGβ (B), and hPL (C) cDNA probes. Four ng of cDNA probe was applied to each slide. This corresponded to 3.2×10^5 cpm for the hCGα probe, 3.5×10^5 cpm for the hCGβ probe, and 2.8×10^5 cpm for the hPL probe. The slides were exposed for one week. Multinucleated syncytial cells (*ST*) with prominent vacuolization show well-localized signals for hCGα and hCGβ but few, if any, signals for hPL. Cytotrophoblastic cells (*CT*) show no signal except for a mononucleated large cell in panel *A* (*M*, see text). Hematoxylin-eosin stain, X170.

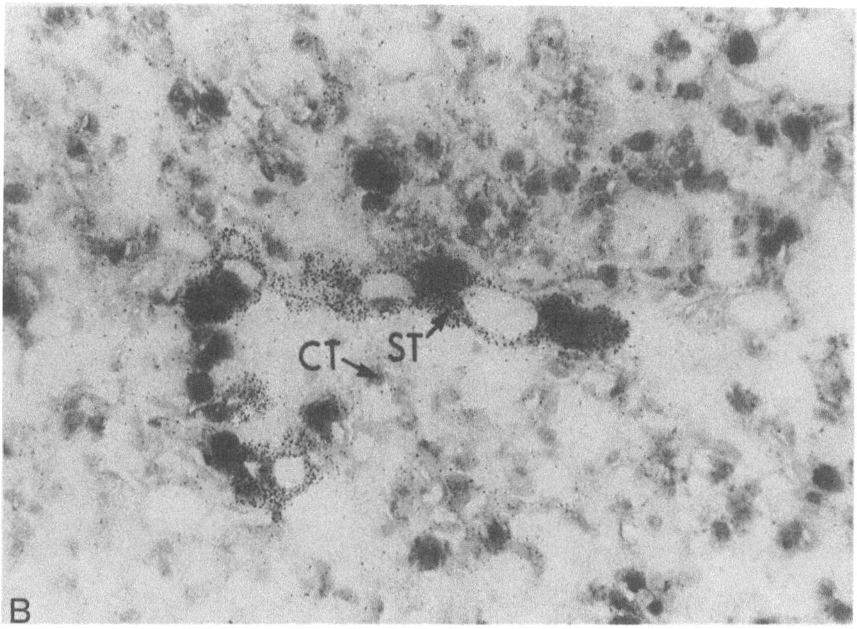
CT
ST
B

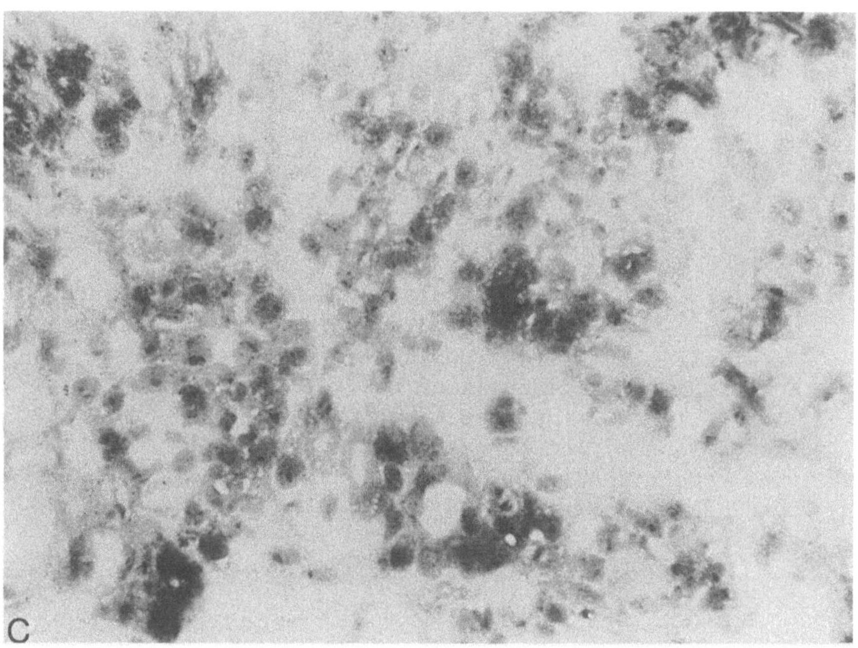
C

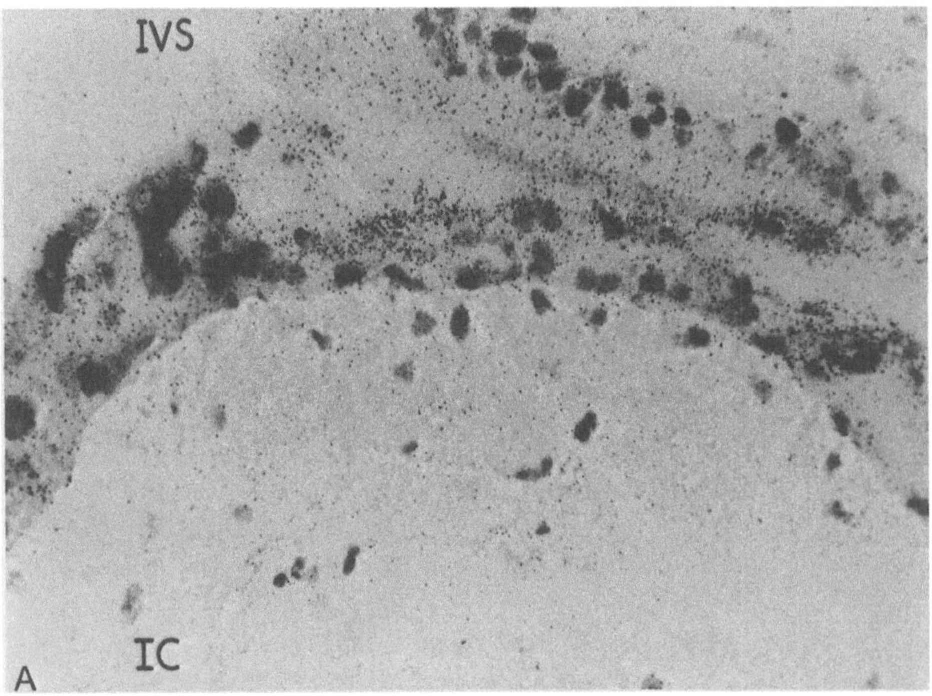

Fig. 4. *In situ* hybridization of sections of hydatidiform mole with hCGα (A), hCGβ (B), and hPL cDNA probes (C). The amount and specific activity of cDNA applied was the same as described for Fig. 3. The molar tissue still maintains a significant villous morphology but there is swelling of the interstitial tissue and a large cystic central area. In mole there is hyperplasia of the trophoblast and a loss of the boundary between syncytiotrophoblast and cytotrophoblast (*i.e.*, *layer*). The hCGα and hCGβ and hPL mRNA signals are distributed rather homogeneously throughout the villi.

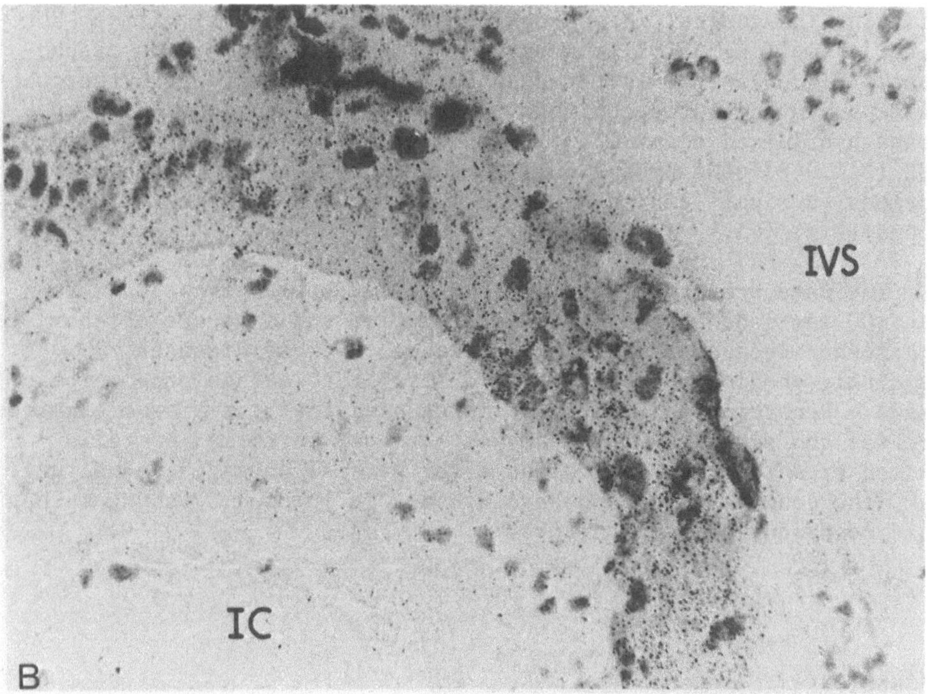
IVS
IC
B

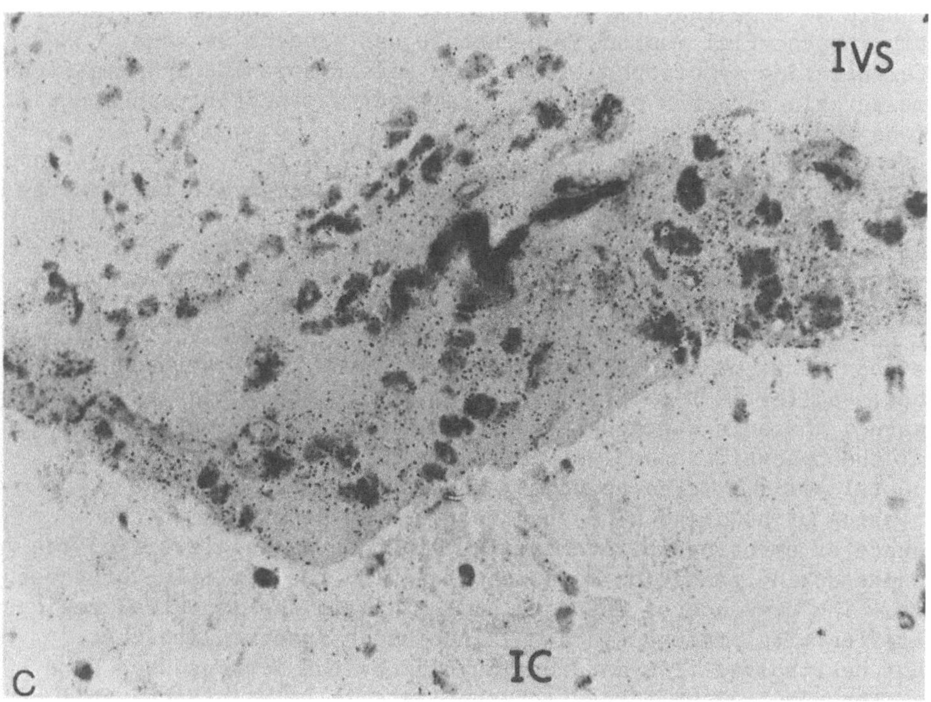
IVS
IC
C

Another form of trophoblast tumor, hydatidiform mole, still maintains the general morphology of a normal placental villus, but there is swelling of villous stroma and hyperplasia of the trophoblasts (Fig. 4). The latter results in the admixture of cytotrophoblasts and syncytiotrophoblasts. As expected, sections of molar tissue hybridized significantly with the hCGα (Fig. 4A) and hCGβ (Fig. 4B) cDNA probes but, in contrast to choriocarcinoma sections, a significant hPL signal was observed relative to background (Fig. 4C).

The data presented here are the results of analyses on more than 100 sections of two hydatidiform moles and one case of choriocarcinoma. Because of the low incidence of these diseases, especially choriocarcinoma, it is difficult to obtain non-necrotic tissue. Regarding this point it is crucial that the tissue examined here was the actual tumor; analyses were not performed on cells derived from the tumors obtained after several passages in culture. Thus, the conclusions drawn here are not influenced by changes that could occur during cell culture.

DISCUSSION

Here we show that the hCGα subunit mRNA was localized predominantly in syncytial regions but that it was present in some differentiating cytotrophoblasts. The signal for hCGβ mRNA in first-trimester placenta was primarily localized to syncytiotrophoblast regions and in a few cytotrophoblasts.

By contrast, hPL mRNA was localized exclusively to the syncytium. These data imply that activation of the hCG subunit and hPL genes occur at different stages of placental differentiation. Previously we demonstrated a six-fold decrease of hCGα mRNA and a decrease, to barely detectable levels, of hCGβ mRNA in term placenta. This was shown by three levels of analysis: (a) translatable levels of steady state mRNAs; (b) quantitation of the mRNAs with cDNA probes; and (c) *in situ* hybridization. It is noteworthy that during pregnancy there is a gradual decrease of cytotrophoblasts until, at term, the syncytiotrophoblast is the major cellular component of placental villi. Taken together, the data suggest that the expression of hCGα and hCGβ subunit genes is dependent on the presence of cytotrophoblasts and that the decreasing levels of the subunits during gestation are associated with the depletion of these cells. The presence of hCGα and hCGβ mRNAs in the syncytial regions may reflect its presence in a multinucleated intermediate that cannot be resolved from mature syncytium by the methods used here. Thus, the requirement for cytotrophoblasts is to maintain a pool of these transient intermediates. Apparently the presence of cytotrophoblasts is not necessary for maintaining the production of hPL in mature syncytium. It is also clear that hPL is expressed only in fully differentiated trophoblast whereas, at least in the case of the hCGα subunit, expression is initiated prior to syncytial formation.

Data obtained from sections of neoplastic trophoblast are consistent with this model. Choriocarcinoma is composed of trophoblasts that are not fully differentiated. There are clusters of cytotrophoblastic cells and multinucleated cells which are apparently immature syncytial elements. In these sections, hCGα and hCGβ mRNA signals were seen in syncytial cells, while the signal for hPL mRNA was almost at background. Nevertheless, it appears that certain cytotrophoblast elements also contain hCGα and hCGβ mRNAs, since some large mononucleated trophoblasts having both syncytiotrophoblastic and cytotrophoblastic morphology showed significant amounts of message. These mononucleated trophoblasts may represent the equivalent of an intermediate cell formed during the development of syncytiotrophoblasts from progenitor cytotrophoblasts.

In the case of hydatidiform mole, the hPL gene, as well as the hCG subunit genes, is expressed. It is significant that one of the distinguishing features of molar tissue compared to choriocarcinoma tissue is that the former retains a significant placental villous morphology. Thus, it seems reasonable that a certain level of differentiation such as that indicated by villus formation is essential for hPL gene expression.

We would propose the following scheme for coupled events of hormone expression and trophoblast differentiation: the hCGα gene is first activated in committed cytotrophoblasts (Langhan cells) that lie beneath the syncytium. Later, as these cells further differentiate, the hCGβ subunit gene begins to be expressed. This intermediate cell thus elaborates both subunits and is similar to the multinucleated structure expressing the hCG subunits in choriocarcinoma. This intermediate cell exists transiently; the population of intermediate cells peaks at 8-10 weeks of pregnancy, and declines thereafter. This intermediate cell cannot be resolved by the method used in the present study. Thus, hCGβ signals seen in placental sections reflect such an intermediate.

Further information regarding how the expression of the hPL and hCG subunit genes is linked to normal trophoblast differentiation and tumorigenesis might be obtained by following the cytotrophoblast/syncytiotrophoblast maturation process *in vitro* with the cDNA probes used here. In addition, isolation and characterization of the genetic regions flanking these genes from choriocarcinoma and molar tissue may provide more information concerning the differences between normal and malignant trophoblast.

SUMMARY

Normal trophoblast of the human placenta elaborates at least two major protein hormones, hCG and hPL. Molar and choriocarcinoma tissues characteristically synthesize large amounts of hCG and small quantities of hPL. To examine the role of trophoblast differentiation in the expression of the hCG and hPL genes, we studied the cytological distribution of their mRNAs in tissue sections of human hydatidiform mole and choriocarcinoma by *in situ* hybridization. Histologically, these tissues are in different stages of cellular differentiation. In normal placenta, hCGα and hCGβ mRNAs can be localized to some cytotrophoblasts and primarily to the syncytium, whereas hPL mRNA appears only in the syncytial layer. In hydatidiform mole, which still retains placental villous morphology, the hPL gene and hCGα and hCGβ genes are expressed but are poorly localized because of the admixture of cyto- and syncytiotrophoblasts. By contrast, choriocarcinoma, which is devoid of placental villous pattern but in which the cyto- and syncytiotrophoblast-like components are distinguishable, expresses hCGα and hCGβ in the syncytial-like areas but little, if any, hPL.

These results suggest that a certain level of trophoblast differentiation, such as villus formation, is associated with hPL expression, while the hCGα gene and the hCGβ gene can be expressed in more disorganized tissues which contain cytotrophoblastic elements.

ACKNOWLEDGEMENTS

This work was preformed while Dr. Hoshina was on leave from the Department of Obstetrics and Gynecology, Kobe University School of Medicine, Kobe, Japan. We are grateful to Dr. Thomas Woolsey for his advice and comments regarding the manuscript. We also thank Mrs. Margaret McHugh for helping us with the photography, and Jacquelyn Udell and Linda Hammond for assisting with the manuscript. This investigation was supported by U. S. Public Health Service grants 13481 and CA23357.

REFERENCES

1. Enders, A. C., Formation of syncytium from cytotrophoblast in the human placenta, Obstet. Gynecol. 25:378 (1965).
2. Pierce, G. B. and Midgley, A. R., The origin and function of human syncytiotrophoblastic giant cell, Amer. J. Pathol. 43: 153 (1963).
3. Wynn, R. M., Cytotrophoblastic specialization: an ultrastructural study of the human placenta, Amer. J. Obstet. Gynecol. 114:339 (1972).

4. Ashitaka, Y., Nishimura, R., Takemori, M., and Tojo, S., Production and secretion of hCG and hCG subunits by trophoblastic tissue, in: S. J. Segal, ed., "Chorionic Gonadotropin," Plenum Press, New York (1980), p. 147.
5. Biswas, S., Hindocha, P., and Dewhust, C. J., Human chorionic somatomammotropin in serum and urine in various states of pregnancy: its correlation with enzymes and oestrogens, J. Endocrinol. 54:251 (1972).
6. Boime, I., McWilliams, D., Szczesna, E., and Camel, M., Synthesis of human placental lactogen as a function of gestation, J. Biol. Chem. 251:821 (1976).
7. Boime, I., Landefeld, T., McQueen, S., and McWilliams, D., The biosynthesis of chorionic gonadotropin and placental lactogen in first- and third-trimester human placenta, in: K. W. McKern, ed., "Structure and Function of the Gonadotropins," Plenum Press, New York (1978), p. 235.
8. Bagshawe, K. D., "Choriocarcinoma, The Clinical Biology of the Trophoblast and its Tumours," The Williams & Wilkins Co., Baltimore (1969), p. 72.
9. Pattillo, R. A., Endocrine and immunological factors in trophoblastic cancers, in: K. W. McKerns, ed., "Hormones and Cancers," Academic Press, New York (1974), p. 363.
10. Hertz, R., "Choriocarcinoma and Related Gestational Trophoblastic Tumors in Women," Raven Press, New York (1978), p. 23.
11. Goldstein, D. P., and Berkowitz, R. S., "Major Problems in Obstetrics and Gynecology, Gestational Trophoblastic Neoplasms, Clinical Principles of Diagnosis and Management," W. B. Saunders Co., Philadelphia (1982), p. 11.
12. Hussa, R. O., Clinical utility of human chorionic gonadotropin and α subunit measurements, Obstet. Gynecol. 60:1 (1982).
13. Seppala, M., Rutanen, E. M., Ranta, T., Aho, I., Nieminen, U., Unnerus, H. A., and Saksela, E., Choriocarcinoma: expression of tumor- and trophoblast-associated antigens in patients with low chorionic gonadotropin excretion, Cancer 38:2065 (1976).
14. Mochizuki, M., Morikawa, H., Kawaguchi, K., and Tojo, S., Growth hormone, prolactin and chorionic somatomammotropin in normal and molar pregnancy, J. Clin. Endocrinol. Metab. 43: 614 (1976).
15. Forest, J. C., Talbot, J., Page, M., and Loiselle, J. M., Tumour antigens associated with primary mediastinal choriocarcinoma, Canad. Med. Assoc. J. 117:1386 (1977).
16. Dawood, M., Saxena, B., and Landesman, R., Human chorionic gonadotropin and its subunits in hydatidiform mole and choriocarcinomas, Obstet. Gynecol. 50:172 (1977).
17. Clayton, L. A., Tyrey, L., Weed, J. C., Jr., and Hammond, C. B., Endocrine aspects of trophoblastic neoplasia, J. Reprod. Med. 26:192 (1981).

18. Boothby, M., Daniels-McQueen, S., McWilliams, D., Zernik, M., and Boime, I., Human chorionic gonadotropin alpha and beta subunit m-RNAs: translatable levels during pregnancy and molecular cloning of DNA sequences complementary to hCG, in: S. J. Segal, ed., "Chorionic Gonadotropin," Plenum Press, New York (1980), p. 253.
19. Boothby, M., Ruddon, R. W., Anderson, C., McWilliams, D., and Boime, I., A singel gonadotropin α-subunit gene in normal tissue and tumor-derived cell lines, J. Biol. Chem. 256: 5121 (1981).
20. Hoshina, M., Boothby, M., and Boime, I., Cytological localization of chorionic gonadotorpin α and placental lactogen mRNAs during development of the human placenta, J. Cell Biol. 93: 190 (1982).
21. Policastro, P., Ovitt, C., Hoshina, M., Fukuoka, H., Boothby, M., and Boime, I., The β subunit of human chorionic gonadotropin is encoded by multiple genes, J. Biol. Chem. 258:11492 (1983).

CLINICAL APPLICATIONS OF hCG

K. D. Bagshawe

Department of Medical Oncology
Charing Cross Hospital
Fulham Palace Road
London, W6 8RF, United Kingdom

INTRODUCTION

The concept of tumor markers has widened in recent years. In the 1950s and 1960s we thought of them primarily as means of detecting and monitoring tumors. In the past decade their potential value at the immunocytochemical level has become more evident, and now the possibilities of in vivo localization with antibodies and of drug targeting have come under serious study. A marker which is ideal for one purpose is not necessarily the best for another; as more trophoblastic products are defined, we may find different markers coming into use for different purposes. The four best known trophoblastic products are human chorionic gonadotropin (hCG), the so-called placenta specific protein (SP_1), human placental lactogen (hPL), and placental alkaline phosphatase (PLAP). The first two of these are secreted freely by trophoblast in the earliest stages of pregnancy, whereas the last two reach their peak values late in pregnancy. As serological markers, hCG and SP_1 are much the better for trophoblastic tumors. SP_1 is a good marker for trophoblastic tumors and only slightly inferior to hCG. For some patients SP_1 may indeed be slightly superior (1-3), but in my experience this was not sufficient to merit measuring SP_1 in all cases. For the concept of serum tumor markers, hCG remains the best model we have. Many other placental products have been described in recent years, but none have so far been shown to be superior to hCG as a marker for trophoblastic tumors.

There have been suggestions that there may be advantage in measuring the α-subunit to detect remission status in choriocarcinoma (4). Our experience with α-subunit assays has not led us to think it is superior to hCG where the assay is sensitive and specific enough to reliably detect 1 IU/l. Nevertheless, this remains an area requiring further study.

Our experience at Charing Cross Hospital with trophoblastic tumors began in 1956. Since that time, more than 8,000 patients with hydatidiform mole have been followed up, and more than 800 patients have been treated for invasive mole or choriocarcinoma. Our early measurements of hCG used urine extraction procedures with bioassays, but by 1961 the first immunoassays were beginning to supplement those results. By 1965, radioimmunoassay was firmly established on a routine basis. It was clear that the scale on which measurements of hCG and other tumor products would be required would increase to high levels, and in 1966 we started laboratory studies to automate these assays. By 1973 all our radioimmunoassays had been automated so that as many tests as needed could be performed at low cost. Since then, the instruments have improved in precision and reliability (5).

The introduction of assays using antisera to hCGβ was a notable step forward, improving effective assay sensitivity by 10 to 50 fold. It would be possible to improve assay sensitivity by a further 100-fold by combining RIA in addition to the urine extraction procedures used for bioassay or by more modern methods of concentration using affinity chromatography. We have not done this, partly because extraction and recovery procedures remain labor intensive. Also, there is variability in the percentage of hCG recovery from such procedures, and this could result in great difficulties in clinical interpretation. Moreover, we would probably again run up against problems of discrimination between hCG and luteinizing hormone (hLH) unless the extraction procedure also discriminated against hLH. Nevertheless, improvements in assay sensitivity, better than the 1 IU/l now obtained with good antisera, are potentially achievable.

At the other end of the technology spectrum there is the question of assays for developing countries. The reagent supply problem should be readily soluble with monoclonal antibodies. Enzyme or fluorescent assays would be advantageous in terms of shelf life, provided adequate sensitivity can be achieved. So far as radioimmunoassay is concerned, the use of complicated autogamma counters requiring reliable servicing arrangements which don't always exist, have resulted in breakdowns and long interruptions in assay performance. Manual gamma counters which are cheap, simple and rugged would seem to be a better solution.

It is worth noting that, although it has become fashionable in recent years to refer to the β-subunit assay, there is much misunderstanding in terminology. Most assays in clinical use employ antisera raised against hCGβ. They are of variable specificity, in that some assays are influenced at the lowest levels of detection by cross-reactivity with hLH. This is, however, less than with antisera raised to intact hCG. However, "β-subunit assays" principally detect intact hCG, although if there are free β-subunits present, these will also contribute to the measured response in the assay. It should be clear that "β-subunit assays" are hCG assays; they do not measure hCGβ exclusively.

HYDATIDIFORM MOLE

Although hCG values are often very high in patients with complete or partial hydatidiform mole, this does not occur with sufficient regularity to be a completely dependable diagnostic aid. Values greater than 100,000 IU/l in serum or urine are exceptional in the absence of hydatidiform mole. On the other hand, hydatidiform mole may be associated with hCG values less than 10,000 IU/l. Ultrasound has proved a more reliable diagnostic aid. Nevertheless, hCG values have been thought to have some prognostic significance with respect to the development of sequelae following hydatidiform mole (6). Published data, however, are scanty. In our series, 6 of 26 patients with pre-evacuation hCG values of greater than 100,000 IU/l urine required chemotherapy by the criteria we use (7), compared with 4 of 72 patients with values less than 100,000 IU/l urine.

The main application of hCG assays in relation to hydatidiform mole lies, of course, in the follow-up of patients after evacuation. The objectives of this follow-up are to select out those patients who require therapeutic intervention from those who do not, and to do this at a time when eradication of the trophoblast can be achieved with confidence. Different centers have applied different criteria for the selection of patients; those used in our center result in 6-10% of all hydatidiform mole patients receiving chemotherapy (8). This may be compared with the 3% of hydatidiform mole patients who develop choriocarcinomas (9), and the 20% or more of hydatidiform mole patients treated in some American series.

Following evacuation of mole, hCG values fall steeply at first, but thereafter the pattern of values is very variable. The maximum rate of fall is determined by the metabolic clearance rate of hCG, and the halving time is usually 24-36 hours. Following the initial fall, values may continue to fall rapidly until hCG becomes undetectable at around 1 IU/l (*i.e.*, about 200 pg/l) by about 20 days post-evacuation. More commonly, however, after the initial drop, values fall more slowly or may plateau or even rise temporarily before falling again. In such patients, hCG remains detectable for variable periods up to about 6-12 weeks post-evacuation before becoming undetectable. These various patterns of hCG excretion occur in about 90% of patients after evacuation of hydatidiform mole.

Up to 10% of patients' values do not fall to this limit in that time, and after an initial fall there may be a variable level of hCG followed by progressively increasing values. Where values persist in excess of 25,000 IU/1 in the serum 4-6 weeks post-evacuation, there is danger of uterine perforation by invasive mole or choriocarcinoma, and therapeutic intervention is indicated in these patients.

Any level of hCG detectable 4-6 months after evacuation has been regarded as one indication for treatment in this series.

The follow-up arrangements in the United Kingdom are based on a Registration scheme supported by the Royal College of Obstetricians and Gynaecologists and the Department of Health. The scheme is voluntary, and patients are registered with one of three laboratories based in London, Sheffield, and Dundee. The laboratory sends the patient instructions for sending a specimen to the laboratory in a reply pre-paid box. Both urine and serum samples are employed. Serum assays still have a slight superiority in terms of sensitivity and freedom from interference, but urine is advantageous in terms of patient compliance.

Tests are performed every two weeks until hCG becomes undetectable, then monthly till one year post-evacuation, and then every three months in the second year. However, patients are advised that they may start another pregnancy when hCG has been undetectable for six months. The risk of developing a trophoblastic tumor in the second year of follow-up is less than 1:1000.

This screening program appears to be highly cost-effective. It spares patients unnecessary chemotherapy and ensures that those who need it can be effectively treated.

Age-related data from 3,000 patients with hydatidiform mole is of interest when compared with maternal age for registered births in England and Wales. The data show that the risk of a pregnancy resulting in hydatidiform mole is about 30 times greater in females under 15 years of age than in patients aged 20-30 years. In women over the age of 50 years, the risk is more than 200 times greater. These data will be published in detail elsewhere.

DIAGNOSIS OF INVASIVE MOLE, CHORIOCARCINOMA, PLACENTAL SITE TUMOR, AND ECTOPIC PRODUCTION OF hCG

Although hCG has proved to be one of the most specific tumor markers yet defined, it is necessary to be aware of its limitations in the diagnostic context. The need to exclude pregnancy, including ectopic pregnancy, as a cause of elevated hCG hardly needs emphasis, yet the occasional presentation of a patient with, for example, metastases in the lungs from an occult carcinoma of the breast and with a very early pregnancy can be a sharp test of clinical acumen. Similarly, we have to make the important distinction between a gestational tumor and a germ cell tumor, which can prove exceedingly difficult, as well as exclude ectopic hCG production by nontrophoblastic tumors.

Invasive mole and choriocarcinoma cannot be distinguished by their hCG production alone, although taken with other clinical features, such as extensive or large metastases, a high hCG is indicative of choriocarcinoma.

A relatively low value in comparison with observed tumor bulk appears to be usual in cases of placental site tumor, and is also usual in ectopic product syndrome. There are also problem cases such as adenocarcinoma of the stomach, showing choriocarcinomatous differentiation, where hCG values may be high. Placental site tumor and ectopic hCG production may be difficult to distinguish in some cases. Even with histological and immunocytochemistry, the ground rules for discrimination have yet to be sharply defined.

Placental site tumor is characterized by a predominance of cytotrophoblastic cells, with only scattered syncytial elements where hCG can be demonstrated by immunocytochemistry (10, 11). In contrast to choriocarcinoma, these lesions are relatively slow to metastasize, but are only moderately sensitive or resistant to chemotherapy. My present view is that they should be removed surgically whenever possible. It also seems possible that there are tumors with characteristics in between those of typical choriocarcinoma and typical placental site tumor. Such tumors have the general morphology of choriocarcinoma, but the cytotrophoblastic elements are dominant. Again, my experience suggests that one should suspect that these tumors have a greater potential for drug resistance, although an attempt we made some years ago to correlate drug resistance with the proportion of cyto- and syncytiotrophoblast in choriocarcinoma did not give a decisive answer.

It has been noted in our series that where resistance occurs and the disease progresses, hCG values are commonly less than when the patient presented with extensive disease. Again, there may be a shift in the histological pattern in these cases, toward cytotrophoblastic dominance, but formal studies are incomplete.

PROGNOSIS

The long-known relationship between hCG values and total body burden of tumor is only partly compromised by the above considerations. Studies in vitro and in vivo have indicated that the mean cell production of hCG is of the order of 10^{-5} IU per day.

Thus, at the time when hCG becomes undetectable, 10^4-10^5 cells may still be present, constituting a volume of viable cells of less than 1 mm^3 (12). Such a figure is useful conceptually, but it should be anticipated that there are wide biological variations as well as significant variations resulting from assay methodology.

Nevertheless, tumor burden as judged by hCG values in serum or urine is a powerful prognostic factor. Analysis of our series up to 1973 showed that the fatality rate for patients with hCG values at the start of treatment in the range of 1,000 to 10,000 IU/1 was about 2.5%. As hCG values increased, the fatality rate increased, and with initial values greater than 10^6 IU/1 the fatality rate overall was 60% (5). Curiously, there was an apparent aberration in the data with respect to hCG values less than 1,000 IU/1. The small number of patients in this category did not permit reliable interpretation, but it was noted that 2 of 18 died from drug-resistant disease. Moreover, there was clinical and radiological evidence of more tumor bulk than was expected for the hCG values observed. In retrospect, it seems likely that these resistant patients were an atypical subset, possibly with placental site tumors or some other variant. In general, however, high hCG values may be regarded as a warning of danger to the patient, either from the initial extent of the disease, or from the risk of drug resistance later. Low values, on the other hand, generally imply a small burden of tumor which is likely to respond well, but there may be exceptions.

Of course, it is essential to distinguish between high values associated with hydatidiform mole in situ which, as already noted, may have significance with respect to the risk of sequelae, and high values due to an established tumor and in particular to choriocarcinoma.

MONITORING INVASIVE MOLE AND CHORIOCARCINOMA

The true test of a good marker is correlation with the course of the disease over a wide range of tumor volumes. It is general experience that patients with clinically evident invasive mole or choriocarcinoma all have detectable levels of hCG by radioimmunoassay. Where treatment has reduced hCG to undetectable levels, and when hCG has remained undetectable, disease progression has not been observed. Where hCG values have increased progressively, either with or without treatment, death has invariably occurred from choriocarcinoma.

When effective chemotherapy is first given to a patient with a trophoblastic tumor, hCG values may increase for a few days before they start to fall. Evidence has been presented that this may be due to promoting the differentiation of non-hCG-producing cytotrophoblast to hCG-producing syncytium (13). It is also possible that some hCG is released by tumor lysis, but evidence for this is less secure. The magnitude of the fall in hCG values following a course of chemotherapy can be measured from the start of the course of chemotherapy to a point where recovery from the associated toxicity allows a subsequent course of treatment to be started. This provides a basis for comparative evaluation of cytotoxic agents and regimen (14). In general, a useful response measured in these terms should exceed a one log fall, although in resistant tumors a response of half that magnitude may be acceptable.

During the early 1960s, when immunoassay provided us with the first readily reproducible assays, I was impressed by the fact that hCG values fell by a constant fraction with each course of chemotherapy. Skipper and associates (16) presented experimental evidence from animal models for the important concept of fractional cell kill. Data from the chemotherapy of choriocarcinomas provide some of the best clinical evidence to support this concept. It has to be remembered that the clearance rate of hCG is sufficiently slow to smooth out the changes in hCG values so that they reflect changes in cell numbers more evenly than they probably occur. It is not uncommon for the hCG curve for a responding tumor, plotted on a log hCG *versus* linear time scale, to be a straight line over the observable range of values.

In cancer chemotherapy generally, treatment tends to be discontinued according to a sort of cook-book formula, such as the number of courses judged to be optimal. With choriocarcinoma, it is possible to be a little more scientific, but clearly the limitation is our inability to detect the smallest amount of tumor which can survive treatment and ultimately lead to clinical recurrence. In attempting to define the endpoint of treatment, we recognize the individuality of each clinical situation. The rate of response, as judged by falling hCG values, is highly variable. The limit of detecting hCG is reached in a few weeks in some patients, but takes several months in others. The residue of undetectable tumor may not require prolonged treatment with the former, but failure to continue treatment long enough in the latter carries a high risk of relapse. Diagrammatically, this can be illustrated by extrapolating the hCG curve down to the "one cell level". This indicates the minimum length of continued treatment which can be expected to eradicate residual disease if it is assumed that the rate of tumor destruction, on a constant fractional kill basis, is not less than it was during the observable part of tumor destruction (14, 15). This assumption may not be justified, since as treatment proceeds, particularly with difficult tumors, the fall of hCG values tends to flatten out.

Therefore, it is wise to continue treatment longer than the minimum, particularly in the higher risk patient. In general, patients in the low risk category (5) have 2-3 courses after hCG has become undetectable, those in the middle risk category have

3-4 courses, and those in the high risk category have 5-8 courses, depending on the protocols in use.

METASTASES IN THE CENTRAL NERVOUS SYSTEM

The risk of brain metastases in choriocarcinoma is well known. They may remain silent until a serious event such as epilepsy or intracranial hemorrhage. When detected at the start of treatment, they can usually be eradicated by chemotherapy, but when they develop during the course of chemotherapy they prove much more difficult (17). Metastases to the brain, arising from cells which have migrated from other sites where they have already encountered cytotoxic agents, tend to be more resistant to eradication. Moreover, brain penetration by cytotoxic agents tends to be poor.

CT scanning makes a most valuable contribution to the detection and localization of brain metastases, and is probably desirable in all high risk patients and in all those with pulmonary metastases. Although lumbar puncture is not a popular activity amongst patients or physicians, measurement of the serum/CSF ratio of hCG has been found to be a sensitive method for detecting brain metastases (18, 19). In our experience, there have been a few instances where hCG has been diagnostic and CT has failed, and others where hCG values were less decisive than the CT scan. In general, we believe that these diagnostic techniques are complementary to each other.

A serum/CSF ratio less than 60:1 is generally found in the presence of brain metastases, and a value greater than 60:1 in their absence. Lumbar punctures cannot be performed, of course, where there is raised intracranial pressure, but otherwise we think the information it yields outweighs the protracted headaches it often causes. Rapid changes in the serum concentration of hCG can lead to transient changes in serum/CSF ratio, so that when in doubt it is desirable to get more than one CSF sample for estimation.

We have to take into account the problem of preventing brain metastases during chemotherapy. Methotrexate remains the principal defense against brain metastases and needs to be given in high intravenous dosage to reach effective concentrations in the central nervous system. Doses of 0.75 or 1 g/m^2, however, are very expensive and need to be followed by another expensive drug, folinic acid. The effective dosage by lumbar puncture is 10.0-12.5 mg. If, therefore, lumbar puncture is performed therapeutically to prevent brain metastases, as I think it should be in high risk patients, then CSF hCG should always be measured. It is also usefully performed in a patient who has persisting elevation of hCG after treatment, and when the site of the disease is unknown. Serum/CSF values can be used to monitor the results of chemotherapy in CNS metastases. It has been noted that CSF values may be higher than serum values, thus indicating that the raised values of CSF are not simply due to the breakdown of the blood-brain barrier, but rather due to direct escape of hCG into the CSF from the tumor.

FOLLOW-UP AFTER TREATMENT FOR TROPHOBLASTIC TUMOR

The need to continue the follow-up of patients after treatment for invasive mole or choriocarcinoma is well known. This is a policy which we follow for all patients, although we have not seen any patient relapse where the lesion was known to be invasive mole. Initially, hCG must be estimated frequently, but can be measured less frequently after defined intervals of time. As a general guide, assays at this center are performed every two weeks up to six months after the end of treatment, then monthly up to two years, then every three months up to five years. Subsequently, assays are performed every six months. In patients who have had a previous relapse, still closer observation may be needed in the early years.

Distinction from a subsequent pregnancy rarely presents a major problem. The rate of increase of hCG values in the early weeks of pregnancy is only rarely seen in patients with choriocarcinoma. When this does happen, it is usually in relapses occurring soon after discontinuation of therapy. With relapses more than 3-4 months after discontinuing therapy, the rate of increase in hCG values shows a longer doubling time. Also, as pregnancy proceeds, α-fetoprotein becomes detectable and ultrasound may confirm the diagnosis at an even earlier stage.

RADIOIMMUNODETECTION

Although most choriocarcinomas are sensitive to, and can be eliminated by, present chemotherapeutic agents (20), there is a small number of patients who develop persisting drug resistant disease. If one continues to treat with chemotherapy alone, the tumor eventually metastasizes further, and death is likely to ensue. At the stage when resistance to all known agents becomes apparent, it is reasonable to ask whether radiotherapy and/or surgery can help. Our experience with radiotherapy has been disappointing, but it is possible that with the more refined localization of brain metastases and the improved planning now possible, better results will be obtained.

Elsewhere, radiological and CT examination may reveal persisting metastases, and in selected cases with only one or a few persisting metastases, surgical intervention may be indicated (21). If the patient has not had hysterectomy, this may be indicated, particularly if arteriography or ultrasound suggest that there is tumor still present in the uterus or adnexae (9).

Part of the problem is that the tumor may be too small to detect by present radiological methods. Even when tumor is demonstrable it is not possible in many cases to determine whether it contains viable tumor or whether it is only dead tumor. Sometimes this can be resolved by needle biopsy, but there are patients where these matters remain unresolved. It is in such situations that the technique of radioimmunolocalization may prove to have a role (22). Radiolabeled, affinity column-purified antibodies to hCG have been injected intravenously and have been demonstrated by external scintigraphy to localize in hCG-producing tumors (23).

When anti-hCG is injected intravenously into a subject with free hCG in the body fluids, immune complexes form, but, presumably because of their association-dissociation behavior, sufficient antibody reaches the tumor to allow discrimination. Images have been obtained in patients with serum hCG values between 50 and 500,000 IU/l. The excess of antibody in the tumor, compared with other tissues, may be very low and it may, in absolute terms, be lower than the concentration in the serum. Nevertheless, pictures can be obtained. The antibody is mainly retained in the extracellular fluid space of the tumor rather than bound to the cells. Theoretically, one might expect localization to define tumors actually secreting the antigen, but antigen retention in dead tumor tissue may occur. Present methods with ^{131}I-labeled antibodies in the human subjects are not without substantial difficulties in the interpretation of the images obtained, yet there have nevertheless been a few patients in our series where clinically useful results have been obtained.

There is reason to be optimistic that the methods of radioimmunolocalization can be substantially improved by using more suitable isotopes, by techniques for reducing the background, by using monoclonal antibodies, and by further refinement of the hardware and programming systems.

REFERENCES

1. Tatarinov, Y. S., Falaleeva, D. M., and Kalashnikov, V. V., Human pregnancy-specific-beta$_1$-globulin and its relation to chorionepithelioma, Int. J. Cancer 17:626 (1976).
2. Searle, F., Leake, B. A., Dent, J., and Bagshawe, K. D., Serum-SP$_1$-pregnancy-specific-β-glycoprotein in choriocarcinoma and other neoplastic disease, Lancet 1:579 (1978).
3. Bagshawe, K. D., Lequin, R. M., Sizaret, Ph., and Tatarinov, Y. S., Pregnancy β_1-glycoprotein and chorionic gonadotrophin in the serum of patients with trophoblastic and non-trophoblastic tumours, Europ. J. Cancer 14:1331 (1978).
4. Quigley, M., Tyrey, L., and Hammond, C. B., Utility of assay of alpha subunit of human chorionic gonadotropin in management of

gestational trophoblastic malignancies, Amer. J. Obstet. Gynecol. 138:545 (1980).
5. Bagshawe, K. D., Risk and prognostic factors in trophoblastic neoplasia, Cancer 38:1373 (1976).
6. Goldstein, D., Berkowitz, and Bernstein, M., Management of molar pregnancy, J. Reprod. Med. 26:208 (1981).
7. Stone, M., Dent, J., Kardana, A., and Bagshawe, K. D., Relationship of oral contraception to development of trophoblastic tumor after evacuation of a hydatidiform mole, Brit. J. Obstet. Gynaecol. 83:913 (1976).
8. Stone, M. and Bagshawe, K. D., An analysis of the influence of maternal age, gestational age, contraceptive method and the mode of primary treatment of patients with hydatidiform mole on the incidence of subsequent chemotherapy, Brit. J. Obstet. Gynaecol. 86:782 (1979).
9. Bagshawe, K. D., "Choriocarcinoma. The Clinical Biology of the Trophoblast and its Tumours," Edward Arnold, London (1969).
10. Scully, R. E. and Young, R. H., Trophoblastic pseudotumor. A reappraisal, Amer. J. Surg. Pathol. 5:75 (1981).
11. Eckstein, R. P., Paradinas, F. J., and Bagshawe, K. D., Placental site trophoblastic tumour (trophoblastic pseudotumor): a study of four cases requiring hysterectomy, including one fatal case, Histopathol. 6:211 (1982).
12. Bagshawe, K. D., Trophoblastic disease, in: "Advances in Obstetrics and Gynecology", R. M. Caplan and W. J. Sweeney, eds., Williams & Wilkins Company, Baltimore (1975).
13. Browne, P. and Bagshawe, K. D., Enhancement of human chorionic gonadotrophin production by antimetabolites, Brit. J. Cancer 46:22 (1982).
14. Bagshawe, K. D., Wilson, H., Dublon, P., Smith, A., Baldwin, M., and Kardana, A., Follow-up after hydatidiform mole studies using radioimmunoassay for urinary human chorionic gonadotrophin (hCG), J. Obstet. Gynaecol. Brit. Comwlth. 80:461 (1973).
15. Bagshawe, K. D., Computer controlled automated radioimmunoassay, Lab. Practice, September, 573 (1975).
16. Skipper, H. E., Schabel, F. M., and Wilcox, W. S., Experimental evaluation of potential anti-cancer agents, Cancer Chemother. Rpts. 35:1 (1964).
17. Athanassiou, A., Begent, R. H. J., Newlands, E. S., Parker, D., Rustin, G. J. S., and Bagshawe, K. D., Central nervous system metastases of choriocarcinoma: 23 years' experience at Charing Cross Hospital, Cancer (In press, 1983).
18. Rushworth, A., Orr, A. H., and Bagshawe, K. D., The concentration of hCG in the plasma and spinal fluid of patients with trophoblastic tumours in the central nervous system, Brit. J. Cancer 22:253 (1968).
19. Bagshawe, K. D. and Harland, S., Immunodiagnosis and monitoring of gonadotrophin producing metastases in the central nervous system, Cancer 38:112 (1976).

20. Begent, R. H. J. and Bagshawe, K. D., The management of high risk choriocarcinoma, Seminars in Oncology 9:198 (1982).
21. Edwards, J. L., Makey, A. R., and Bagshawe, K. D., The role of thoracotomy in the management of pulmonary metastases of gestational choriocarcinoma, Clinical Oncology 1:329 (1975).
22. Goldenberg, D. M., Deland, K. F., and Kimm, E. E., Use of radiolabeled antibodies to carcinoembryonic antigen for detection and localization of diverse cancers by external photoscanning, New Engl. J. Med. 298:1384 (1978).
23. Begent, R. H. J., Searle, F., Stanway, G., Jewkes, R. F., Jones, B. E., Vernon, P., and Bagshawe, K. D., Radioimmuno-localisation of malignant teratoma using radiolabelled anti-body directed against human chorionic gonadotrophin, in: "Germ Cell Tumours," C. K. Anderson, W. G. Jones, and A. Milford-Ward, eds., Taylor and Francis, London (1981).

CLINICAL STAGING

Insights into the biological evolution of the disease process may be gained by careful study of the primary tumor source, followed by study of the anatomic distribution of the growth process. Clinical staging will add this significant dimension of the natural history of growth and dissemination of the trophoblast neoplasm. At the same time, a clearer understanding of the treatment field may be obtained by more quantitative tabulation of areas of disease spread.

Prognostic indicators of potential survival, surgical resectability, or curability are among the advantages to be found in uniform staging criteria for this disease process. A standard basis for comparing outcome, statistics, and predictability of response to various treatment programs will accrue from the adaptation of such fundamental staging criteria as those outlined in the following chapter.

A PROPOSAL ON THE CLINICAL STAGING OF MALIGNANT TROPHOBLASTIC NEOPLASMS BASED ON THE STUDY OF PROCESS OF DEVELOPMENT OF THE DISEASE

Hung-Chao Sung, Pao-Chen Wu, Yuan-E Wang,
Ming-Yi Tang, and Hsiou-Yu Yang

Department of Obstetrics and Gynecology
Capital Hospital
Chinese Academy of Medical Sciences
Beijing, China

INTRODUCTION

An agreement on the criteria of diagnosis of malignant trophoblastic neoplasms has been reached in recent years. Outstanding achievements have been made in the treatment causing a dramatic improvement in prognosis. However, there still lacks a satisfactory clinical staging which may be used to designate the extent and development of this group of tumors. Without a universally accepted method of staging, the clinical materials from various sources cannot be compared, the prognosis of patients cannot be correctly predicted, and the therapeutic results of different methods of treatment cannot be accurately evaluated. Therefore, in 1962, based on the careful analysis of a large series of cases, a preliminary proposal of clinical staging of malignant trophoblastic tumors was reported (1). Through years of trial in patients, it was found that this staging method is very practical for clinical use and correlates well with the prognosis of the disease (2). Recently, it has been re-evaluated on the basis of an intensive study of the process of development of the diseases in 870 patients. The results are reported below.

MATERIALS AND METHODS

From 1949 through 1975, 429 cases of choriocarcinoma and 441 cases of invasive mole were admitted to the Capital Hospital. The clinical course of development of the disease was carefully observed in all patients. The abdominal viscera were carefully explored in all surgically treated cases to evaluate the extent of metastases and their relationships. Autopsy was available in 60 cases of choriocarcinoma and 4 cases of invasive mole, of which all organs were subjected to both macroscopic and microscopic studies. Particular attention was given to the early metastases to uncover the initial changes. In all cases operated upon and autopsied, the resected lymph nodes were examined histologically. In the surgically removed specimens of pelvic organs, both ovarian and uterine arteries and veins were segmentally ligated before fixation and serial sections of the vessels were carried out to seek the possible existence of tumor emboli and/or free tumor cells. Because the lungs are the most common sites of tumor spreading, a special study was carried out (3). Correlation of different forms of metastases on the chest films to the underlying pathological changes was made to elucidate the nature of various roentgenological manifestations. In addition, pulmonary arteriography of resected lung specimens was performed in a few autopsied cases to study the vascular changes and the formation and development of metastases. Because of its serious outcome, brain metastasis was also specially studied and the results were reported in a previous article (4). Metastases to other organs such as liver, spleen, kidney, intestine, etc., were also carefully studied both clinically and pathologically.

RESULTS

Route of Metastasis of Malignant Trophoblastic Tumors

Among 428 cases of surgery and 64 cases of autopsies, direct invasion of the adjacent organs from the primary foci of the uterus or secondary foci of the pelvis was found in only 9 cases (1.8%), of which bladder invasion occurred in 6 and bowel invasion in 3. Lymph node metastasis was found in another 9 cases, of which multiple-site metastases occurred in one and single-site metastasis in 8. All lymph node metastases were discovered at autopsy except one in which mediastinum node spreading was confirmed during pneumonectomy. On the other hand, in contrast to the rarity of local invasion and lymph node spreading, tumor emboli were the frequent findings in the blood vessels adjacent to sites of secondary tumors, indicating that the main route of metastases of malignant trophoblastic neoplasms is through blood circulation.

Clinico-Pathological Findings of Primary and Various Metastatic Foci

Primary tumor of the uterus and secondary tumor of parametrium. The primary tumor of the uterus was found in 90% of gestational malignant trophoblastic neoplasms. It appeared either as a single large mass bulging into the uterine cavity or as multiple foci invading the myometrium and serosa. Sometimes the above two types were present in the same specimen. On pathological examination a mass of necrotic tissue as well as hemorrhage was found in the center of the lesion. Massive infiltration of trophoblast was usually located at the junction between the tumor mass and the myometrium. Tumor cells were found frequently, invading the blood sinuses of the uterine wall (Fig. 1).

In the presence of primary uterine foci the ovarian and uterine veins were usually engorged. Large quantities of tumor cells and tumor emboli were frequently identified in the veins, giving an appearance of a grayish tortuous cord (Fig. 2). As the tumor cell mass in the uterine vein grew in size and penetrated through the vascular wall, the parametrial metastatic tumor was formed. This type of spreading was found in about 10% of the cases, including 41 cases of choriocarcinoma and 47 cases of invasive mole. Most of the lesions were unilateral. The continuous growth of the parametrial metastasis might result in a huge tumor mass extending either laterally to the pelvic wall or downward to the vaginal vault.

Vaginal metastases. Vaginal metastases occurred in 112 of 429 cases of choriocarcinoma (26.1%) and in 70 of 441 cases of invasive mole (15.9%). Most of the tumors were located at the lower part of the vagina, particularly beneath the anterior vaginal wall close to the external urethral meatus. Exceptions were 9 cases of choriocarcinoma and 5 cases of invasive mole, in which the tumors were in the fornices of the vagina. The lesions varied in size, and were either single or multiple. The metastasis usually began in the small vein of the submucous connective tissue. Upon microscopic

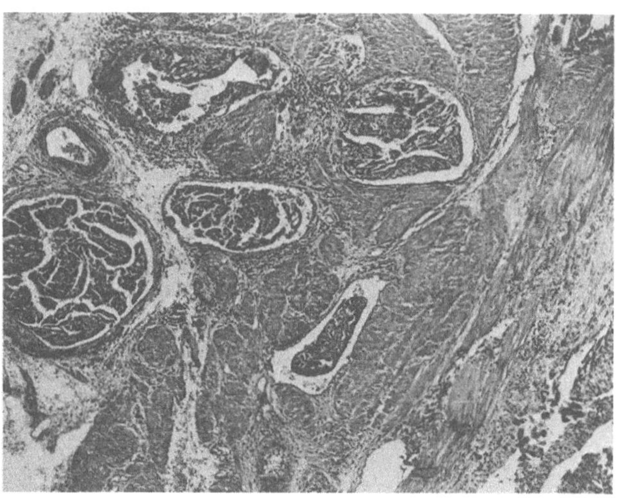

Fig. 1. Choriocarcinoma of the uterus. The blood sinuses of the myometrium are filled with tumor cells (x50).

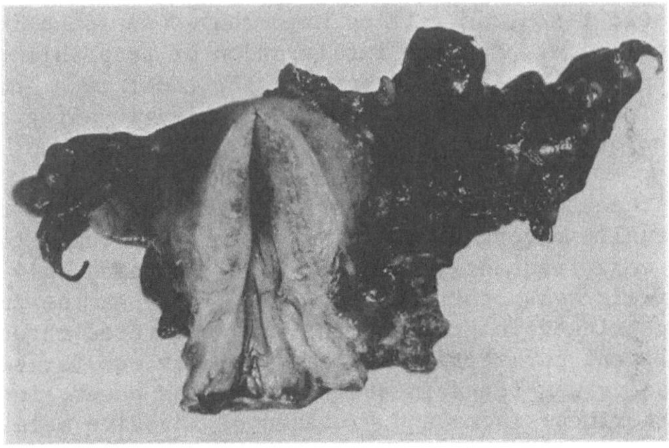

Fig. 2. Surgically removed uterus, revealing engorged uterine and ovarian veins with tumor emboli inside the vessels.

examination, the grain-sized nodules were found to be tumor emboli inside the dilated veins, while the larger nodules were formed from ruptured veins containing actively growing tumor cells (Fig. 3), usually with part of the wall of the vein still identifiable at the periphery of the tumor. All these observations indicate that the vaginal metastases are initiated from within the veins. Because of

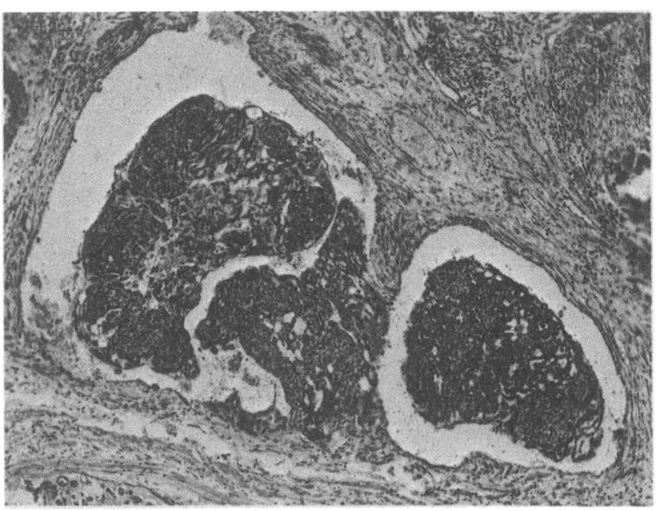

Fig. 3. Vaginal metastasis of choriocarcinoma. Tumor emboli are shown inside the dilated veins (x230).

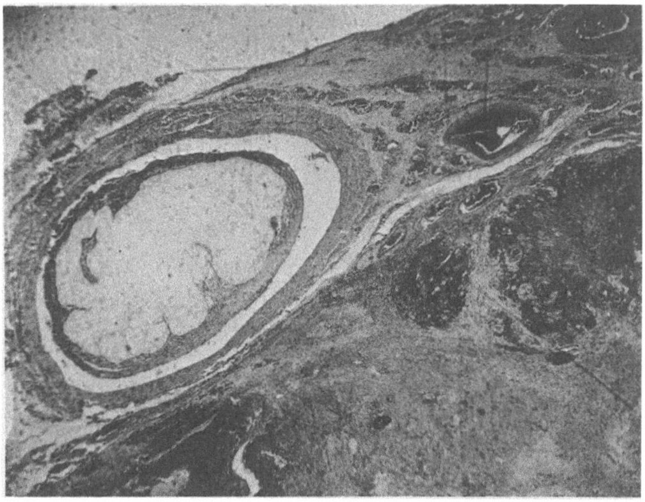

Fig. 4. Tumor emboli in the mesosalpingeal vein with degenerated villi (x125).

the frequently coexisting vaginal nodules and parametrial metastases it is possible that the tumor cells were carried to the veins of the vaginal wall retrograde to those located in the uterine veins, as a result of the blockage of the normal venous blood return.

Adnexal metastases. Metastases to the ovary were found in 4 cases, and metastases to both ovary and tube were found in one case. However, tumor emboli could be demonstrated in the ovarian veins or veins of the mesosalpinx (Fig. 4) in 25 cases of choriocarcinoma (5.8%) and in 5 cases of invasive mole (1.1%). This indicates that metastasis to uterine appendages also occurs mainly through the venous route.

Lung metastases. Pathological study of 64 cases of autopsies and 29 surgically removed specimens indicated that lung metastases began with the formation of tumor emboli in small pulmonary arteries. The continuous growth of tumor cells in the emboli caused local distention and subsequent rupture of the blood vessels, and infiltration of the adjacent lung tissues, resulting in the formation of pulmonary metastatic tumors (Fig. 5). This process could be clearly demonstrated by arteriography of the resected lung specimens. In early pulmonary metastases, showing patchy forms of shadows on the chest film, small irregular sacculations along the small arteries could be seen in the pulmonary arteriograph (Fig. 6). In certain advanced cases showing round form metastatic shadows on the chest film, pulmonary arteriography usually revealed embolic blockage of the terminal arteries (Fig. 7). Therefore, it is evident

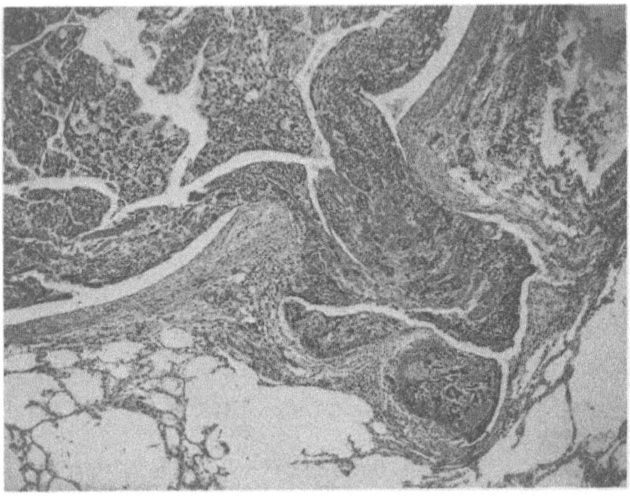

Fig. 5. Tumor emboli in small pulmonary arteries, showing erosion of blood vessels and invasion of parenchyma and alveoli by tumor cells (x50).

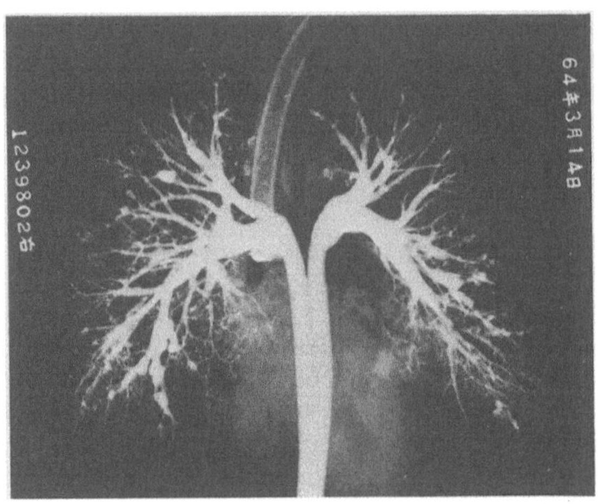

Fig. 6. Arteriograph of resected lung specimen showing irregular sacculation of arterial wall.

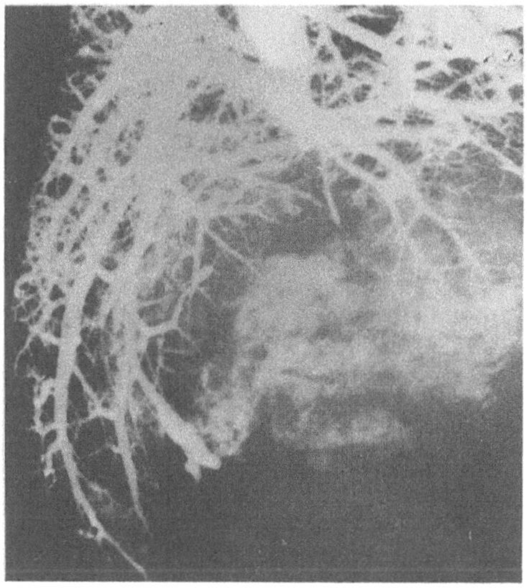

Fig. 7. Arteriograph of resected lung specimen showing drumstick-like enlargement at the end of the small arteries.

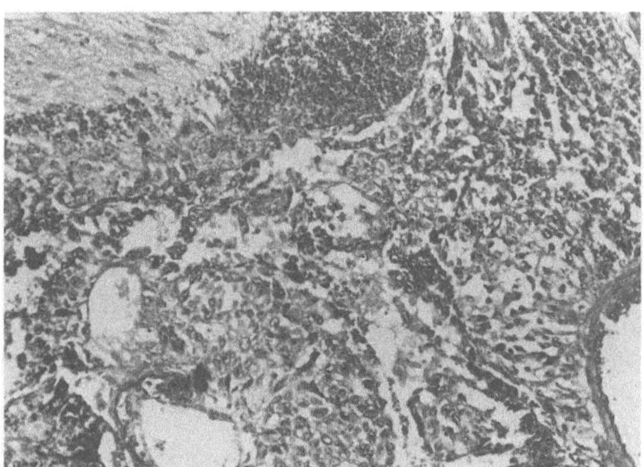

Fig. 8. Brain metastasis of choriocarcinoma. Tumor cells are found around the small arachnoid arteries (x125).

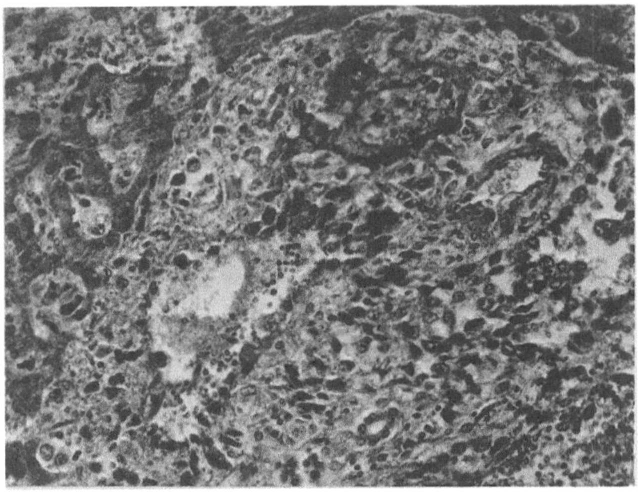

Fig. 9. Liver metastasis of choriocarcinoma. The lesions are located mainly in the periportal space surrounding the hepatic arteries (x250).

that metastases of malignant trophoblastic tumors to the lungs are initiated in the arterial system.

Brain metastases. In an analysis of 98 cases (4), all brain metastases were preceded by pulmonary metastases, without exception. Simultaneous spreading of the tumors to the liver, spleen, kidney, and other organs occurred in about 60% of the cases. Upon microscopic examination of 36 autopsy cases with brain metastases and 5 surgically removed specimens, tumor emboli could be demonstrated in the small arteries of arachnoid in small, early metastatic lesions. As the disease advanced, the tumor cells eroded the blood vessels and invaded into brain tissues, thus resulting in hemorrhage and tumor formation (Fig. 8). The above findings indicate that brain metastasis is secondary to pulmonary metastasis and that tumor cells are carried to the brain through the arterial route via the general circulation.

Liver metastases. Liver metastases occurred in 48 of 429 cases of choriocarcinoma (11.2%), but in none among 441 cases of invasive mole. The reason for the latter is still obscure. As in the case of brain metastases, liver metastases were also invariably preceded by pulmonary metastases. As the early lesions always started in the periportal space and arterial embolism was frequent, it is reasonable to assume that the main route of metastasis to the liver is also through the arterial blood flow (Fig. 9).

Other metastases. Less frequent were metastases to the kidney (33 cases), spleen (30 cases), and gastrointestinal tract (23 cases). These metastases occurred exclusively in patients with choriocarcinoma, and were invariably preceded by pulmonary metastases. Pathological examination of 26 cases of splenic metastasis revealed trophoblastic invasion of the central arteries of the Malpighian bodies of the spleen (Fig. 10), with partial destruction of the vascular wall in 5 early cases and acute infarction without apparent embolism of the arteries in another 5.

In 23 cases of renal metastasis examined pathologically, trophoblastic embolism was found in the glomerulus of 5 early cases (Fig. 11). In 2 cases, infarction and hemorrhage without apparent arterial embolism were found.

In 18 cases of gastrointestinal metastasis, trophoblastic embolism was found in the mesenteric arteries in 5 cases and in the arteries of the submucous layer of the intestine in 11 cases (Fig. 12).

Therefore, the discovery of tumor emboli in small arteries in early cases also indicates that metastases to these organs are mainly initiated in the arterial system.

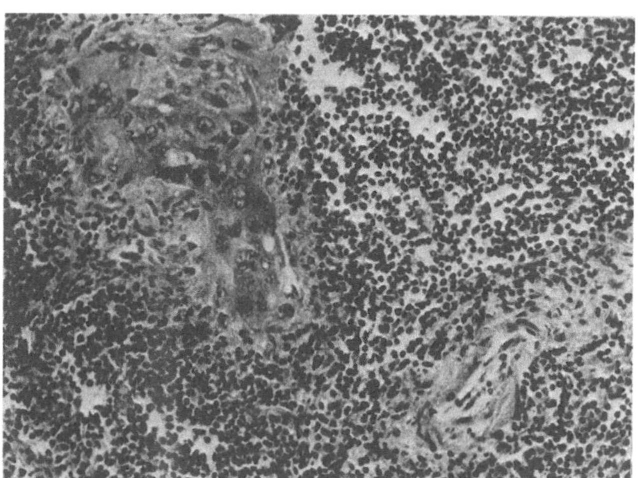

Fig. 10. Spleen metastasis of choriocarcinoma. Tumor emboli are found in the central arteries of the Malpighian body (x250).

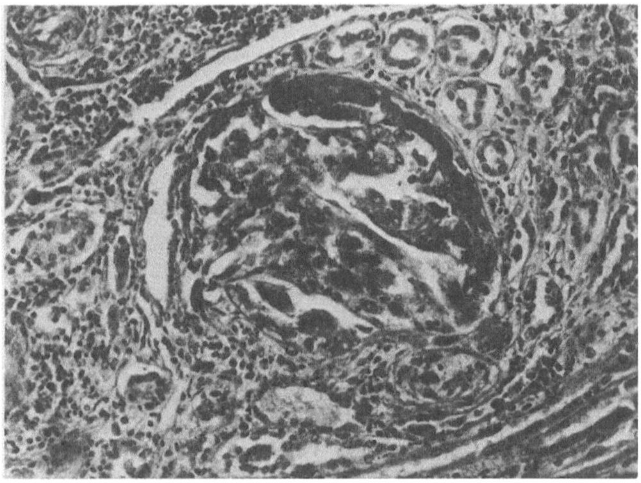

Fig. 11. Kidney metastasis of choriocarcinoma. Tumor emboli are found in the glomerulus (x250).

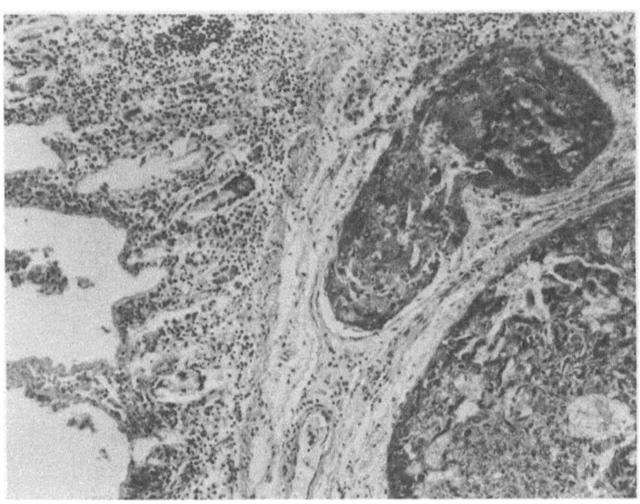

Fig. 12. Intestinal metastasis of choriocarcinoma. Tumor emboli are found in the small submucosal arteries (x125).

Process of Development of Malignant Trophoblastic Neoplasms and Criteria of Clinical Staging

On the basis of unequivocal clinico-pathological evidence, the process of development of malignant trophoblastic tumors can be summarized as in Fig. 13. In almost all gestational trophoblastic tumors, the lesions begin in the uterus and spread widely in a short period of time. The spreading is almost exclusively through the

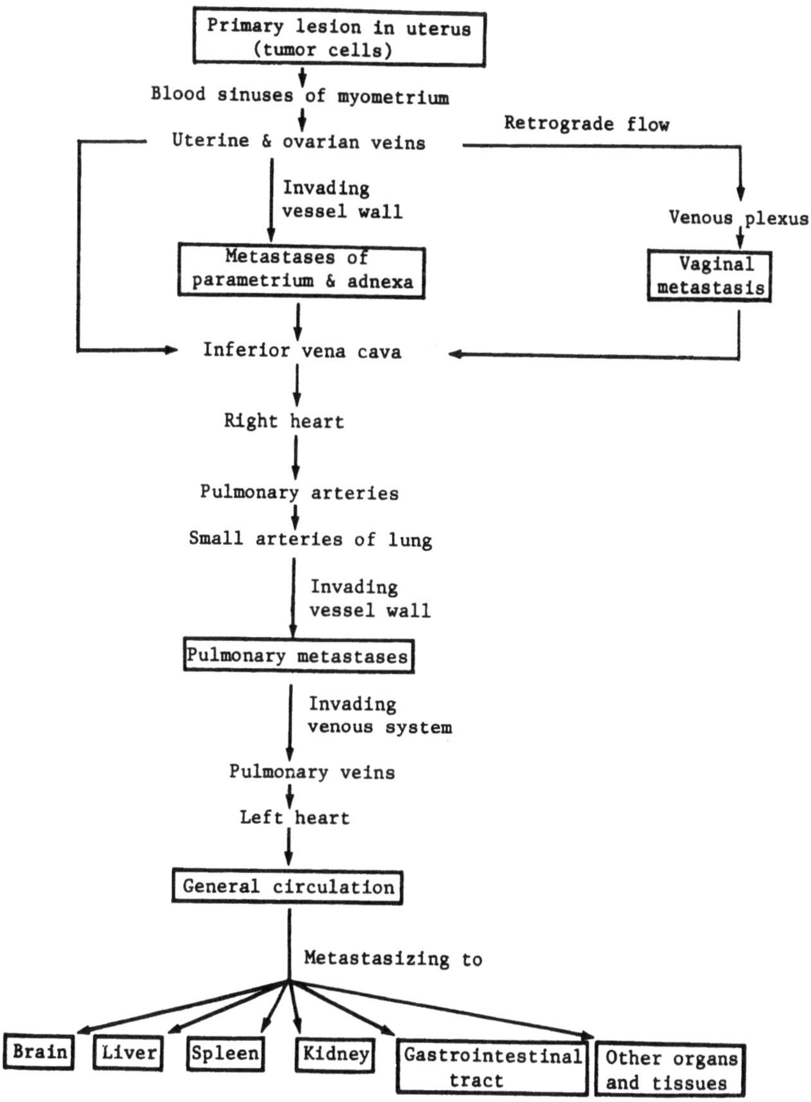

Fig. 13. Diagram showing route of spreading and process of development of malignant trophoblastic neoplasms.

blood stream. The tumor cells invade the blood sinuses of the myometrium first, and then gain access to the uterine or ovarian veins or both, in which tumor emboli are frequently formed. On further development, the tumor cells may penetrate the wall of the vein and invade the parametrium or adnexa to form metastatic lesions in the respective tissues and organs. In some cases, the tumor cells may be transported in retrograde fashion into the venous plexus of the vaginal wall, resulting in formation of tumor emboli and vaginal metastasis. When the tumor cells are dislodged from the primary uterine or secondary pelvic lesions, they are transported along the venous blood flow via the right heart to the pulmonary arteries, resulting in embolism of the arterioles and subsequent metastasis of the lungs.

After remaining in the lungs for different periods of time, the tumor cells finally invade the venous system, move to the left side of the heart and aorta, and disseminate through the general circulation to any part of the body, giving rise to generalized metastases. During the process of development the parametrial, adnexal, and vaginal metastases were almost always initiated in the veins and may thus be designated as "venous metastases". On the other hand, metastases to the lungs, brain, liver, spleen, kidney, and other organs usually begin in the arteries of these organs and may be designated as "arterial metastases". The difference in the nature of these two types of metastasis is obvious.

In addition, a marked difference was observed between pulmonary metastases and generalized metastases in the sequence of occurrence. Prospective and retrospective study of the clinico-pathological data showed that the generalized metastases were invariably preceded by pulmonary metastases. Furthermore, had there been no lung metastases, metastases to the brain, liver, kidney, spleen, and gastrointestinal tract would never have occurred.

In summary, the whole process of development of malignant trophoblastic neoplasms may be clearly divided into 4 steps: 1) primary disease in the uterus without metastasis; 2) venous metastasis to genital organs; 3) arterial metastasis to the lungs; and 4) generalized metastasis. Based on these observations, we propose a clinical staging system corresponding to the 4 steps of development, as shown in Fig. 14.

When the lesion is confined to the uterus, it is categorized as Stage I. When the lesion has extended outside the uterus but is still confined to the genital organs, it is defined as Stage II. When the lesion has extended to the parametrium or the adnexa on one or both sides, it is defined as Stage IIA; if it has metastasized to the vagina it is defined as Stage IIB. If the tumor spreads to the lungs, it is categorized as Stage III. Because the clinical course, treatment, and prognosis vary with the size and

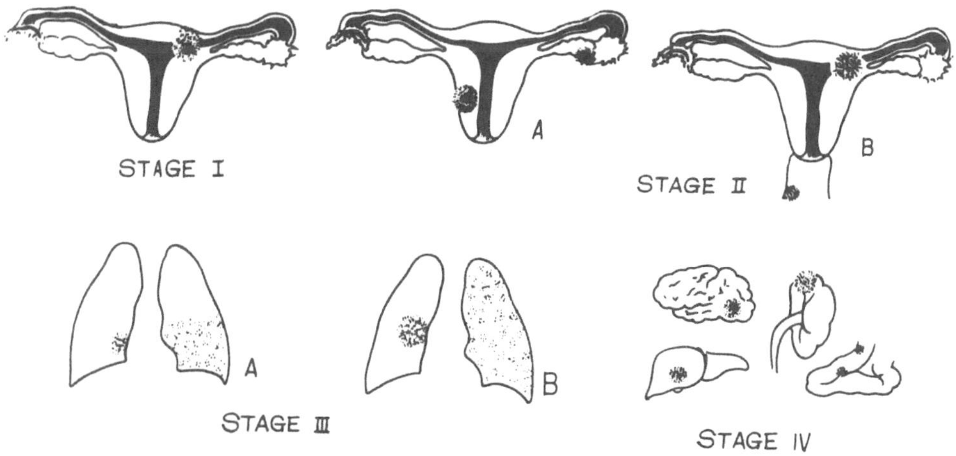

Fig. 14. Diagram showing criteria of clinical staging.

extent of the pulmonary metastases seen on the chest films, Stage III is further divided into substages. Substage IIIA denotes patchy shadows or ball-like shadows not exceeding 3 cm in diameter, while IIIB denotes ball-like shadows exceeding 3.0 cm. When the tumor develops into generalized metastases and spreads to organs such as brain, liver, kidney, spleen, gastrointestinal tract and the like, it is categorized as Stage IV.

DISCUSSION

The extent of disease is generally decided on the basis of the results of clinical studies on admission. These include symptoms, signs, hCG radioimmunoassay, roentgenography of the chest, ultrasonic and isotopic scanning of the liver, and other procedures. Nevertheless, some early minimal lesions may still be missed regardless of painstaking investigation. Therefore, if a patient undergoes operation or dies soon after admission (i.e., within two weeks), the staging should be revised according to exploratory or autopsy findings. For example, if the lesion of a patient is categorized as Stage IIIB on admission but liver metastasis is revealed during subsequent laparotomy, the staging should revised to Stage IV. If this information is obtained later than 2 weeks after admission, however, no re-staging should be made because of the possible progression of disease during this period.

Through years of clinical use, it has been found that this staging system for malignant trophoblastic neoplasms has the following advantages over other staging methods. First, the staging system describes clearly and concisely the degree of development of the disease and is easily understood. Second, the criteria of the staging system are simple, easy to handle, and can be favorably used for the selection of appropriate therapeutic regimen and for comparison of clinical materials from different sources. Third, the staging system bears a close relationship to the prognosis of the disease: the later the staging, the worse the prognosis (2). This relationship holds regardless of the dramatic improvement in therapeutic results achieved in recent years.

Based on our long-term clinical experience, some remarks should be made about certain special conditions. For instance, during the process of development of the disease certain complications may occur, such as hemothorax or massive hemoptysis in the case of pulmonary metastases, or hematoma in the pelvis following rupture of parametrial tumors. These complications may deteriorate the general condition of the patient and exert unfavorable effects on the prognosis, and so should be noted during staging. Next, in the present staging system patients with lung metastasis as well as those with both pulmonary and pelvic metastases are categorized alike under Stage III. We recommend further differentiating the latter group by noting the site of pelvic metastasis (e.g., Stage IIIA-vagina, Stage IIIB-parametrium). Finally, because the prognosis may vary with site of metastasis in Stage IV patients, we suggest that the organ(s) involved be noted at the time of staging (e.g., Stage IV-liver, Stage IV-kidney and spleen).

REFERENCES

1. Sung, H. C., Wu, P. C., and Ho, T. H., Treatment of choriocarcinoma and chorioadenoma destruens with 6MP and surgery, in: "Selected Papers on Cancer Research," edited by the Chinese Academy of Medical Sciences, Shanghai Sci. Tech. Publ. (1962), p. 441. Republished in Acta Unio International Contra Cancerum 20:493 (1964).
2. Sung, H. C., Hsia, T. F., Wu, P. C., and Wang, Y. E., 20 years experience in chemotherapy of choriocarcinoma and malignant mole, Chinese Medical Journal 92:677 (1979).
3. Sung, H. C., Wu, P. C., Hu, M. H., and Su, H. T., Roentgenological manifestations of pulmonary metastases in choriocarcinoma and invasive mole, based on a study of 3915 chest films, Amer. J. Obstet. Gynecol., In Press.
4. Sung, H. C. and Wu, P. C., Brain metastasis in choriocarcinoma and malignant mole, a study of 98 cases, Chinese Medical Journal 92:164 (1979).

CHEMOTHERAPY AND CLINICAL MANAGEMENT

Chemotherapy of the trophoblastic neoplasms was initiated by Li and Hertz, and has been expanded beyond the initial single agent, methotrexate, to more and more specific management schedules. Methotrexate remains the first drug of choice for trophoblast neoplasms, particularly with the safety of high-dose methotrexate and leucovorum factor rescue. This capacity to protect the patient from toxicity of methotrexate made the administration of this drug far more tolerable than at any time in the past. This is a distinct advantage of its use. At the same time, multi-agent chemotherapy has been developed and is used effectively in many of the regimens outlined in the chapters that follow. A comprehension of mechanism of action of the assorted drugs combined in multi-agent protocols -- to be outlined in the following chapters -- will give the reader insight into the great diversity to be found among trophoblastic tumors. At the same time, a constant awareness of this fact must be kept in mind in order to be prepared for the rapid development of resistance frequently observed in the treatment of these neoplasms.

THE ROLE OF METHOTREXATE IN THE CHEMOTHERAPY OF GESTATIONAL TROPHOBLASTIC NEOPLASMS

Alberto Sobrero and Joseph R. Bertino*

Departments of Pharmacology and Medicine
Yale University
School of Medicine
333 Cedar Street
New Haven, Connecticut 06510, USA

INTRODUCTION

The successful use of methotrexate in metastatic choriocarcinoma in 1956 (1) marked a milestone in the history of curative cancer chemotherapy. The survival of patients with widespread disease increased from 10% in the pre-chemotherapy era (2) to 47% in 1961 (3), 74% in 1965 (4), and to about 90% at the present time (5-7). These improvements in survival resulted from improved chemotherapeutic regimens for a disease which presents certain unique features. Methotrexate has played a central role in these regimens, most of the time being the only drug used. The work of centers for the study and treatment of gestational trophoblastic neoplasms, established in the mid-1960s, has also contributed to the more rational use of this drug as new knowledge of clinical pharmacology was developed (8). In this paper, drug treatment for gestational trophoblastic neoplasms is reviewed, with emphasis on the use of methotrexate.

Unique Features of Gestational Trophoblastic Neoplasms

The peculiar characteristics of this tumor must not be underestimated as determinants of successful chemotherapy. First, the conventional criteria for malignancy are very difficult to apply to any form of trophoblastic growth (9). Second, "gestational choriocarcinoma is a tumor of one individual that invades the tissues of another" (10), therefore the host immune response may theoretically

*American Cancer Society Professor

be directed against not only tumor-associated antigens, but also against histocompatibility antigens. Third, all trophoblastic tumors secrete human chorionic gonadotropin (hCG) which has been defined as "the ideal tumor marker" (11), because of the correlation between its level in the serum and the number of viable tumor cells (12). Lastly, the rapidly proliferating cells of this tumor are uniquely sensitive to methotrexate and to actinomycin D.

Definitions and Pathologic Considerations

Gestational trophoblastic neoplasms include hydatidiform mole, invasive mole, and choriocarcinoma. Persistent trophoblastic disease indicates the presence of more or less differentiated trophoblastic tissue in the body which occurs after a molar pregnancy in 50% of cases, after a normal pregnancy in 25% of cases, or after an abortion or ectopic gestation in 25% (13). The majority (80%) of persistent trophoblastic disease cases regress spontaneously, usually within 2 or 3 months. This elimination is likely the result of the balance between tumor aggressiveness and host defenses (14). In the other 20% of cases the disease remains localized to the uterus (15%) or metastasizes (5%) to lungs (80%), vagina (30%), pelvis (20%), brain (10%), bowel, kidney and spleen (<5%)(13). Invasive mole is more frequently found in localized persistent trophoblastic disease, and choriocarcinoma in widespread disease, but the opposite may occur in a significant number of women. However, even if the importance of histopathology in determining the prognosis of persistent trophoblastic disease treated with hysterectomy was clear in the past, since the advent of methotrexate this distinction is no longer of crucial importance, because both forms are now primarily treated with chemotherapy (5).

Historical Aspects of Chemotherapy Use in Gestational Trophoblastic Neoplasms

In the early 1950s it was well known that adequate dietary intake of folic acid was necessary for normal embryonal development and growth of the female genital tract in the rat (15, 16), and that the ingestion of methotrexate markedly reduced the estrogen-induced growth of the chick oviduct (17). These observations, along with the experimental (18) and clinical (19) evidence of the embryotoxic effects of aminopterin, constituted the theoretical background for the use of methotrexate in the first patients with bleeding pulmonary metastasis from choriocarcinoma in 1956 (1). Methotrexate was initially given in two single intravenous injections and then in five fractionated courses orally and intramuscularly over the following two months with complete remission. This initial success was followed by other reports on the cure of metastatic choriocarcinoma with methotrexate (20, 21), and its use was successfully extended to patients with limited disease, allowing them to preserve their reproductive potential (22). Two problems became evident soon: resistance and toxicity. Despite the almost invariable initial response to methotrexate, demonstrated by a fall in the hCG titer, prolonged complete remission was achieved in only 50% of patients with metastatic disease (3). The biological similarities of gestational choriocarcinoma with testicular choriocarcinoma and the effectiveness of the combination of methotrexate, actinomycin D and chlorambucil (MAC)(23), led investigators at the National Cancer Institute to study actinomycin D initially on 13 women who were resistant to methotrexate (24), and then as the primary agent (25). Its efficacy was equal to that of methotrexate, and cross-resistance was not observed regardless of the sequence of administration of the two drugs (4). The result was the introduction of sequential use of actinomycin D and methotrexate with a 74% complete remission rate. The developing principles of combination chemotherapy of those years were applied also to gestational trophoblastic neoplasms (26). The antimetabolite, 6-mercaptopurine, known to be toxic on fetal tissues (23), was introduced in combination with methotrexate, and chlorambucil was added in case of resistance to these drugs (26). Subsequently this triple regimen was shown to be useful in patients with choriocarcinoma no longer responsive to methotrexate (27). Toxicity of methotrexate was severe, with a 10% drug-related mortality rate in the first ten-year experience (27). In addition, when combined agents were given to patients whose reserves had been depleted by several courses of single agent chemotherapy, mortality was as high as 30% with a disappointing remission rate of less than 20% (7, 27). The very high (95-100%) percentage of cases with limited disease cured with single-agent chemotherapy on one hand (8, 28), the very low response rate of resistant patients to additional more potent regimens on the other hand, and the overall significant toxicity of chemotherapy, induced investigators to focus on individualization of therapy. This concept emerged from the observation that a successful response to chemotherapy was dependent on certain prognostic variables identified as the "age" of the tumor, as measured by duration of the disease prior to the onset of chemotherapy, the pretreatment level of the serum hCG titer, and the presence or absence of widespread metastasis (4). The recognition of these factors led to a new classification of gestational trophoblastic neoplasm which was no longer based on morphologic criteria, but separated gestational trophoblastic neoplasms into nonmetastatic and metastatic disease, with the latter group subsequently divided into low and high risk (10, 29).

According to this staging system, Hammond (29) treated low-risk patients with either methotrexate (15-25 mg intramuscularly each day for five days per course), or actinomycin D (10 to 13 micrograms per kg intravenously, daily for five days per course), obtaining a complete remission in 70 of 71 patients. Ten patients in the high-risk group were treated initially with the MAC regimen while 7 other high-risk patients were given the triple regimen only after failure of single agent chemotherapy. Seven patients of the former group were cured, while only one of the latter group survived; drug toxicity was much more severe in this group as well. These data, confirmed by subsequent studies (28, 30), led to a new crucial therapeutic concept: intensive chemotherapeutic regimens are more effective and less toxic if given to patients with high-risk disease as primary therapy. The above-mentioned classification has been recently modified to the present form of staging of gestational trophoblastic neoplasms (Table 1)(13). In addition, several other prognostic factors have been identified (10, 31), promoting a system of mathematical quantitation of the patient's risk for failure of treatment (10, 13) (Table 2). This approach has resulted in a further individualization of treatment and in the development of multi-drug regimens for more aggressive treatment of high-risk patients.

Methotrexate with Leucovorin "Rescue"

Despite the emergence of these regimens, reserved for high-risk patients in Stage II, III, and IV, the great majority of women with gestational trophoblastic neoplasms still benefit from single agent chemotherapy with methotrexate. The importance of methotrexate in this field has increased even more since the introduction of the "rescue" with citrovorum factor (32). Initially suggested in 1969 (33), this regimen subsequently appeared to be as effective as methotrexate alone, actinomycin D alone, or the sequence of the two drugs (3, 4, 34). Furthermore, methotrexate with citrovorum factor rescue (MTX-CF) has been demonstrated to reduce the number of courses necessary to induce complete remission (55, 56) in comparison to methotrexate without citrovorum factor (27, 34) or actinomycin (25) and, most importantly, the moderate to severe hematological, epithelial, or hepatic toxicity of the two drugs is significantly lower in patients receiving MTX-CF (35).

Table 1. Staging of Gestational Trophoblastic Neoplasms[a]

Stage	Characteristics
0	Molar pregnancy
A	Low-risk
B	High-risk
I	Confined to uterine corpus
II	Metastases to pelvis and vagina
III	Metastases to lung
IV	Distant metastases

[a]From reference 13.

Table 2. Risk Factors in Gestational Trophoblastic Neoplasms

	Prognostic score[a]			
Risk factor	0	1	2	3
Antecedent pregnancy	Hydatidiform mole	Nonmole abortion; ectopic	Term pregnancy	
Interval in months between end of antecedent pregnancy and initial therapy	<3	3-6	7-12	>12
hCG value (mIU/ml) at time of initial therapy	<10	10^3-10^4	10^4-10^5	>10^5
ABO blood group of patients			A or AB	
Largest tumor (cm)	<2		2-5	>5
Site of metastasis		Lung	GI tract; kidney; spleen	Brain; liver
Number of metastases identified		1-4	4-8	>8
Previous chemotherapy			Failed prophylactic chemotherapy	Failed therapeutic chemotherapy

[a]From reference 13.

Quite recently, a retrospective study of 58 patients with gestational trophoblastic neoplasia confirmed this last observation, but the direct comparison of activity of methotrexate alone *vs* MTX-CF favored the drug without rescue (36). Despite this latest report, because of its low toxicity MTX-CF is now recommended as the first line of treatment for all patients in Stage I and for low risk women in Stage II or Stage III (13, 37).

Table 3. Treatment of Patients with GTN[a] with Various Therapeutic Regimens: Summary of Results

Regimen	Year	Patients No.	Patients %CCA	Remission %	Final % remission	Reference
Nonmetastatic GTN						
MTX	1967	58	28	93	99	34
MTX or ACT	1970	29		89	100	27
MAC	1971	80	24	100	100	8
ACT	1975	31	10	94	100	25
MTX-CF	1978	35	9	91	100	55
MTX-CF	1979	41		88	100	56
MTX-CF	1982	29		72	100	36
MTX	1982	39		92	100	36
Metastatic GTN: All Patients						
MTX(VLB)	1961	63	70	47	47	3
MTX or ACT	1965	50	58	74	74	4
ACT	1975	39	46	67	82	25
MAC	1971	71	75	(87)	87	8
Various agents	1982	29	83	48	(48)	7
Metastatic GTN: Low-Risk Patients						
MTX or ACT	1970	27		77	100	27
MTX or ACT	1973	79		91	98	29
MTX or ACT	1982	95		87	100	38

[a]Abbreviations: GTN, gestational trophoblastic neoplasms; MTX, methotrexate; ACT, actinomycin D; MAC, triple therapy with methotrexate, actinomycin D, and cyclophosphamide, used after failure with methotrexate and actinomycin D as single agents; MTX-CF, methotrexate with citrovorum factor rescue; VLB, vinca leucoblastine; CCA, choriocarcinoma.

Current Therapeutic Regimens for Low-Risk Patients

A comparison of results of different regimens for metastatic and nonmetastatic disease is shown in Table 3. Remission rates are generally lower in those patients with histologically documented choriocarcinoma as opposed to invasive mole, but the importance of histology in influencing the outcome of therapy remains an unsettled matter (5, 7). Actinomycin D is preferred to MTX-CF only when liver function tests are abnormal at the time of pretreatment evaluation (25), while hysterectomy, although equally effective as the former two drugs (13), is suggested as initial therapy only for patients who no longer wish to preserve fertility. In this latter circumstance, one course of MTX-CF at the time of surgery is recommended (38). The still controversial rationale for this approach lies mainly on the prevention of dissemination of viable tumor cells at surgery (39). For the same reason, any surgical procedure aimed at elimination of resistant tumor foci in resectable sites should be performed under appropriate cover of chemotherapy (40, 41). The small percentage of patients resistant to single agent chemotherapy or hysterectomy uniformly respond well to treatment with multi-agent therapy; the cure rate for these patients is now around 100% (41, 42).

The use of prophylactic chemotherapy at the time of molar evacuation is still highly controversial. The rationale for its use (39), and several reports on lower incidence of gestational trophoblastic disease in patients prophylactically treated with MTX (50-52) or actinomycin D (53), seem to favor this approach. However, substantial drug toxicity and the danger of selecting resistant cells are arguments against prophylactic chemotherapy (54).

Treatment of High-Risk Patients

The role of methotrexate in the management of patients in Stage IV and high-risk Stage II and III is limited to its contribution to the multi-agent regimens (Table 4). The seven-drug protocol, CHAMOCA (41), and its modification (42), were developed as an alternative to the widely used MAC program. These combination programs may be used as second line of treatment in patients after failure of previous regimens (13), or as initial chemotherapy for high-risk patients (40, 41). Quite recently, Surwit suggested a further modification employing *cis*-platinum and bleomycin in place of cytoxan and adriamycin, and claimed it is particularly valuable for patients who can no longer receive the seven-drug regimen because of chronic marrow suppression (40).

The combination of MTX-CF, high-dose *cis*-platinum (120 mg/m^2), and vincristine was reported to induce complete response in 35% of patients who failed CHAMOCA (43). Vinblastine, bleomycin, and *cis*-platinum have shown encouraging results in two patients resistant to MAC (44). VP 16-213 is also being evaluated alone or integrated in the above protocols (41, 45). These regimens have warranted some improvement in response rate, but this has been achieved at the cost of severe toxicity (25% incidence of severe pancytopenia and sepsis) (40). Nevertheless, the recurrence rate for patients at highest risk still remains close to 100% (10). This group of women may still benefit from special uses of methotrexate in certain particular situations. Development of central nervous system and liver metastasis is a very bad prognostic sign which almost invariably leads to death (46). Bagshawe (41) reported that the CHAMOCA

Table 4. Treatment of High-Risk Patients with Metastases

Regimen[a]	Year	No. patients	% Remission	Ref.
MAC initially	1973	10	70	29
MAC after failure of MTX, ACT	1973	7	14	29
MAC, CHAMOCA, VP-BC	1979	51	72	42
MAC after failure of MTX and/or ACT	1982	18	17	7
VP-16 alternating with CHAMOCA	1982	40	Too early	41
MTX-CF, Plat-HD, VCR	1982	24	33	45
VP-16 (previously treated patients)	1982	37	19	45

[a]New abbreviations: Plat-HD, high-dose *cis*-platinum; VCR, vincristine; CHAMOCA, cyclophosphamide, hydroxyurea, adriamycin, methotrexate, oncovin, citrovorum factor, and actinomycin D; VP-BC, VP-16, bleomycin, and *cis*-platinum.

regimen combined with a high level of methotrexate in the cerebrospinal fluid obtained by either intrathecal administration (12.5 mg each course) or high-dose (greater than 1 g/m^2) systemic methotrexate induced sustained complete remission in 7 of 12 patients with cerebral metastasis. Because the patients who died developed central nervous system metastasis while under treatment, Bagshawe advocates the prophylactic intrathecal administration of methotrexate to patients who are at high risk to develop central nervous system metastasis during systemic treatment. Other authors (46, 47) do not recognize the value of prophylactic intrathecal administration of methotrexate or its role as first line of treatment of central nervous system metastasis. Rather, they suggest the combination of radiotherapy (3000 R whole brain irradiation) and intensive systemic chemotherapy, reporting response rates of 62% (47), 50% (46), and 43% (48).

When liver metastases fail to respond to multi-agent chemotherapy, methotrexate alone or in combination with actinomycin D has been locally infused via a hepatic artery catheter (27, 49), but this approach is not at present included in the standard guidelines of management of advanced choriocarcinoma.

CONCLUSIONS

While more effective regimens are still needed in the treatment of the advanced stages of gestational trophoblastic neoplasms, choriocarcinoma remains the best example of curability of human malignancies with drugs. The successful use of chemotherapy in this disease has provided guidelines to the use of drug therapy in other cancers, and the principles established for treatment of this disease have had a major impact on cancer treatment in general.

ACKNOWLEDGEMENT

This work was supported by USPHS Grants CA-08010 and CA-08341.

REFERENCES

1. Li, M. C., Hertz, R., and Spencer, D. B., Effect of methotrexate therapy upon choriocarcinoma and chorioadenoma, Proc. Soc. Exptl. Biol. Med. 93:361 (1956).
2. Brewer, J. I., Smith, R. T., and Pratt, G. B., Choriocarcinoma, absolute 5 year survival rates of 122 patients treated by hysterectomy, Amer. J. Obstet. Gynecol. 85:841 (1963).
3. Hertz, R., Lewis, J., Jr., and Lipsett, M. B., Five years experience with the chemotherapy of metastatic choriocarcinoma and related trophoblastic tumors in women, Amer. J. Obstet. Gynecol. 82:631 (1961).
4. Ross, G. T., Goldstein, D. P., Hertz, R., Lipsett, M. B., and Odell, W. D., Sequential use of methotrexate and actinomycin D in the treatment of metastatic choriocarcinoma and related trophoblastic diseases in women, Amer. J. Obstet. Gynecol. 93: 223 (1965).
5. Lewis, J. L., Jr., Treatment of metastatic gestational trophoblastic neoplasms, Amer. J. Obstet. Gynecol. 136:163 (1980).
6. Newlands, E. S. and Bagshawe, K. D., International symposium on gestational trophoblastic tumours, Brit. J. Cancer 41:144 (1980).
7. Lurain, J. R., Brewer, J. I., Torok, E. E., and Halpern, B., Gestational trophoblastic disease: treatment results at the Brewer Trophoblastic Disease Center, Obstet. Gynecol. 60:354 (1982).
8. Brewer, J. I., Eckman, T. R., Dolkart, R. E., Torok, E. E., and Webster, A., Gestational trophoblastic disease. A comparative study of the results of therapy in patients with invasive

mole and with choriocarcinoma, Amer. J. Obstet. Gynecol. 109: 335 (1971).
9. Hreshchyshyn, M. M., Trophoblastic neoplasia, in: "Cancer Medicine," J. F. Holland and E. Frei, eds., Lea and Febiger, Philadelphia (1981).
10. Bagshawe, K. D., Risk and prognostic factors in trophoblastic neoplasia, Cancer 38:1373 (1976).
11. Jones, W. B., Gestational trophoblastic disease: Is human chorionic gonadotropin the ideal tumor marker: in: "Gynecologic Oncology," S. C. Ballon, ed., G. K. Hall, Boston (1982).
12. Lewis, J. L., Jr., Chemotherapy of gestational choriocarcinoma, Cancer 30:1517 (1972).
13. Goldstein, D. P. and Berkowitz, R. S., Management of gestational trophoblastic neoplasms, Curr. Probl. Obstet. Gynecol. 3:1 (1980).
14. Pattillo, R. A., Immunology of gestational trophoblastic neoplasms, Semin. Oncol. 9:157 (1982).
15. Nelson, M. M., and Evans, H. M., Pteroylglutamic acid and reproduction in the rat, J. Nutr. 38:11 (1948).
16. Hertz, R. and Tullner, W. W., Quantitative interference with estrogen-induced tissue growth by folic acid antagonists, Endocrinology 44:278 (1949).
17. Hertz, R., Interference with estrogen-induced tissue growth in the chick genital tract by a folic acid antagonist, Science 107:300 (1948).
18. Thiersh, J. B. and Phillips, F. S., Effect of 4-amino pteroylglutamic acid (aminopterin) on early pregnancy, Proc. Soc. Exptl. Biol. Med. 74:204 (1950).
19. Thiersh, J. B. and Phillips, F. S., Therapeutic abortion with a folic acid antagonist, 4-amino pteroylglutamic acid administered by oral route, Amer. J. Obstet. Gynecol. 63: 1298 (1952).
20. Li, M. C., Hertz, R., and Bergenstal, D. M., Therapy of choriocarcinoma and related trophoblastic tumors with folic acid and purine antagonists, New Engl. J. Med. 239:66 (1958).
21. Hertz, R., Bergenstal, D. M., Lipsett, M. B., Parke, E. B., and Hilbish, T. F., Chemotherapy of choriocarcinoma and related tumors in women, J. Amer. Med. Assoc. 168:845 (1958).
22. Hertz, R., Ross, G. T., and Lipsett, M. B., Primary chemotherapy of nonmetastatic trophoblastic disease in women, Amer. J. Obstet. Gynecol. 86:808 (1963).
23. Li, M. C., Management of choriocarcinoma and related tumors of uterus and testis, Med. Clin. North Amer. 45:661 (1961).
24. Ross, G. T., Stolbach, L. L., and Hertz, R., Actinomycin D in the treatment of methotrexate-resistant trophoblastic disease in women, Cancer Res. 22:1015 (1962).
25. Osathanondth, R., Goldstein, D. P., and Pastorfide, G. B., Actinomycin D as the primary agent for gestational trophoblastic disease, Cancer 36:863 (1975).

26. Bagshawe, K. D. and McDonald, J. M., Treatment of choriocarcinoma with a combination of cytotoxic drugs, Brit. Med. J. 426 (1960).
27. Hammond, C. B. and Parker, R. T., Diagnosis and treatment of trophoblastic disease, Obstet. Gynecol. 35:132 (1970).
28. Goldstein, D. P., The chemotherapy of gestational trophoblastic disease, J. Amer. Med. Assoc. 220:209 (1972).
29. Hammond, C. B., Borchert, L. G., Tyrey, L., Creasman, W. T., and Parker, R. T., Treatment of metastatic trophoblastic disease: good and poor prognosis, Amer. J. Obstet. Gynecol. 115:451 (1973).
30. Jones, W. B. and Lewis, J. L., Jr., Treatment of gestational trophoblastic disease, Amer. J. Obstet. Gynecol. 120:14 (1974).
31. Miller, J. M., Surwit, E. A., and Hammond, C. B., Choriocarcinoma following term pregnancy, Obstet. Gynecol. 53:207 (1979).
32. Djerassi, I., Methotrexate infusions and intensive supportive care in the management of children with acute lymphocytic leukemia: Follow up report, Cancer Res. 27:2561 (1967).
33. Bagshawe, K. D., "Choriocarcinoma," Edward Arnold, Ltd., London (1969).
34. Hammond, C. B., Hertz, R., Ross, G. T., Lipsett, M. B., and Odell, W. D., Primary chemotherapy for nonmetastatic gestational trophoblastic neoplasms, Amer. J. Obstet. Gynecol. 98:71 (1967).
35. Berkowitz, R. S., Goldstein, D. P., Miles, J. A., Marean, A. R., and Bernstein, M. R., Methotrexate with citrovorum factor rescue, Cancer 45:423 (1980).
36. Smith, E. B., Weed, J. C., Tyrey, L., and Hammond, C. B., Treatment of nonmetastatic gestational trophoblastic disease: Results of methotrexate alone versus methotrexate-folinic acid, Amer. J. Obstet. Gynecol. 144:88 (1982).
37. Perez, C. A., Knapp, R. C., and Young, R. C., Trophoblastic tumors, in: "Cancer Principles and Practice of Oncology," V. T. DeVita, Jr., S. Hellman, and S. A. Rosenberg, eds., Lippincott, Philadelphia (1982).
38. Goldstein, D. P. and Berkowitz, R. S., Non-metastatic and low risk metastatic gestational trophoblastic neoplasms, Semin. Oncol. 9:191 (1982).
39. Lewis, J., Jr., Gore, H., Hertig, A. T., and Goss, D. A., Treatment of trophoblastic disease, Amer. J. Obstet. Gynecol. 96:710 (1966).
40. Surwit, E. A., The management of poor prognosis trophoblastic disease, Semin. Oncol. 9:204 (1982).
41. Begent, R. H. J. and Bagshawe, K. D., The management of high risk choriocarcinoma, Semin. Oncol. 9:198 (1982).
42. Surwit, E. A., Sucio, T. N., Schmidt, H. J., et al., A new combination chemotherapy for resistant trophoblastic disease, Gynecol. Oncol. 8:110 (1979).
43. Newlands, E. S. and Bagshawe, K. D., Activity of high dose *cis*-platinum in combination with vincristine and methotrexate

in drug resistant gestational choriocarcinoma. A report of 17 cases, Brit. J. Cancer 40:943 (1979).

44. Shlaerth, J. B., Morrow, C. P., and Depetrillo, A. D., Sustained remission of choriocarcinoma with *cis*-platinum, vinblastine and bleomycin after failure of conventional chemotherapy, Amer. J. Obstet. Gynecol. 136:983 (1980).

45. Newlands, E. S., New chemotherapeutic agents in the management of gestational trophoblastic disease, Semin. Oncol. 9:239 (1982).

46. Weed, J. C. and Hammond, C. B., Cerebral metastatic choriocarcinoam: Intensive therapy and prognosis, Obstet. Gynecol. 55:89 (1980).

47. Surwit, E. A. and Hammond, C. B., Treatment of metastatic trophoblastic disease with poor prognosis, Obstet. Gynecol. 55:565 (1980).

48. Weed, J. C., Woodward, K. T., and Hammond, C. B., Choriocarcinoma metastatic to the brain, therapy and prognosis, Semin. Oncol. 9:208 (1982).

49. Goldstein, D. P., Couch, N. P., and Hall, T. C., Infusion therapy in the treatment of patients with choriocarcinoma and related trophoblastic tumors, Surg. Forum 18:426 (1967).

50. Goldstein, D. P., Berkowitz, R. S., and Cohen, S. M., The current management of molar pregnancy, Curr. Probl. Obstet. Gynecol. 3:4 (1979).

51. Koga, K. and Maeda, K., Prophylactic chemotherapy with amethopterin for prevention of choriocarcinoam following removal of hydatidiform mole, Amer. J. Obstet. Gynecol. 100:270 (1968).

52. Fasoli, M., Ratti, E., Franceschi, S., et al., Management of gestational trophoblastic disease: Results of a cooperative study, Obstet. Gynecol. 60:205 (1982).

53. Goldstein, D. P., Prevention of gestational trophoblastic disease by use of actinomycin D in molar pregnancies, Obstet. Gynecol. 43:475 (1974).

54. Lewis, J. L., Jr., Current status of gestational trophoblastic disease, Cancer 38:620 (1976).

55. Goldstein, D. P., Saracco, P., Osathanondth, R., et al., Methotrexate with citrovorum factor rescue for gestational trophoblastic neoplasms, Obstet. Gynecol. 51:93 (1978).

56. Berkowitz, R. S., Goldstein, D. P., and Bernstein, M. R., Methotrexate with citrovorum factor rescue as primary therapy for gestational trophoblastic disease, Cancer 50:2024 (1982).

RE-EVALUATION OF 5-FLUOROURACIL AS A SINGLE AGENT FOR GESTATIONAL MALIGNANT TROPHOBLASTIC NEOPLASMS

Hung-Chao Sung, Pao-Chen Wu, and Yuan-Bh Wang

Department of Obstetrics and Gynecology
Capital Hospital
Chinese Academy of Medical Sciences
Peking, China

INTRODUCTION

It has been more than 20 years since 6-mercaptopurine was successfully used for the first time in the treatment of malignant trophoblastic neoplasms in the Capital Hospital in 1958. Since then, a total of four effective drugs have been found, and a dramatic improvement in prognosis of the patients has been achieved, resulting in permanent cure of this group of tumors. The overall results of treatment were reported in 1979 (1). To provide a general principle for the selection of a proper chemotherapeutic agent for clinical use, it is mandatory to evaluate each drug individually. The purpose of this paper is to present the therapeutic results of 5-fluorouracil used as a single agent in the treatment of malignant trophoblastic neoplasms.

MATERIALS AND METHODS

The trial of 5-fluorouracil in patients with malignant trophoblastic neoplasms was initiated in 1963. The rationale for the trial was based on the fact that both 5-fluorouracil and 6-mercaptopurine are antimetabolites, and that the latter had been proven to be effective in the treatment of this group of tumors. Initially, a routine method of administration was used, namely 12-15 mg/kg/day by intravenous bolus injection for 5 consecutive days, followed by half dosage every other day until toxic effects appeared. No notable therapeutic effects were observed, and the toxic reactions were so severe that few patients could tolerate the drug. We later tried to improve the method of administration by using slow intravenous drip instead of bolus injection. This modification resulted in a significant reduction in toxic effects. By gradually increasing the drug dosage, a satisfactory therapeutic result was eventually obtained. From 1964 through 1975, 5-fluorouracil was used as a single agent in the treatment of 312 cases of malignant trophoblastic neoplasms comprising 173 cases of invasive mole and 139 cases of choriocarcinoma. This series of patients was further divided into Group A, in which 5-fluorouracil was used as initial therapy, and Group B, in which 5-fluorouracil was given to those who developed resistance to 6-mercaptopurine and/or to methotrexate. The number of patients included in each group is shown in Table 1. The details of diagnostic criteria and method of clinical staging were previously described (2).

RESULTS

Immediate Results

Therapeutic results were classified as either complete remission, partial remission, or no response. In complete remission, there was no residual tumor detectable by the currently available methods. No clinical symptoms of trophoblastic disease remained, pulmonary metastatic shadows were completely absorbed, and hCG levels were undetectable. Partial remission was defined as partial or complete resolution of pulmonary metastases but lack of favorable

Table 1. Two Groups of Patients Treated with 5-Fluorouracil[a]

Neoplasm	Group A	Group B	Total
Invasive mole	126	47	173
Choriocarcinoma	86	53	139
Total	212	100	312

[a]Protocol for 5-fluorouracil therapy: 28-30 mg/kg/day dissolved in 500 ml 5% dextrose was given by slow intravenous drip over a period of 8 hours, for 10 consecutive days. The interval between courses of therapy was generally 2 to 3 weeks, depending on the rate of subsidence of toxic effects. 5-Fluorouracil was replaced by other drugs only after repetition of two to three courses without apparent therapeutic effect.

Table 2. Therapeutic Results, Group A Patients

	Invasive mole		Choriocarcinoma	
Therapeutic result	No.	%	No.	%
Complete remission	107	84.9	51	59.3
Partial remission	17	13.5	29	33.7
No response	2	1.6	6	7.0
Total	126	100.0	86	100.0

response in the hCG level, or the converse in which the hCG level decreased ten fold or became undetectable but the pulmonary metastases failed to respond favorably. If, after two or three courses of 5-fluorouracil therapy there was still only partial remission, the 5-fluorouracil treatment was replaced by another agent or by combination therapy. The therapeutic results for Group A and Group B patients are presented in Tables 2 and 3, respectively.

The overall remission rate in Group A patients was 98.4% for invasive mole and 93.0% for choriocarcinoma. In Group B patients, the overall remission rate was 93.6% and 71.7%, respectively, for invasive mole and choriocarcinoma, indicating that 5-fluorouracil is effective not only in patients receiving this agent as initial therapy, but also in those who develop resistance to other drugs.

Table 3. Therapeutic Results, Group B Patients

	Invasive mole		Choriocarcinoma	
Therapeutic result	No.	%	No.	%
Complete remission	38	80.8	20	37.7
Partial remission	6	12.8	18	34.0
No response	3	6.4	15	28.3
Total	47	100.0	53	100.0

Table 4. Rate of Complete Remission in Relation to Clinical Staging in Choriocarcinoma

Stage	Percent remission	
	Group A	Group B
I	92.9	
II	85.7	66.7
IIIA	56.0	50.0
IIIB	39.1	40.0
IV	30.0	22.2
Overall	59.3	37.7

The complete remission rates in relation to clinical staging of both Group A and B choriocarcinoma patients are summarized in Table 4. It is noteworthy that complete remission was achieved with 5-fluorouracil therapy in seven Stage IV patients with widespread metastases all over the body.

Follow-Up Studies

After 5-fluorouracil therapy a total of 216 patients, consisting of 145 invasive mole and 71 choriocarcinoma cases, achieved complete remission. The results of long-term follow-up of these patients are shown in Table 5.

All three cases of recurrence belonged to Group B and occurred in the early period of trial of 5-fluorouracil therapy. Of these three patients, two were cured by further chemotherapy. One patient died of the recurrent disease, providing a 0.5% death rate due to

Table 5. Follow-Up Results of Patients Achieving Complete Remission

Neoplasm	Cases	No. lost	No. recurrences		No. surviving	
Invasive mole	145	2	1	(0.7%)	142	(97.9%)
Choriocarcinoma	71	1	2	(2.8%)	68	(95.8%)
Overall	216	3	3	(1.4%)	210	(97.2%)

Table 6. Duration of Follow-Up of Surviving Patients

Neoplasm	5-10 yr	10-15 yr	15-20 yr	Total
Invasive mole	51 (35.9%)	64 (45.0%)	27 (19.0%)	142
Choriocarcinoma	26 (38.2%)	32 (47.0%)	10 (14.7%)	68
Overall	77 (36.7%)	96 (45.7%)	37 (17.6%)	210

recurrence. The duration of follow-up of the living patients is shown in Table 6. All patients had survived for more than 5 years up to the end of 1981.

Number of Courses of Chemotherapy

The average number of courses of 5-fluorouracil required to achieve complete remission is summarized in Table 8 . Generally, patients with choriocarcinoma required more courses than those with invasive mole, and patients who developed drug resistance before 5-fluorouracil therapy required more courses than those who received the drug as initial therapy.

Toxic Reactions

Generally, 5-fluorouracil is less toxic than either 6-mercaptopurine or methotrexate by the method and dosage currently used. The suppression of white and platelet counts after the first course of 5-fluorouracil therapy in 212 Group A patients is compared with that of 6-mercaptopurine and methotrexate in Table 7. After a course of 5-fluorouracil, the white count remained at a level of 4000 per ml

Table 7. Average Number of 5-Fluorouracil Courses Required for Complete Remission

Neoplasm	Group A	Group B
Invasive mole	3.0	3.2
Choriocarcinoma	3.8	4.3

Table 8. Bone Marrow Suppression by 5-Fluorouracil (FU), 6-Mercaptopurine (MP), and Methotrexate (MTX)

White blood cell and platelet count	Percent distribution		
	FU	MP	MTX
White blood cells per ml:			
<1,000	0.5	5.1	9.1
1,000-2,000	4.2	31.2	30.4
2,000-3,000	13.7	47.1	30.4
3,000-4,000	17.5	10.1	15.1
>4,000	64.1	6.5	15.1
Total	100	100	100
Platelets per ml:			
<10,000	0.5	8.0	7.6
20,000-30,000	2.4	34.0	28.8
30,000-50,000	5.7	26.1	22.7
50,000-100,000	24.5	24.6	30.3
>100,000	67.0	7.2	10.6
Total	100	100	100
Total no. patients	212	138	66

or higher, and the platelet count remained at 100,000 per ml or higher, demonstrating that there was no apparent bone marrow suppression in more than 60% of the cases. The corresponding percentages were only 10-15% for methotrexate, and less than 10% for 6-mercaptopurine.

Hepatic toxicity of 5-fluorouracil is also less severe. After the first course of 5-fluorouracil therapy only 7.1% of the 212 Group A patients showed elevation of serum glutamate-pyruvate transaminase (SGPT). By contrast, 42.7% and 22.7% of the Group A patients had elevated SGPT after the first course of 6-mercaptopurine and methotrexate, respectively (Table 9).

Other toxic effects were also milder and less frequent in patients treated with 5-fluorouracil. Severe stomatitis occurred in only 3.2% of the patients, in which the ulceration was mostly confined to the oral cavity. The mucous membrane of the deep pharynx was rarely involved. Alopecia was less severe, and complete loss of hair from the scalp was uncommon.

Table 9. Liver Toxicity from 5-Fluorouracil, 6-Mercaptopurine, and Methotrexate

Drug	No. patients	Elevated SGPT[a]	
		No. cases	%
5-Fluorouracil	212	15	7.1
6-Mercaptopurine	138	59	42.8
Methotrexate	66	15	22.7

[a]Serum glutamate-pyruvate transaminase.

The toxic reactions specific to 5-fluorouracil were abdominal colic and diarrhea, which occurred in about 20% of the cases. These symptoms began on the eighth or ninth day of medication, and subsided spontaneously two or three days after cessation of chemotherapy. Improper management of the diarrhea, however, can occasionally result in life-threatening pseudomembranous colitis. Among 312 patients in the present series, there were two deaths related to drug toxicity, of which one died of pseudomembranous colitis. The other succumbed to septicemia resulting from repeated severe bone marrow suppression from previous chemotherapy. In addition, the skin can become pigmented after 5-fluorouracil along the veins of medication and/or on the face, giving rise to the appearance of the mask of pregnancy. In severe cases, pigmentation can occur all over the body. All these changes gradually disappear after cessation of chemotherapy.

DISCUSSION

5-Fluorouracil treatment of malignant tumors began as early as 1957 (3). Nevertheless, effective treatment of malignant trophoblastic neoplasms with 5-fluorouracil has never been reported. According to our experience, after improving the method of administration and increasing the dosage, we have found 5-fluorouracil to be an effective chemotherapeutic agent for choriocarcinoma and invasive mole, and superior to 6-mercaptopurine or methotrexate by its better therapeutic effect and milder toxic reactions (Figs. 1 and 2). Furthermore, there seems to be no cross-resistance between 5-fluorouracil and the other two antimetabolites, so that patients who develop resistance to 6-mercaptopurine and methotrexate may still be treated by 5-fluorouracil with favorable results.

Another advantage of 5-fluorouracil is its outstanding effect

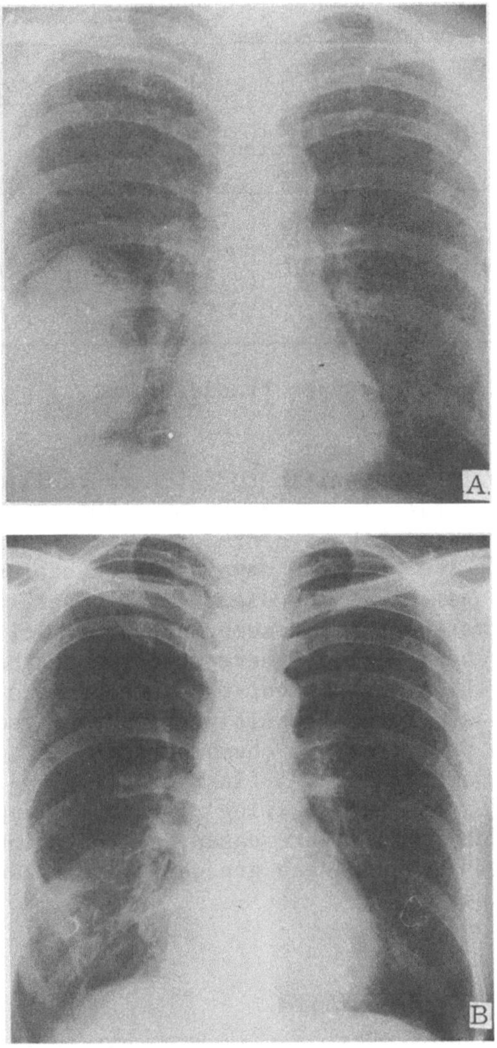

Fig. 1. Case of choriocarcinoma with huge metastatic mass in the right lower lung. The patient was admitted in December 1966 as a case of primary carcinoma of the lung. Surgical intervention was intended, but failed because of extensive adhesions. The biopsy proved to be choriocarcinoma. The patient was then treated with 5-fluorouracil, and responded well. The pulmonary shadows disappeared completely after 7 courses of 5-fluorouracil, leaving only some fibrotic changes in this area. The patient is currently in remission. *A*, chest X-ray taken before treatment; *B*, chest X-ray taken after the patient had gone into remission.

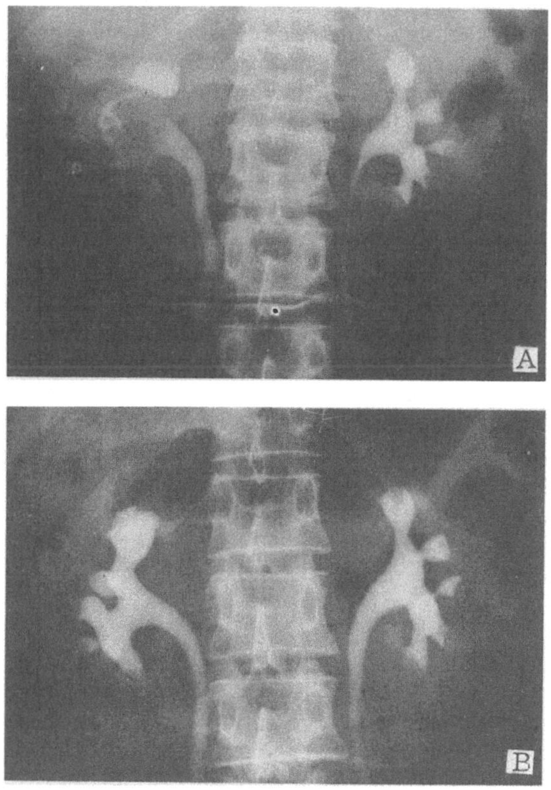

Fig. 2. A case of choriocarcinoma with metastases of both lungs, right kidney, and right lower gum. The patient was treated in 1975 with 5-fluorouracil alone, and responded well. Complete remission was achieved after four courses of 5-fluorouracil. Long-term follow-up revealed no recurrence or residual disease. *A*, intravenous pyelography taken before treatment, showing the filling defect of the right renal calyx; *B*, intravenous pyelography after patient had achieved remission.

on the metastatic tumors of genitourinary tract, gastrointestinal tract, and liver. Most impressive is its effect on vaginal metastasis which is a frequent occurrence in this group of diseases. In the case of vaginal metastatic nodule with ulceration and severe hemorrhage, intravenous infusion of 5-fluorouracil should be given immediately after packing. Generally the bleeding will be stopped within 4 or 5 days and the tumor will totally disappear after one or two courses of therapy. This occurs without scar formation no matter how large the original mass might have been. 5-Fluorouracil can be administered through a variety of routes in addition to intravenous administration. These include intra-arterial infusion, intracavitary instillation, intratumor injection, as well as oral medication owing to its negligible irritating effect at the local sites.

The therapeutic effect and toxic reaction of 5-fluorouracil are closely related to the dosage and method of administration. When 5-fluorouracil is used as a single agent given for 10 days at a daily dose less than 25 mg per kg, both effects are negligible. On the other hand, at doses greater than 30 mg per kg the toxic reactions may become overwhelming and intolerable for most patients. Therefore, the dosage recommended (Tables 1 and 10), which has been formulated through repeated trials, should not be changed without adequate justification. For patients weighing less than 40 kg, however, the daily dose per kg can be increased slightly, and for patients weighing more than 60 kg the dose per kg should be reduced. The total daily dosage should not exceed 1,750 mg for any patient.

At a constant dose level, the rate of administration is crucial. While 500 mg of 5-fluorouracil given daily by single-bolus intravenous injection for five consecutive days may cause profound suppression of bone marrow, most patients can tolerate a dosage of 1,500 mg daily for 10 days if administered by slow infusion. We have found it optimal to dissolve the 5-fluorouracil in 500 ml of 5% dextrose solution and to instill it into the patient over an 8-hour period.

The mortality rate due to toxic reactions in 5-fluorouracil chemotherapy of other malignant tumors has been reported to be as high as 9.8% (3). However, the incidence of death due to toxicity in our series was only 0.6%, *i.e.*, two deaths in a total of 950 courses given to 312 patients who received far larger dosages of the drug than described in the literature. Our results are not in accordance with Sullivan (4), who claims that slow intravenous infusion of 5-fluorouracil might reduce the therapeutic effect as well as the toxic reactions of the drug. It seems likely that the gratifying results of the present series were achieved by the significantly lower toxicity of even high doses of 5-fluorouracil when administered by slow intravenous drip.

Table 10. Routes and Methods of Administration of 5-Fluorouracil in Relation to Varying Indications

Route	Indication	Dose and method	Remarks
Intra-arterial infusion	Brain, liver, or pelvic metastasis	Same as for intravenous infusion (Table 1)	Use intra-arterial catheter
Intra-cavitary injection	Hemothorax	1,000-1,500 mg once or twice per week	No dilution required
Intratumor injection	Pelvic metastasis	250-1,000 mg once or twice per week, varying with size of tumor	No dilution required
Oral	Gastro-intestinal or liver metastasis	½ of daily i.v. dose in 2 divided doses for 8-10 days (i.v. dosage remains unchanged and is given simultaneously)	Solution is preferable to tablets
Combined therapy	Advanced and/or resistant cases		
1. 5FU		26 mg/kg/day i.v. infusion	12 hours for medication
KSM[a]		300 μg/day i.v. infusion for 8 days	
2. 5FU		26 mg/kg/day i.v. infusion	8 hours for medication
Nitrocaphane		30 mg/day i.v. for 8 days	

[a]Kengshengmycin

Most of the toxic manifestations of 5-fluorouracil are mild. The most troublesome toxic reaction is diarrhea, which may result in dangerous pseudomembranous colitis. Therefore, once diarrhea occurs during chemotherapy with 5-fluorouracil, the medication should be withdrawn immediately and the frequency of bowel movement and stool characteristics should be watched carefully. For the early detection of pseudomembranous colitis, it is necessary to monitor the bacterial flora by Gram stain of the fecal smear.

If Gram-negative bacilli are found to be decreasing and Gram-positive cocci (in clumps) increasing, appropriate treatment with antibiotics should be instituted immediately. We recommend the oral administration of *Lactobacillus*, and antibiotics effective against *Staphylococcus aureus* (Gentamycin, Kanamycin, Erythromycin, or Methicillin). Generally, combined treatment with antibiotics in sufficient dosage is preferred. Once the diarrhea is under control, the antibiotics should be discontinued in time to prevent secondary fungal infection resulting from imbalance of the intestinal flora.

Regardless of the discovery of new drugs such as Kengshengmycin, Tisupurine, and Nitrocaphane, all of which are effective in treating malignant trophoblastic neoplasms, 5-fluorouracil has remained the agent of first choice or the major therapeutic agent when used singly or in combination with other drugs. Table 10 summarizes the indications for using 5-fluorouracil, and the routes and methods of administration of the drug.

SUMMARY

Large doses of 5-fluorouracil, administered by slow intravenous drip, have proven to be very effective in the treatment of malignant trophoblastic tumors. From 1964 through 1975, 5-fluorouracil was used as a single chemotherapeutic agent in 173 cases of invasive mole and 139 cases of choriocarcinoma. This series of patients was further divided into Group A (212 cases) in which 5-fluorouracil was used as initial therapy, and Group B (100 cases) in which 5-fluorouracil was given to those who developed resistance to 6-mercaptopurine and/or to methotrexate. The overall remission rate in Group A patients was 98.4% for invasive mole and 93.0% for choriocarcinoma. In Group B patients the corresponding remission rate was 93.6% and 71.7%, respectively, indicating that 5-fluorouracil is effective in patients who develop resistance to other antimetabolic agents. The rate of recurrence among 213 patients achieving complete remission during follow-up was 1.4% (3 cases). All of the remaining 210 patients had survived for more than 5 years up to the end of 1981, and 96 patients (45.7%) had survived for more than 10 years. In comparison with other antimetabolites, 5-fluorouracil has the advantages of being more effective and less toxic, and can be administered through multiple routes. Therefore, it has remained the agent of first choice in the chemotherapy of malignant trophoblastic neoplasms.

REFERENCES

1. Sung, H. C., Xia, Z. F., Wu, P. C., and Wang, Y. E., 20 years experience in chemotherapy of choriocarcinoma and malignant mole, Chinese Medical Journal 92:677 (1979).

2. Sung, H. C., Wu, P. C., and Ho, T. H., Treatment of choriocarcinoma and chorioadenoma destruens with 6MP and surgery, a clinical report of 67 cases, in: "Selected Papers on Cancer Research," edited by Chinese Academy of Medical Sciences, Shanghai Sci. Tech. Publ. (1962), p. 441; republished in Acta Unio Inter-nationalis Contra Cancerum 20:491 (1964).
3. Zubrod, C. G., Effects of 5FU and 5FUDR on G-I cancer, J. Amer. Med. Assoc. 178:832 (1961).
4. Sullivan, R. D., "Clinical Cancer Chemotherapy Including Ambulatory Infusion," Charles C. Thomas, Publisher, Springfield, Ill. (1970), p. 50, p. 87.

MANAGEMENT OF PATIENTS WITH GESTATIONAL TROPHOBLASTIC NEOPLASIA: EXPERIENCE OF THE SOUTHEASTERN REGIONAL CENTER

Charles B. Hammond, Daniel L. Clarke-Pearson
and John T. Soper

The Southeastern Regional Center
for Trophoblastic Disease
Department of Obstetrics and Gynecology
Duke University Medical Center
Durham, North Carolina
USA

INTRODUCTION

Gestational trophoblastic neoplasia (GTN), a group of the more virulent malignant tumors in humans, is derived from the trophoblast of human pregnancy. Prior to 1956, the prognosis for these patients was exceedingly poor, regardless of the surgical or irradiation therapies utilized (1). Since that time and the advent of systemic chemotherapy as the primary therapeutic modality for these patients, results have become exceedingly good (2). Sequential reports have been published documenting increasingly good remission rates (3-6). Cure rates now approach 100% for patients without metastases and those with "good" prognosis metastatic disease. Even in patients with "poor" prognosis GTN, high rates of remission have been achieved with vigorous multi-modality therapy.

From 1956 through 1966, workers at the National Institutes of Health provided significant progress in the treatment of patients with GTN (3-5). Work by Drs. Brewer and Bagshawe at other institutions added to and extended these accomplishments (7, 8). Through these efforts, the responsiveness of trophoblastic neoplasms to systemic chemotherapy was well documented and provided the basic concepts of today's treatment. Since 1966, accomplishments include the introduction of the categorization of patients to allow individualization of therapy; the use of initial multi-agent chemotherapy for patients with "poor" prognosis, a technique which yields enhanced survival; redefinition of the role of surgery and irradiation therapy for these patients; studied the value of arteriography in the diagnosis of these diseases plus further defined the role of infusion chemotherapy; developed regimens of therapy with reduced toxicity; and enhancement of our understanding of the basic precepts of the disease. The present report will summarize the experience of a regional center for the diagnosis and therapy of patients with GTN during the interval from 1966 through 1982.

MATERIALS AND METHODS

The Southeastern Regional Center for Trophoblastic Disease was established in the Department of Obstetrics and Gynecology July 1, 1966. All patients are included in this report who were admitted to this center from that opening date through December 31, 1982. Patients were included if they had entered the treatment course after the 1966 date and if therapy was terminated, either with remission or death, prior to December 31, 1982. During this interval of sixteen and one-half years, 361 patients were treated by the physicians of this center for malignant gestational trophoblastic disease. In addition to these patients, the staff provided consultation and sensitive hCG assay support for over 700 other patients with malignant trophoblastic disease who were treated elsewhere, and laboratory support and clinical consultation for in excess of 2,000 patients who had primary hydatidiform moles and whose care was provided by physicians in other localities. Only the former group of 361 patients treated for malignant GTN at this institution is included in this report.

All 361 patients had a diagnosis of malignant trophoblastic disease based upon the pathologic documentation of choriocarcinoma or invasive mole (chorioadenoma destruens) or hydatidiform mole. All had elevated hCG levels. If a patient had only the pathologic diagnosis of hydatidiform mole, then hCG was required to be either plateaued or rising, or the patient had metastases at the time of diagnosis.

Once the diagnosis of GTN was established, the patient was admitted to hospital for staging studies and treatment. Studies included a complete history and physical examination, chest X-ray, isotopic liver and brain scans (replaced by computerized axial tomography scanning in 1978), intravenous pyelogram, hematologic and serum chemistry determinations, thyroid panel, and an immediate pretreatment hCG assay. For the interval 1966 through 1973, hCG was determined by the Klinefelter mouse uterine weight assay (4) on concentrates of 24-hour urines. Since 1973, sensitive radioimmunoassay determination of hCG has been done with the beta-subunit radioimmunoassay being utilized entirely since 1976 (10). In recent years, patients have routinely undergone pelvic ultrasound. Selected patients also underwent selective arteriography, lung tomography, uterine curettage, and/or other studies as deemed appropriate by clinical findings. Based upon all of these studies, patients were then categorized as having *nonmetastatic* GTN, or "good" or "poor" prognostic *metastatic* GTN (11). The patient with metastases was categorized as having "poor" prognostic metastatic GTN if there was evidence of at least one of the following: (a) brain metastasis; (b) liver metastasis; (c) an initial pretreatment urinary hCG titer in excess of 100,000 IU/24 hours, or serum beta-hCG titer in excess of 40,000 mIU/ml; (d) significant unsuccessful prior chemotherapy; (e) symptoms of malignancy in excess of four months; or (f) as recently demonstrated, choriocarcinoma following term gestation (12). All other patients with metastatic disease demonstrated on staging evaluation were considered as having "good" prognosis GTN. The remainder of patients without demonstrable metastases was classified as having nonmetastatic GTN. Table 1 illustrates the number of patients in the various categories of staging who were treated at this institution during this interval.

RESULTS

Nonmetastatic GTN

Until January 1978, patients without metastases and without evidence of impaired liver or renal function were treated with methotrexate (0.4 mg/kg given daily by intramuscular injection) for five days per treatment course (4). This was recycled on the seventh day after completion of the previous course, as long as hCG remained elevated, or unless prohibited by toxicity. If the patient had hepatic or renal dysfunction or the hCG titer failed to regress with repetitive methotrexate, an alternative therapeutic program consisted of actinomycin D (10 to 13 μg/kg by intravenous injection) for five

Table 1. GTN Patients Treated at Duke Regional Center from 1966 to 1982

Category	No. of patients
Nonmetastatic GTN	195
Metastatic GTN	
"Good" prognosis	81
"Poor" prognosis	85
Total	361

days per treatment course (5, 6). Courses of actinomycin D were repeated in a similar fashion and under similar restrictions as for methotrexate. Remission was diagnosed only after three consecutive, weekly negative hCG assays. Patients usually received one complete treatment course after receipt of the first negative hCG titer. If the patient no longer desired to maintain childbearing capability, total abdominal hysterectomy was done in the first course of treatment. In patients in whom disease could not be totally eradicated through the use of methotrexate or actinomycin D, total abdominal hysterectomy was done at a later date during a cycle of chemotherapy in an attempt to extirpate the disease resistant to systemic chemotherapy. In a small number of selected patients, with disease resistant to systemic single agent therapy, pelvic arterial infusion (methotrexate or actinomycin D) or multi-agent systemic chemotherapy was used prior to hysterectomy in a final attempt to preserve their reproductive capacity.

Since January 1978, patients with nonmetastatic GTN who had no evidence of abnormal liver or renal function have been primarily treated with methotrexate, 1 mg/kg intramuscularly daily, on Days 1, 3, 5, and 7 of an eight-day protocol. Folinic acid, 0.1 mg/kg intramuscularly daily, was administered on Days 2, 4, 6, and 8. The regimen was repeated seven days after completion of the previous course for as long as the hCG titer remained elevated. With this technique, toxicity from methotrexate has been nearly completely avoided. This regimen, as initially advocated by Bagshawe and Wilde (13) and modified by Goldstein and associates (11), was originally given only once, and the hCG levels were subsequently determined without further therapy unless an hCG titer plateau occurred. At this institution, however, we have consistently treated patients with repetitive courses of the drugs and usually give one additional course after the first negative hCG assay has been determined (14). At our center, failure of a weekly significant decline of hCG (>25%) resulted in a change of therapy to single agent actinomycin D or to other choices of therapy as noted above for GTN resistant to single agent chemotherapy. Techniques for all of these regimens have previously been reported (2, 6, 12, 15). During this therapy, hCG is measured by sensitive radioimmunoassay for the beta-subunit of hCG at least weekly, along with chest roentgenography, physical examination, and other studies as needed, to monitor induced toxicity as well as the status of the disease. After remission status has been achieved, follow-up is initiated (see below).

Table 2 illustrates our experience in the 195 patients who were treated for nonmetastatic trophoblastic malignancy at this center from 1966 through 1982. Of the 195 patients treated, all but one have achieved remission, which has been sustained until the present time. The one patient who died received primary chemotherapy for nonmetastatic disease at another institution. After metastatic

Table 2. Nonmetastatic GTN: Results of Therapy at Duke University Center from 1966 to 1982

	Total no.	No. survived
Patients treated	195	194 (99.5%)
Primary therapy at this center	180	180 (100%)
Secondary therapy at this center	15	14 (33%)
Recurrences after remission	8 (14%)	8 (100%)
Died	1[a] (0.5%)	0

157 of 175 patients (89.7%) who desired to retain their uterus were able to avoid hysterectomy.

[a]Patient died of drug-resistant metastatic disease. The patient was referred after failure to achieve remission for recurrence at another institution and with metastases present.

recurrence had occurred, refractory to systemic chemotherapy, she was referred for further treatment. Despite vigorous efforts, including multi-agent chemotherapy, hysterectomy, and significant further therapy, she succumbed to progressive disease resistant to all forms of treatment. Eight of these 194 patients (4%) have had recurrences despite achievement of negative hCG titers during initial therapy and receiving one additional course of therapy after the first negative hCG titer. All eight have been successfully re-entered into remission (four by hysterectomy plus chemotherapy, and four by chemotherapy alone). Of the 175 patients who desired to preserve childbearing ability, 157 (89%) have been able to do so.

Metastatic GTN

Patients with trophoblastic neoplasia who are demonstrated by staging studies to have any metastases are categorized as having "metastatic GTN", and are then subdivided into "good" or "poor" prognosis categories. The latter category is identified by the presence of one or more of the six characteristics noted above.

"Good" prognosis metastatic GTN. Methotrexate was used as the drug of choice to initiate therapy in these "good" prognosis metastatic patients, and they were treated with repetitive five-day courses of 0.4 mg/kg intramuscularly per day if liver and renal function permitted. Chemotherapy was repeated on the seventh day after treatment, toxicity permitting, until a negative hCG titer was obtained. One additional treatment course was then given. If resistance to methotrexate developed, as indicated by plateauing or rising titers or the development of new metastases, or if a negative titer was not achieved after five courses of the agent, therapy was changed to actinomycin D. Patients with liver or renal dysfunction who should not be given methotrexate were started initially on a regimen of actinomycin D as outlined above for nonmetastatic disease. If resistance developed to both drugs, the patient was then switched to one of the multi-agent protocols (see below) and/or considered for hysterectomy if all evidence of metastatic disease had been cleared and there was evidence of persistent uterine disease. Pelvic arterial infusion was also utilized for a few of these patients (15). Currently, the regimen of alternating methotrexate and folinic acid (as in nonmetastatic GTN, above) is considered still to be investigational at this institution and is not yet felt to be the treatment of choice for patients with earlier, "good" prognosis metastatic disease.

Results of treatment in patients with "good" prognosis metastatic disease are illustrated in Table 3. As noted, all 81 of these patients with "good" prognosis metastatic disease achieved remission.

Table 3. "Good" Prognosis Metastatic GTN: Results of Therapy at Duke University Center from 1966 to 1982

	Total no.	No. survived
Patients treated	81	81 (100%)
Sites of metastases		
Lung alone	65	
Vagina alone	3	
Lung and vagina	4	
Other	9 (none liver or brain)	
Recurrences after remission	4 (5%)	4 (100%)

57 of 63 patients (90.3%) who desired to retain their uterus were able to avoid hysterectomy.

Sixty-three of these patients desired to preserve childbearing capability, and 57 patients (90.5%) were able to do so. Metastases were confined to the lung in 65 patients, the vagina only in 3 patients, the vagina and lung in 4 patients, and other sites (except liver or brain) in 9 patients. Four patients (5%) had recurrence after initial remission status had been achieved. All were successfully returned to remission status with systemic chemotherapy.

Metastatic "poor" prognosis disease. Patients with "poor" prognosis gestational trophoblastic neoplasia present difficult and challenging problems for the physician and the patient. It has been our consistent recommendation that these patients can best be treated at one of the trophoblastic disease centers, where their chances for achieving remission are likely to be maximized.

Prior to 1969, patients with "poor" prognosis metastatic GTN were treated in a fashion similar to that outlined above for "good" prognosis metastatic disease. Such single-agent methotrexate or actinomycin D therapy yielded poor results in these high risk patients (6).

Since 1969, patients with "poor" prognosis metastatic GTN have initially been treated with combination chemotherapy. For the first eight years of this experience, such treatment has included triple agent chemotherapy (MAC) given daily in five-day courses which includes methotrexate (0.3 mg/kg intramuscularly per day), actinomycin D (10-12 μg/kg intravenously per day), and chlorambucil (10 mg orally per day)(6). Courses were repeated at 10 to 14 days after completing the previous treatment, depending upon hematopoietic recovery and other toxicity. Cerebral or hepatic metastases were treated simultaneously with a single course of whole organ (brain or liver) irradiation of 2,000 to 3,000 rads, delivered in ten fractions. The MAC chemotherapy regimen was subsequently changed to other regimens if the hCG titer plateaued or rose after two courses of the MAC triple chemotherapy, or if toxicity precluded adequate frequency of therapy. Prior to 1976, such alternative chemotherapy consisted primarily of either actinomycin D alone (10 to 13 μg/kg intravenously per day for five days) or a combination of Velban (3 mg intravenously twice daily for three days) and actinomycin D (as given alone). Courses were again repeated at 7 to 12 day intervals (4, 6).

Since 1976, patients resistant to the standard MAC triple agent chemotherapy have been treated with the modified Bagshawe regimen (16), with courses being repeated at 7 to 14 day intervals. Most recently, patients with poor prognosis metastatic disease resistant to MAC therapy are treated with chemotherapy consisting of either the modified Bagshawe regimen, the Einhorn regimen (18), or courses which alternate VP-16 (19) with the modified Bagshawe protocol. Patients not responding to these regimens have been treated with either single-agent methotrexate or actinomycin D therapy or with newer Phase II experimental drugs given at weekly intervals or as marrow toxicity permits. Adjuvant hysterectomy, resection of metastases, or radiation of other nonresectable metastases were often done for failure of response to more traditional therapy.

Complete remission was diagnosed only after three consecutive normal weekly hCG assays. Most of these "poor" prognosis patients had at least one to three courses of chemotherapy after the initial negative titer was first achieved.

In all of these patients with metastatic GTN, intensive support and vigorous therapy have been required to enhance the likelihood of obtaining remission. Surgical intervention was often carried out to deal with complications of disease or treatment or to attempt removal of a residual focus of additional disease. More recently, supportive techniques including hyperalimentation and the in-dwelling Hickman catheter have been utilized.

For the interval 1966 through 1982, 86 patients have been treated for "poor" prognosis metastatic trophoblastic disease at this center (Table 4). Fifty-seven of these patients have survived (67.3%), while 28 patients have died. Death was due to progressive, drug-resistant disease in 21 patients, and to toxicity of therapy in the face of drug-resistant disease in 7 patients.

Poor prognostic factors in these 86 patients with "poor" prognosis GTN at the time of admission included the following: high initial pretreatment hCG titer in 46, the presence of brain or central nervous system metastasis in 22, liver metastasis in 15, duration of symptoms of disease for greater than four months in 49, prior unsuccessful therapy in 26, and previous antecedent pregnancy of term gestation in 24. Multiple factors were present in many patients.

In review of these data, other items of significance may be noted. Eighteen of 25 patients (69.2%) who were referred for treatment of "poor" prognosis malignant GTN after failure of initial therapy elsewhere ultimately expired with drug-resistant disease. In comparison, among the 59 patients who initially began their therapy for "poor" prognosis disease at this center, only ten (16.9%) died.

Surgery was required in a number of these patients. These included elective hysterectomy, bowel resection, craniotomy, thoracotomy, laparotomy, or nephrectomy for control of hemorrhage, or delayed surgery for resistant foci which could not be eradicated by systemic treatment.

Table 4. "Poor" Prognosis Metastatic GTN: Results of Therapy at Duke University Center from 1966 to 1982

	Total no.		No. survived
Patients treated	85		57 (67.3%)
Patients died	28		
Resistant disease		21	
Drug/therapy toxicity		7	
Poor prognostic criteria[a]			
High pretreatment hCG titer	46		
Brain/CNS lesions	22		
Hepatic lesions	15		
Duration of symptoms >4 months	49		
Prior term gestation	24		
Prior unsuccessful therapy	26		
Recurrences[b]			
15/66 (22.6%) of patients who achieved remission had subsequent recurrences.			
7 - Successfully retreated with long-term remission			
8 - Died of resistant disease			

[a]All patients had metastases. Multiple factors were present in some patients.
[b]Since 1979 the recurrence rate has only been 11.6%, suggesting additional treatment after remission is of benefit (see text).

Toxicity from chemotherapy was a major factor in the therapy of these high risk patients. Hematopoietic suppression with resultant thrombocytopenia or leukopenia was often severe. The former of these problems was usually treated with platelet transfusion for levels below 15,000 mm^3 or hemorrhage due to thrombocytopenia. Bleeding, so managed, was rarely a problem. Leukopenia, however, was often prolonged and severe. Isolation, antibiotics, leukocyte transfusions were occasionally utilized. Recently, we are beginning to utilize lithium carbonate as prophylaxis for leukopenia (20, 21). These problems, plus oral and cutaneous toxicity, are often formidable and require diligent care to reduce morbidity and mortality.

Remission has only been diagnosed after three consecutive weekly negative hCG titers (less than 5 mIU/ml, beta-subunit radioimmunoassay). Subsequent follow-up includes hCG assays at two-week intervals for three months, then monthly for three months, then bimonthly for six months and every six months thereafter, indefinitely. Re-evaluation of hCG titer results in prompt evaluation, exclusion of intercurrent pregnancy, and prompt retreatment if indicated. Pregnancy is prohibited for at least one year after the diagnosis of remission, and oral contraceptives are advised if there are no other contraindications.

We have always felt that chemotherapy should be continued for some interval after the initial diagnosis of remission. Usually this consists of one additional course. Since 1979 we have increased the duration of this therapy to one course for nonmetastatic disease, two courses for "good" prognosis metastatic GTN, and three or more courses for patients with "poor" prognosis metastatic disease. Data presented in Table 4 illustrate the benefit of such additional therapy.

DISCUSSION

Since the introduction of systemic chemotherapy in 1956, gestational trophoblastic neoplasia has evolved into one of the most curable gynecologic malignancies. This has occurred predominantly through the intrinsic sensitivity of these tumors to a variety of anti-neoplastic agents. Other factors affecting this success rate for treatment have been the effective use of sensitive assays for the monitoring of hCG and the identification of high-risk factors that allow for individualization of therapy. The present series compares favorably with other published results of treatment in patients with trophoblastic neoplasia, in that an overall remission rate of 92% was achieved. In patients with less extensive disease (nonmetastatic or "good" prognosis metastatic disease), the remission rate should approach 100%. The evolution of chemotherapeutic modalities to include systemic single-agent chemotherapy, multi-agent combined chemotherapy, arterially infused chemotherapy, and the advent of newer drugs and techniques, all have enhanced the responsiveness to treatment in this group of patients. The integration of radiation therapy to selected sites of metastases and the appropriate use of indicated surgery have improved the prognostic expectations and reduced the duration and amount of therapy required. Even in the group of patients with "poor" prognostic metastatic trophoblastic disease, one can expect a good response with vigorous therapy. If one considers only the past three years of experience at this center with patients with "poor" prognostic disease, remission has been achieved in 17 of 23 patients (73.9%)

Chemotherapy remains the single most effective method of treatment for patients with trophoblastic disease. The intrinsic sensitivity of these tumors to various chemotherapeutic agents offers not only a unique opportunity to eradicate localized uterine disease, but also to treat disseminated lesions. While the original results with these agents were encouraging, and many of these agents remain useful in the treatment of appropriately selected patients, the advent of multi-agent protocols has increased the remission rate for patients at greater risk. Thus, in any discussion of the treatment of trophoblastic disease, primary attention should be focused on the various types of therapy used, the frequency of administration, and the integration of all other approaches to that particular treatment modality.

We consider the individualization of therapy and the vigorous approach to therapy to be the two most important factors in achieving high rates of remission. Regionalization of care has enhanced our efforts to deliver the individualization of vigorous therapy. Presently, we feel that all patients with "poor" prognosis metastatic disease should be treated in centers by physicians intimately familiar with these diseases. Patients with less extensive disease may be adequately treated in local areas, provided that attention to care and vigorous therapy is carried out. The present report documents again the extreme responsiveness of patients with these lesions to the appropriate therapies. The utilization of the center concept, the vigorous administration of systemic chemotherapy, the appropriate integration of surgery and irradiation, excellence in supporting facilities, and the continuation of chemotherapy after remission has been established are all allowing an increased salvage of these patients. With continued efforts, we anticipate that the near complete control of this disease can be achieved with the techniques that are currently available.

ACKNOWLEDGEMENTS

This work was supported in part by NIH Grant #2 R18 CA 19272-04.

REFERENCES

1. Brewer, J. I., Halpern, B., and Torok, E. E., Gestational trophoblastic disease: selected clinical aspects and chorionic gonadotropin test methods, in: "Current Clinical Problems in Cancer," R. C. Hickey, ed., Year Book Medical Publishers, Chicago (1979), p. 5.
2. Hammond, C. B., Weed, J. C., and Currie, J. L., The role of operation in current therapy of gestational trophoblastic disease, Amer. J. Obstet. Gynecol. 136:844 (1980).
3. Li, M. D., Hertz, R., and Spencer, D. B., Effects of methotrexate upon choriocarcinoma and chorioadenoma, Proc. Soc. Exptl. Med. 93:361 (1956).

4. Hertz, R., Lewis, J. L., Jr., and Lipsett, M. B., Five years' experience with chemotherapy of metastatic choriocarcinoma and related trophoblastic tumors in women, Amer. J. Obstet. Gynecol. 82:631 (1961).
5. Ross, G. T., Goldstein, D. P., Hertz, R., Lipsett, M. B., and Odell, W. D., Sequential use of methotrexate and actinomycin D in the treatment of metastatic choriocarcinoma and related trophoblastic diseases in women, Amer. J. Obstet. Gynecol. 93:223 (1965).
6. Hammond, C. B. and Parker, R. T., Diagnosis and management of trophoblastic disease, Obstet. Gynecol. 35:132 (1970).
7. Brewer, J. I., Eckman, T. R., Dolkart, R. E., Toruk, E. E., and Webster, A., Gestational trophoblastic disease - a comparative study of the results of therapy in patients with invasive mole and with choriocarcinoma, Amer. J. Obstet. Gynecol. 109:335 (1971).
8. Bagshawe, K. D., Treatment of trophoblastic tumors, Ann. Acad. Med. 5:273 (1976).
9. Klinefelter, H. F., Albright, F., and Griswold, G. C., Experience with a quantitative test for normal or decreased amounts of follicular stimulating hormone in the urine in endocrinological diagnosis, J. Clin. Endocrinol. 3:529 (1943).
10. Vaitukaitis, J. L., Braunstein, G. D., and Ross, G. T., A radioimmunoassay which specifically measures human chorionic gonadotropin in the presence of human luteinizing hormone, Amer. J. Obstet. Gynecol. 113:751 (1972).
11. Goldstein, D. P., Saracco, P., Osathanondh, R., Goldstein, P. R., Mareau, A. R., and Bernstein, M. R., Methotrexate with citrovorum factor rescue for gestational trophoblastic neoplasms, Obstet. Gynecol. 51:93 (1978).
12. Miller, J. M., Jr., Surwit, E. A., and Hammond, C. B., Choriocarcinoma followign term pregnancy, Obstet. Gynecol. 53:207 (1979).
13. Bagshawe, K. D. and Wilde, C. E., Infusion therapy for pelvic trophoblastic tumors, Brit. J. Obstet. Gynecol. 71:565 (1964).
14. Smith, E. B., Weed, J. C., Tyrey, L., and Hammond, C. B., Treatment of nonmetastatic trophoblastic disease: results of methotrexate alone versus methotrexate-folinic acid, Amer. J. Obstet. Gynecol. 144:88 (1982).
15. Maroulis, G. B., Hammond, C. B., Johnsrude, I. S., Weed, J. C., Jr., and Parker, R. T., Arteriography and infusional chemotherapy in localized trophoblastic disease, Obstet. Gynecol. 45:397 (1945).
16. Surwit, E. A., Suciu, T. N., Schmidt, H. J., and Hammond, C. B., A new combination chemotherapy for resistant trophoblastic disease, Gynecol. Oncol. 8:110 (1979).
17. Einhorn, L. H. and Donohue, J. H., Cis-diamine dichloroplatinum, vinblastine, and bleomycin. Combination chemotherapy in disseminated testicular cancer, Ann. Intern. Med. 87:293 (1967).

18. Newlands, E. S., The activity of epipodophyllis derivative VP 216-213, and cis-platinum in combination in drug resistant choriocarcinoma. International Symposium on Gestational Trophoblastic Tumors, London, May 1979.
19. Begent, R. H. J. and Bagshawe, K. D., The management of high risk choriocarcinoma, Semin. Oncol. 9:198 (1982).
20. Rothstein, G., Clarkson, D. R., Larson, W., et al., Effect of lithium on neutrophile mass and production, New Engl. J. Med. 298:178 (1978).
21. Lyman, G. H., Williams, C. C., and Preston, D., The use of lithium carbonate to reduce infection and leukopenia during systemic chemotherapy, New Engl. J. Med. 302:257 (1980).

THE ROLE OF REGIONAL CENTERS FOR GESTATIONAL TROPHOBLASTIC DISEASE

Donald P. Goldstein and Ross S. Berkowitz

New England Trophoblastic Disease Center
Department of Obstetrics and Gynecology
Harvard Medical School
Boston, Massachusetts 02115, USA

INTRODUCTION

The concept of establishing regional centers for the management of patients with gestational trophoblastic disease (GTD) evolved as a direct result of the success of the program established by Dr. Roy Hertz at the National Cancer Institute. A number of individuals trained in the field of obstetrics and gynecology emerged from the clinical fellowship program at that institution who recognized that they had both an obligation and an opportunity to create in their own academic centers the type of facility which had functioned so well on a national level for over 10 years. Decentralization, as it were, would at the same time make available this new therapeutic modality to the largest number of patients and provide an adequate source of material for expanded clinical and laboratory research and teaching programs.

The purpose of this paper is to illustrate the role that a regional center of this type can play in fulfilling the goals outlined above. We have used our own experience at the New England Trophoblastic Disease Center as the model because of our personal involvement and because we feel that its evolution as a clinical, research and teaching resource in the Department of Obstetrics and Gynecology at Harvard Medical School reaffirms the wisdom of this concept.

ADMINISTRATIVE ASPECTS, PERSONNEL, AND FACILITIES

The New England Trophoblastic Disease Center was organized in 1965 at Harvard Medical School within the Department of Obstetrics and Gynecology when the senior author (DPG) returned to that institution after completing a two-year clinical fellowship at the National Cancer Institute. From its inception until 1975 it functioned more or less as an independent unit within the department and comprised a considerable part of the senior author's clinical activities. Support for the Center was obtained in part from a five-year grant from the National Cancer Institute, in part from the Boston Lying-In Hospital, and in part from third party and patient reimbursement to cover laboratory expenses, inpatient costs, and physician fees. Personnel of the Center included the director, a nurse-administrator, a fellow, and the resident staff. Patients were admitted for treatment to the Boston Lying-In Hospital, where a specially designated area was made available so as to centralize patient care. Laboratory facilities for hCG testing were located in the Gynecologic-Endocrine Laboratory at the Peter Bent Brigham Hospital, also a Harvard teaching affiliate.

In 1975 the Center became incorporated into the newly organized Division of Gynecologic Oncology and moved its administrative office to the Parkway Hospital, which served as the Gynecologic Service of the newly renamed Boston Hospital for Women. This move provided the Center with stronger clinical support from the Gynecologic-Oncology Training Program. Laboratory facilities for hCG testing were also moved to the newly organized Gynecologic-Endocrine Laboratory located at the Boston Lying-In Division.

In 1979 the Center moved to its present location in the newly constructed Brigham and Women's Hospital, a 700-bed teaching facility affiliated with Harvard Medical School, which merged the Boston Hospital for Women, the Peter Bent Brigham and Robert Breck Brigham Hospitals. This move resulted in strengthened clinical services, access to a wider range of consultants, centralization of clinical, laboratory and research facilities, stronger administrative ties to the Division of Gynecologic Oncology and the Department of Obstetrics and Gynecology, and improved teaching opportunities because of an expanded residency program, gyn-oncology fellowship program, and easier access to medical students.

PATHOLOGY

Accurate and reliable interpretation of pathologic material is a vital component of any trophoblast tumor service. At the New England Trophoblastic Disease Center we were fortunate to have Dr. Arthur T. Hertig, Shattuck Professor of Pathology, Emeritus, Harvard Medical School, and his assistant at the time, Dr. Hazel

Gore, available to review all specimens referred to our Center, as well as all surgical specimens obtained during inpatient therapy. In 1975 when the move to the Parkway Hospital was accomplished, and following Dr. Hertig's retirement, Dr. Shirley G. Driscoll, Department of Pathology, Boston Hospital for Women, took over these responsibilities and since that time has provided continuity of morphologic diagnosis. Many of the cases ultimately admitted to our service for treatment are referred to us by Dr. Driscoll after she has received outside slides for review as consultative material. Dr. Driscoll, in conjunction with our group, established a monthly clinicopathology trophoblast conference for the pathology and the gyn-oncology staff members, at which time all cases accessioned during the previous month are presented and clinical management discussed. In addition to reviewing all pathologic specimens, Dr. Driscoll has undertaken an intensive review of all placentas submitted to the Center which resulted from subsequent live births following either hydatidiform mole or gestational trophoblastic tumor.

hCG TESTING

The measurement of hCG is probably the single most important component of any program designed to identify and treat patients with gestational trophoblastic disease. hCG serves as a reliable tumor marker used for diagnosis, monitoring of therapy, and follow-up to ensure remission and detect recurrences. Thus, a reliable laboratory for measurement of hCG must be a vital component of any regional trophoblastic tumor center.

In 1965, the state of the art for hCG testing was the semi-quantitative mouse uterine weight bioassay which measured FSH, LH, and hCG. This assay had been used by Dr. Hertz from the inception of the National Cancer Institute program in 1955. A number of limitations of this assay system were widely recognized. First, it was semiquantitative. Second, it required a 24-hour urine collection. Third, one week was required to complete the assay. Fourth, the bioassay depended on a stable supply of immature rats. Finally, the bioassay lacked specificity. The advent of the technique of radioimmunoassay in the mid-1960's opened up a new era in the measurement of polypeptide hormones. Between 1968 and 1972 the radioimmunoassay for LH was utilized as the main hCG testing system in our laboratory. Although not specific for hCG, this assay had many advantages over the mouse uterine weight bioassay in that it was more specific, quantitative, and readily performed. It was possible to use this system to identify remission by using the endogenous LH level as the level at which remission was indicated by the absence of hCG. In 1972, the so-called beta subunit radioimmunoassay proved to be a more satisfactory technique for measuring hCG. A modified assay for this subfraction was developed in our laboratory in 1973 and has been in use since that time. The beta subunit radioimmunoassay provides a sensitive and reasonably specific tool for the management of patients with molar pregnancy and persistent trophoblastic tumors. Since hCG is measurable in small aliquots of serum within one working day, serum levels can be determined on a daily basis if desired, thus permitting more frequent testing to determine tumor doubling time and to assess the slope of the regression curve as the most reliable indication of response to therapy.

This improved method of monitoring allowed us to develop treatment protocols which were based on tumor growth and regression rather than more rigid protocols which administer drugs at specific time intervals. This resulted in a decrease in the total dose of drugs required for treatment as well as shortened hospital stays and significantly reduced toxic side effects.

Approximately 2500 hCG assays are performed annually at our laboratory on patients who are undergoing therapy and in patients who are being followed post-therapy for remission. Newer assay techniques are currently under investigation, particularly those which can be performed on aliquots of urine which would simplify gonadotropin testing for our patients.

REGISTRY

The establishment of a registry for patients with trophoblastic tumors should be regarded as a primary obligation of any regional center. This can be accomplished by establishing and maintaining excellent relations with clinicians in the region served by the center. The purpose of the registry is to accumulate a large body of clinical material including history, pathology, hCG titers, course of disease, therapy utilized, and follow-up. Physicians are requested to submit a history on all patients accessioned, slides for pathologic review by our pathology service to establish a uniform pathologic diagnosis, and to submit serum for hCG testing, and keep us informed regarding outpatient follow-up. In return, we offer the clinician advice regarding optimal management, and when it appears that the patient will require therapy we offer the services of our Center for that purpose. We have found that many of the patients who are ultimately admitted to the Center come to us referred by pathologists in the referring hospital who have, in turn, advised their clinical colleagues to contact us for advice regarding treatment.

The patients accessioned to the registry represent an accurate cross section of the type of gestational trophoblastic tumor problems which exist in our community. Between 1965 and 1983 a total of 2004 patients were accessioned to the New England

Trophoblastic Disease Center registry. These include approximately 1600 patients with hydatidiform mole, and 400 patients with persistent gestational trophoblastic disease. These patients have been the basis on which a wealth of clinical material has emerged, allowing us to carry on a number of retrospective clinical studies.

PATIENT CARE

The rationale for the existence of any regional center for gestational trophoblastic disease is founded on the Osterian triad of patient care, teaching, and research. The philosophy of the New England Trophoblastic Disease Center since its inception has been the principle of bringing science to the bedside, and the bedside to the laboratory.

Patients with Molar Pregnancy

Molar pregnancy is the most important patient group, not only because it represents the largest source of clinical material, but also because it is the most common gestation to precede the development of persistent gestational trophoblastic disease. Our approach to the management of molar pregnancy emphasizes early detection to reduce the morbidity of evacuation and prophylactic chemotherapy to minimize the incidence of persistent gestational trophoblastic disease. Initially, all patients admitted with molar pregnancy were treated with prophylactic actinomycin D (1). As our experience with these patients grew, a scoring system was devised which separated a group of patients with molar pregnancy who were at high risk for developing persistent gestational trophoblastic disease. Patients with high-risk molar pregnancy are characterized as having a serum hCG level greater than 100,000 mIU/ml, uterine size larger than dates, ovarian cysts larger than 6 cm in diameter, and associated medical and epidemiologic factors including maternal age over 40, toxemia, hyperthyroidism, and trophoblastic embolization (2). Following evacuation in patients with high-risk molar pregnancy, nonmetastatic and metastatic gestational trophoblastic disease developed in 31% and 8.8% of the patients, respectively (Table 1) (3). In contrast, nonmetastatic and metastatic gestational trophoblastic disease developed in only 3.4% and 0.6% of patients with low-risk molar pregnancy. Prophylactic chemotherapy is now administered only to patients with high-risk molar pregnancy, particularly when there is concern for the reliability or availability of hormonal follow-up. Prophylactic actinomycin D prevents the development of metastatic gestational trophoblastic disease and reduces the incidence of nonmetastatic disease to 4% (4).

Following molar evacuation, patients are monitored with weekly hCG values until they are normal for three consecutive weeks, and then with monthly levels until they are normal for six consecutive

Table 1. Sequelae of Low- and High-Risk Complete Hydatidiform Mole

	Number of patients	
Outcome	Low-risk	High-risk
Normal involution	486/506 (96%)	212/352 (60.2%)
Persistent GTT[a]		
Nonmetastatic	17/506 (3.4%)	109/352 (31.0%)
Metastatic	3/506 (0.6%)	31/352 (8.8%)
Totals	506/858 (59%)	352/858 (41%)

All patients were managed by evacuation with no prophylactic chemotherapy.
[a]GTT, gestational trophoblastic tumor.

months. The necessity for careful hCG follow-up cannot be over-emphasized because hormonal monitoring is the only method that can accurately detect the early development of persistent gestational trophoblastic disease (5). Patients are encouraged to use effective contraception during the interval of hormonal follow-up. We believe that oral contraceptives may be safely prescribed without increasing the risk of persistent gestational trophoblastic disease (6).

After molar evacuation, patients are readmitted to the New England Trophoblastic Disease Center for further evaluation and chemotherapy for the following indications: 1) the hCG level plateaus for three or more weeks, or re-elevates; 2) metastases develop; and 3) the curetted tissues demonstrate myometrial invasion or choriocarcinoma in a patient who did not receive prophylactic chemotherapy.

Staging of Gestational Trophoblastic Disease (GTD)

An anatomic staging system for GTD was adopted by the FIGO Cancer Committee in 1982 to enable the uniform reporting of data on an international basis for inclusion in the FIGO Cancer Registry (Table 2)(7). Stage I includes all patients with persistently elevated hCG titers and trophoblastic tumor limited to the uterine corpus. Stage II includes all patients with tumor outside the uterus but localized to the vagina or pelvic structures. Stage III includes all patients with pulmonary

Table 2. Staging of Gestational Trophoblastic Tumors

Stage	Location of tumor
I	Confined to uterine corpus
II	Metastases to pelvis and/or vagina
III	Metastases to lung
IV	Distant metastases

metastases with or without uterine, pelvic, or vaginal lesions. Patients with involvement of all other distant sites are categorized as having Stage IV disease. These patients have far-advanced tumor with involvement of brain, liver, spleen, kidney, and/or gastrointestinal tract.

In addition to anatomic staging, a prognostic scoring system is also used to help select treatment appropriate for individual patients (2, 7). The prognostic scoring system includes such variables as tumor burden (hCG level, number of metastases, size of metastases), delay in diagnosis, type of antecedent pregnancy, sites of metastatic involvement, and failed prior therapy (8). For all practical purposes, all Stage I patients have a low-risk score, and all Stage IV patients have a high-risk score. Therefore, the prognostic scoring system only applies to patients with Stages II and III GTD in whom the selection of single agent or multiple agent protocols may prove to be decisive in affecting outcome.

Management of Stage I GTD

Single agent chemotherapy is the treatment of choice in patients with Stage I disease who desire to preserve fertility (Table 3). Methotrexate and citrovorum factor is our preferred regimen because it achieves a high cure rate while limiting toxicity (9-11). When patients are resistant to methotrexate, actinomycin D is promptly substituted (12). Our method of administering chemotherapy has been described in detail in other publications from our Center (11, 13). If patients are resistant to single agent chemotherapy, they are then treated with either combination chemotherapy or surgical intervention. When a patient does not want to retain fertility, primary hysterectomy may be performed with adjuvant single agent chemotherapy (14).

Table 3. Treatment Protocol for Stage I Gestational Trophoblastic Tumor (New England Trophoblastic Disease Center)

Initial	
	Sequential MTX/Act D[a] or
	Hysterectomy with adjunctive chemotherapy
Resistant	
	MAC or
	Hysterectomy with adjunctive chemotherapy
	Local resection
	Pelvic infusion
Follow-up	
	hCG weekly until normal for 3 weeks, then
	Monthly until normal for 12 months
Contraception	
	12 consecutive months of normal hCG titers

[a]Abbreviations: MTX, methotrexate; Act D, actinomycin D; MAC, methotrexate, actinomycin D, and cyclophosphamide.

Between July 1965 and December 1982, 253 patients with Stage I GTD were managed at the New England Trophoblastic Disease Center. The results of therapy in these patients are shown in Table 4.

Management of Stage II GTD

Patients with Stage II disease are separated into high- and low-risk groups based upon their prognostic score. While low-risk patients are treated with primary single agent chemotherapy, high-risk patients are managed with primary combination chemotherapy (Table 5)(15). Surgical resection or packing of vaginal metastases may be required in selected patients to control bleeding.

Twenty-five patients with Stage II disease have been treated at the New England Trophoblastic Disease Center, and all have achieved complete remission. Table 6 reviews the outcome of therapy in these patients.

Management of Stage III GTD

Patients with Stage III GTD are also categorized as being

Table 4. New England Trophoblastic Disease Center, July 1965 to December 1982: Stage I GTD (Confined to Uterine Corpus)

Remission therapy	No. patients	No. remissions
Initial	243 (96.0%)	
Sequential MTX/Act D[a]		223 (91.8%)
Hysterectomy		20 (8.2%)
Resistant	10 (4.0%)	
MAC		5 (50.0%)
Hysterectomy		2 (20.0%)
Local uterine resection		2 (20.0%)
Pelvic infusion		1 (10.0%)
Totals	253	253 (100%)

[a]Abbreviations: MTX, methotrexate; Act D, actinomycin D; MAC, methotrexate, actinomycin D, and cyclophosphamide.

Table 5. Treatment Protocol for Stage II GTD (New England Trophoblastic Disease Center)

Low-risk[a]	
Initial	Sequential MTX/Act D[b]
Resistant	MAC
High-risk[a]	
Initial	MAC
Resistant	CHAMOCA, VBP
Follow-up	
hCG	Weekly until normal for 3 weeks, then monthly until normal for 12 months
Contraception	12 consecutive months of normal hCG levels

[a]Local resection optional.
[b]Abbreviations: MTX, methotrexate; Act D, actinomycin D; MAC, methotrexate, actinomycin D, and cyclophosphamide; VBP, vinblastine, bleomycin, *cis*-platinum; CHAMOCA, Bagshawe multi-agent regimen (pps. 349, 350, this book).

Table 6. New England Trophoblastic Disease Center, July 1965 to December 1982: Stage II GTD (Metastases to Pelvis and Vagina)

Remission therapy	No. patients	No. remissions
Low-risk	17 (68.0%)	
Initial: Sequential MTX/Act D[a]		15 (88.2%)
Local resection	3	
Resistant: MAC		2 (11.8%)
Local resection	2	
High-risk	8 (32.0%)	
Initial: Sequential MTX/Act D		2 (25.0%)
MAC		4 (50.0%)
Local resection	2	
Resistant: MAC		1 (12.5%)
CHAMOCA		1 (12.5%)
Local resection	1	
Totals	25	25 (100%)

[a]Abbreviations: MTX, methotrexate; Act D, actinomycin D; MAC, methotrexate, actinomycin D, and cyclophosphamide; CHAMOCA, Bagshawe multi-agent regimen (pps. 349, 350, this book).

high- or low-risk based upon their prognostic score. High-risk patients are treated with primary combination chemotherapy, and low-risk patients are managed with primary single agent chemotherapy (Table 7). Infrequently, pulmonary resection is performed to remove a site of resistant tumor (16).

At the New England Trophoblastic Disease Center, 87 patients with Stage III GTD have been managed, and all attained complete remission. The results of treatment in our patients with Stage III disease are reviewed in Table 8.

Management of Stage IV GTD

All patients with Stage IV GTD are treated with intensive combination chemotherapy and the selective use of radiation therapy and surgical intervention (Table 9). When cerebral metastases are detected, whole head irradiation is promptly instituted (17).

Table 7. Treatment Protocol for Stage III GTD (New England Trophoblastic Disease Center)

Low-risk[a]	
Initial	Sequential MTX/Act D[b]
Resistant	MAC
High-risk[a]	
Initial	MAC
Resistant	CHAMOCA, VBP
Follow-up	
hCG	Weekly until normal for 3 weeks, then monthly until normal for 12 months
Contraception	12 consecutive months of normal hCG levels

[a]Local resection optional.
[b]Abbreviations: MTX, methotrexate; Act D, actinomycin D; MAC, methotrexate, actinomycin D, and cyclophosphamide; VBP, vinblastine, bleomycin, and *cis*-platinum; CHAMOCA, Bagshawe multi-agent regimen (pps. 349, 350, this book).

Table 8. New England Trophoblastic Disease Center, July 1965 to December 1982: Stage III GTD (Metastases to Lung)

Remission therapy	No. patients	No. remissions
Low-risk	63 (72.5%)	
Initial: Sequential MTX/Act D[a]		56 (88.9%)
Local resection	5	
Resistant: MAC		7 (11.1%)
Local resection	3	
High-risk	24 (27.5%)	
Initial: Sequential MTX/Act D		13 (54.2%)
MAC		8 (33.3%)
Local resection	6	
Resistant: MAC		2 (8.3%)
CHAMOCA		1 (4.2%)
Local resection	2	
Totals	87	87 (100%)

[a]Abbreviations: MTX, methotrexate; Act D, actinomycin D; MAC, methotrexate, actinomycin D, and cyclophosphamide; CHAMOCA, Bagshawe multi-agent regimen (pps. 349, 350, this book).

Table 9. Treatment Protocol for Stage IV GTD (New England Trophoblastic Disease Center)

Initial	
MAC[a]	
Brain	Whole head irradiation (3,000 rad) Craniotomy to manage complications
Liver	Resection to manage complications
Resistant[b]	
CHAMOCA	
VBP	
Hepatic arterial infusion	
Follow-up	
hCG	Weekly until normal for 3 weeks, then Monthly until normal for 24 months
Contraception	24 consecutive months of normal hCG levels

[a]Abbreviations: MAC, methotrexate, actinomycin D, cyclophosphamide; VBP, vinblastine, bleomycin, and *cis*-platinum; CHAMOCA, Bagshawe multi-agent regimen (pps. 349, 350, this book).

The concurrent use of combination chemotherapy and brain irradiation reduces the risk of spontaneous bleeding in cerebral metastases. Surgical procedures may be required to manage acute complications such as craniotomy to control intracranial bleeding or to relieve intracranial pressure, hepatic resection to control bleeding from hepatic rupture, or bowel resection to treat bleeding or obstruction.

Since 1975, 15 patients with Stage IV disease have been treated at the New England Trophoblastic Disease Center with aggressive multi-modality therapy, and 11 patients (73%) attained remission. The outcome of treatment in patients with Stage IV GTD is shown in Table 10.

Table 10. New England Trophoblastic Disease Center, July 1965 to December 1982: Stage IV GTD (Distant Metastases)

Remission therapy[a]	No. of remissions	
Before 1975		
Initial: Sequential MTX/Act D[b]	5	
Resistant: MAC	1	6/20 (30%)
1975 and later		
Initial: Sequential MTX/Act D	2	
MAC	2	
Resistant: High-dose MTX/Act D	4	11/15 (73.3%)
MAC	1	
CHAMOCA	1	
VBP	1	

[a]Radiotherapy and surgery were utilized when indicated.
[b]Abbreviations: MTX, methotrexate; Act D, actinomycin D; MAC, methotrexate, actinomycin D, and cyclophosphamide; VBP, vinblastine, bleomycin, and *cis*-platinum; CHAMOCA, Bagshawe multi-agent regimen (pps. 349, 350, this book).

Subsequent Pregnancies

One of the main concerns expressed by patients after treatment for molar pregnancy and gestational trophoblastic disease is their outlook for normal pregnancy in the future. Patients with molar pregnancy and gestational trophoblastic disease who were managed at the New England Trophoblastic Disease Center had 919 and 222 subsequent pregnancies, respectively, between June 1965 and June 1983 (Tables 11 and 12). These later pregnancies had no increased risk of spontaneous abortion, prematurity, or stillbirths (19-21). It is particularly reassuring that the frequency of later congenital malformations is not increased because the chemotherapy employed is potentially teratogenic and mutagenic. The subsequent pregnancies also have no increased risk of obstetrical complications. Patients with molar pregnancy and gestational trophoblastic disease should be reassured that in general they can anticipate a normal reproductive outcome in the future.

However, when a patient has had a molar pregnancy, there is an increased risk of molar gestation (1:120) in subsequent conceptions.

Table 11. Subsequent Pregnancies in Patients with Hydatidiform Mole: New England Trophoblastic Disease Center, 1965 to 1983

Outcome	Number
Term delivery	618 (67.2%)
Stillbirth	4 (0.5%)
Premature delivery	79 (8.6%)
Spontaneous abortion	
First trimester	162 (17.6%)
Second trimester	14 (1.5%)
Therapeutic abortion	22 (2.4%)
Ectopic	7 (0.8%)
Repeat mole	13 (1.4%)
Total number of pregnancies	919
	No./deliveries
Congenital malformations	32/701 (4.5%)
Primary cesarean section	14/110 (12.7%)[a]

[a]January 1979 to June 1983.

Table 12. Subsequent Pregnancies in Patients with Gestational Trophoblastic Disease: New England Trophoblastic Disease Center, 1965 to 1983

Outcome	Number
Term delivery	153 (68.9%)
Stillbirth	5 (2.2%)
Premature delivery	10 (4.5%)
Spontaneous abortion	
First trimester	37 (16.6%)
Second trimester	7 (3.1%)
Therapeutic abortion	6 (3.0%)
Ectopic pregnancy	3 (1.3%)
Repeat molar pregnancy	1 (0.4%)
Total number of pregnancies	222
	No./deliveries
Congenital malformations	5/168 (3.0%)
Primary cesarean section	7/73 (9.6%)[a]

[a]January 1979 to June 1983.

We therefore think that it is prudent to obtain an ultrasound in later pregnancies to confirm normal gestational development. The presence of occult trophoblastic neoplasia should also be excluded by sending the placenta or products of conception for pathologic review and obtaining an hCG level six weeks after completing any future pregnancy.

CONCLUSION

Dramatic advances have occurred in the treatment of molar pregnancy and gestational trophoblastic disease during the past 25 years. The concentration of patient care in regional centers has been essential to enable the development of improved therapy. The recent adoption of a uniform staging system by FIGO represents an important step in the management of gestational trophoblastic disease. The use of a uniform staging system will hopefully encourage prospective multi-institutional treatment trials to assess new therapies as well as the relative merits of current therapies and to suggest new areas for clinical and basic research.

REFERENCES

1. Goldstein, D. P., Prevention of gestational trophoblastic disease by use of actinomycin D in molar pregnancies, Obstet. Gynecol. 43:475 (1974).
2. Goldstein, D. P., and Berkowitz, R.S., "Gestational Trophoblastic Neoplasms -- Clinical Principles of Diagnosis and Management," W. B. Saunders Company, Philadelphia, 1982.
3. Goldstein, D. P., Berkowitz, R. S., and Bernstein, M. R., Management of molar pregnancy, J. Reprod. Med. 26:208 (1981).
4. Goldstein, D. P., Berkowitz, R. S., and Cohen, S. M., The current management of molar pregnancy, Curr. Probl. Obstet. Gynecol. 3:1 (1979).
5. Goldstein, D. P., Chorionic gonadotropin, Cancer 38:453 (1976).
6. Berkowitz, R. S., Goldstein, D. P., Marean, A. R., and Bernstein, M. R., Oral contraceptives and postmolar trophoblastic disease, Obstet. Gynecol. 58:474 (1981).
7. Goldstein, D. P., and Berkowitz, R. S., The management of gestational trophoblastic neoplasms, Curr. Probl. Obstet. Gynecol. 3:1 (1980).
8. Bagshawe, K. D., Risk and prognostic factors in trophoblastic neoplasia, Cancer 38:1373 (1976).
9. Berkowitz, R. S., and Goldstein, D. P., Methotrexate with citrovorum factor rescue and non-metastatic gestational trophoblastic neoplasms, Obstet. Gynecol. 54:725 (1979).
10. Berkowitz, R. S., Goldstein, D. P., Jones, M. A., Marean, A. R., and Bernstein, M. R., Methotrexate with citrovorum factor rescue: reduced chemotherapy toxicity in the management of gestational trophoblastic neoplasms, Cancer 45:423 (1980).
11. Berkowitz, R. S., Goldstein, D. P., and Bernstein, M. R., Methotrexate with citrovorum rescue as a primary therapy for gestational trophoblastic disease, Cancer 50:2024 (1982).
12. Osathanondh, R., Goldstein, D. P., and Pastorfide, G. B., Actinomycin D as the primary agent for gestational trophoblastic disease, Cancer 36:863 (1975).
13. Goldstein, D. P., The chemotherapy of gestational trophoblastic disease: principles of clinical management, J. Amer. Med. Assocn. 220:209 (1972).
14. Berkowitz, R. S., Goldstein, D. P., and Bernstein, M. R., Management of nonmetastatic trophoblastic tumors, J. Reprod. Med. 26:219 (1981).
15. Goldstein, D. P., and Berkowitz, R. S., Nonmetastatic and low risk metastatic gestational trophoblastic neoplasms, Seminars in Oncology 9:191 (1982).
16. Shirley, R. L., Goldstein, D. P., and Collins, J. J., Jr., The role of thoracotomy in the management of patients with chest metastases from gestational trophoblastic disease, J. Thor. Cardio. Surg. 63:545 (1972).

17. Brace, K. C., The role of irradiation in the treatment of metastatic trophoblastic disease, Radiology 91:540 (1968).
18. Hammond, C. B., Weed, J. C., Jr., and Currie, J. L., The role of operation in the current therapy of gestational trophoblastic disease, Amer. J. Obstet. Gynecol. 136:844 (1980).
19. Pastorfide, G. B., and Goldstein, D. P., Pregnancy after hydatidiform mole, Obstet. Gynecol. 42:67 (1973).
20. Goldstein, D. P., Berkowitz, R. S., and Bernstein, M. R., Reproductive performance after molar pregnancy and gestational trophoblastic tumors, Clin. Obstet. Gynecol. 27:221 (1984).
21. Federschneider, J. M., Goldstein, D. P., Berkowitz, R. S., Marean, A. R., and Bernstein, M. R., Natural history of recurrent molar pregnancy, Obstet. Gynecol. 55:457 (1980).

THE STUDY AND TREATMENT OF GESTATIONAL TROPHOBLASTIC DISEASES AT THE BREWER TROPHOBLASTIC DISEASE CENTER, 1962 - 1979

John R. Lurain and John I. Brewer

The John I. Brewer Trophoblastic Disease Center
Department of Obstetrics and Gynecology, and
Cancer Center
Northwestern University Medical School and
Northwestern Memorial Hospital
Chicago, Illinois, USA

INTRODUCTION

The John I. Brewer Trophoblastic Disease Center of Northwestern University Medical School was founded in 1962 for the study and treatment of gestational trophoblastic diseases. From 1962 to 1984, the Center has received referrals of 4,461 patients from 42 states and 7 foreign countries. Experience gained at the Center in the management of these patients provides the basis for this report. Only patients managed at the Center up to 1979 are analyzed here in order to provide for five-year follow-up (1).

TREATMENT RESULTS

From 1962 through 1978, 399 patients with invasive mole or choriocarcinoma were admitted to the Center for treatment with chemotherapy. Of these, 359 patients received complete treatment at the Center, 37 patients had received chemotherapy elsewhere before referral to the Center, and three patients died before one complete course of chemotherapy could be administered.

Chemotherapy was the main form of treatment, usually involving methotrexate, actinomycin D, or a combination of these agents and cyclophosphamide (MAC). Whole brain irradiation of 3,000 to 4,000 rads was given to patients with cerebral metastases. Adjuvant surgery and radiation therapy to sites other than the brain were used in selected patients.

Table 1. Results of Treatment of 359 Patients with Choriocarcinoma and Invasive Mole

Diagnosis	No. of patients	Remissions
Choriocarcinoma	159	129 (81%)
Metastatic	105	75 (71%)
Nonmetastatic	54	54 (100%)
Invasive mole	200	200 (100%)
Metastatic	69	69
Nonmetastatic	131	131
Total	359	329 (92%)
Metastatic	174	144 (83%)
Nonmetastatic	185	185 (100%)

Table 1 presents the results for 359 patients who received their entire treatment at the Center. The overall cure rate was 92%. The data are shown for invasive mole and choriocarcinoma as well as for the presence or absence of metastases.

Five factors were determined to significantly influence response to treatment in patients with metastatic disease: 1) clinicopathologic diagnosis; 2) height of the pretreatment hCG titer along with duration of disease; 3) metastatic site; 4) antecedent pregnancy; and 5) prior unsuccessful therapy. There was a significant effect of clinicopathologic diagnosis on survival ($P<0.0005$). All 69 patients with metastatic invasive mole were cured compared to 71% (75/105) of patients with metastatic choriocarcinoma (Table 1).

As seen in Table 2, 93% of patients with both an hCG titer of 100,000 IU/l or less and a duration of disease of four months or less entered remission, whereas only 62% of patients with hCG titers greater than 100,000 IU/l and an interval of greater than four months from antecedent pregnancy to treatment were cured ($P<0.0005$). The effect of sites of metastases on survival is shown in Table 3. If metastatic disease was confined to the lung and/or vagina, survival was 92% *versus* 37% for all other sites ($P<0.0005$). There was a significant difference ($P<0.02$) in remission rates in patients with metastatic choriocarcinoma following term gestation (19/34, 56%) as compared with combined rates for disease following abortion, ectopic pregnancy and hydatidiform mole (56/71, 79%). Of 37 patients initially treated elsewhere before referral to the authors' center, the remission rate

Table 2. Effect of Duration of Disease and hCG Titer on Response to Therapy in Metastatic Gestational Trophoblastic Disease

Duration of disease	hCG titer[a] ≤100,000 IU/l	hCG titer[a] >100,000 IU/l	Total
≤4 months	70/75 (93%)	32/39	102/114
>4 months	24/32	15/24 (62%)	36/56
Total	94/107	47/63	141/170 (83%)

[a]Remission/total no. of patients.

Table 3. Effect of Metastatic Site on Response to Therapy in Metastatic Gestational Trophoblastic Disease (N = 174)

Metastatic site(s)	No. of patients	No. of survivals	No. of deaths
Lung	122	113 (93%)	9
Vagina	8	8 (100%)	0
Lung and vagina	14	12 (86%)	2
Pelvis ± lung	7	3 (43%)	4
Brain[a]	13	8 (62%)	5
Brain and liver	3	0	3
Liver[b]	3	0	3
Intra-abdominal[c]	4	0	4
Total	174	144 (83%)	30 (17%)

[a]Eleven patients also had lung metastases.
[b]Two patients also had lung metastases.
[c]Three patients also had lung metastases and one had liver metastases.

Table 4. Results of Treatment of 37 Patients with Gestational Trophoblastic Disease Referred after Failure of Treatment Elsewhere

Diagnosis	No. of patients	No. of remissions
Choriocarcinoma	26	11 (42%)
Metastatic	24	9 (38%)
Nonmetastatic	2	2
Invasive mole	11	11 (100%)
Metastatic	5	5
Nonmetastatic	6	6
Total	37	22 (59%)
Metastatic	29	14 (48%)
Nonmetastatic	8	8 (100%)

was 59%, whereas the rate for patients treated totally at the center was 92% ($P<0.005$)(Table 4).

Secondary treatment with other chemotherapeutic agents including the modified Bagshawe protocol (CHAMOCA) and combinations of vinblastine, bleomycin and *cis*-platinum, was given to 34 patients after failure of initial therapy to cure the disease. Only three of these patients (8.8%) achieved remission. Adjuvant radiation therapy to sites other than the brain, did not yield any significant responses.

Sixteen patients (4.5%) relapsed from one to 11 months following remission. The relapse rate decreased from 18.2% to 3.1% when additional courses of chemotherapy (usually two) were given following the first normal hCG level. Four patients died after achieving one or more remissions and 12 were apparently cured, two by hysterectomy, one by chemotherapy and thoracotomy, and nine by additional chemotherapy alone. Forty-one patients died without ever attaining remission.

ANALYSIS OF DEATHS

Of 399 patients referred to the Center from 1962 to 1979 for treatment of gestational trophoblastic disease, 48 (12%) died (2, 3). Three patients died before receiving any treatment, 15 patients received treatment elsewhere before referral, and 30 patients received all of their treatment at the Center (Table 5).

Table 5. Deaths from Gestational Trophoblastic Disease at the Brewer Trophoblastic Disease Center, 1962 - 1979

Treatment category	Patients	Deaths
Complete treatment at Center	359	30 (8%)
Initial treatment elsewhere	37	15 (41%)
No treatment	3	3 (100%)
Total	399	48 (12%)

Table 6. Sites of Metastasis at Diagnosis in 48 Patients with Fatal Gestational Choriocarcinoma

	Patients	
Metastatic site	No.	%
None	4	8
Lung only	14	29
Lung and vagina	2	4
Lung and pelvis	3	6
Pelvis only	1	2
Brain and lung	8	17
Liver	9[a]	19
Intraperitoneal	7[b]	15

[a]Two patients, liver only; five patients, liver and lung; two patients, liver and bowel.
[b]Two patients with liver and bowel not included; five patients additionally with lung.

Table 7. Causes of Death in 48 Patients with Metastatic Gestational Choriocarcinoma

Cause of death	Patients No.	%
Hemorrhage	20	42
Pulmonary insufficiency	15	31
Drug toxicity	5	10
Sepsis	1	2
Uremia	1	2
Acute tubular necrosis (postoperative)	1	2
Pulmonary embolism (postoperative)	1	2
Unknown	4	8

All patients who died had histologically documented choriocarcinoma. The time from pregnancy event to treatment was greater than four months and/or the pretreatment hCG titer was greater than 100,000 IU/l in 64% of these patients. Seventy-one percent of fatal cases developed in association with term pregnancies, abortions, or ectopic pregnancies rather than hydatidiform mole. Fifty percent of patients who died had metastases to the brain, liver, and/or peritoneal cavity when they first presented for treatment (Table 6). As noted in Table 7, the most common causes of death were hemorrhage from one or more metastatic sites (42%) and pulmonary insufficiency (31%). Factors primarily responsible for the treatment failures in these patients were: 1) the presence of extensive disease at the time of initial treatment; 2) inadequate initial treatment; and 3) failure of presently used chemotherapy protocols in advanced disease.

REPEAT GESTATIONAL TROPHOBLASTIC DISEASE

During a ten-year period from 1969 to 1979, 22 of 1,648 patients referred to the Center had repeat gestational trophoblastic disease, an incidence of 1.33% (4). A total of 52 trophoblastic disease episodes occurred in these 22 patients. There were five patients (23%) who had more than one trophoblastic disease event; one of these patients had six consecutive hydatidiform moles. Invasive mole or choriocarcinoma occurred as the first trophoblastic disease episode in only three patients (14%), whereas one of these sequelae was the second trophoblastic disease event in seven patients (32%). Seventeen patients (77%) had consecutive trophoblastic disease episodes. After a second trophoblastic disease episode, the risk for a subsequent event rose to 28%; however, 44% of these patients delivered viable infants. There was no difference in outcome of subsequent pregnancies with respect to previous chemotherapy.

NATURAL HISTORY OF HYDATIDIFORM MOLE AFTER PRIMARY EVACUATION

From 1962 to 1978, 738 patients with hydatidiform mole were referred to the Center for follow-up and hCG testing after evacuation (5). Spontaneous regression of trophoblastic disease occurred in 596 (80.8%) of the patients, and treatment with chemotherapeutic agents was required in 142 (19.2%) of the 738 patients. Of the 596 patients in whom spontaneous regression occurred, hCG titers reached normal levels in 135 (22.7%) by 30 days after evacuation, in 255 (42.8%) between days 31 and 60, and in 206 (34.6%) between days 61 and 170. Of the 142 patients requiring treatment, 125 (16.9%) of these had invasive mole (107 nonmetastatic and 18 metastatic) and 17 (2.3%) had choriocarcinoma (13 nonmetastatic and four metastatic). Therefore, 15.5% of the 142 treated patients or 3% of the 738 total patients had metastatic disease to the lung and/or vagina.

All 596 patients in whom hCG titers declined spontaneously to normal levels have remained well and free from disease. All of the 142 patients who were treated with chemotherapy experienced permanent remission. Thus, all 738 patients, those treated and those not treated, are well and free from disease five to 19 years after evacuation of the hydatidiform mole. No patient in whom the hCG titer declined each time it was tested (every 10 to 14 days) developed evidence of disease progression, and none required treatment. A consistent decline in hCG values thus indicates spontaneous regression of disease. In all patients with progressive disease, a rise in hCG titer more accurately and rapidly identified the presence of disease than physical or roentgenologic examinations.

EARLY DEVELOPMENT OF CHORIOCARCINOMA

A study has been made by one of the authors (JIB) of the origin and development of choriocarcinoma in seemingly normal placentas (6, 7). Histologically, the tumors all appear to arise from the cytotrophoblastic cells covering the stromal portion of chorionic villi, and in some areas the involved villi retain a portion of normal investing trophoblast. This finding indicates that gestational choriocarcinoma unassociated with hydatidiform mole does have an early stage in which chorionic villi are present. Spontaneous degeneration involving both the abnormal trophoblast and villous stroma is consistently present in regions of the tumor. Localized necrosis and fragmentation of the malignant trophoblast may lead to deportation of the trophoblast into the intervillous space and myometrial venous channels and thus to myometrial or more distant sites. This spontaneous and progressive degeneration of the stromal portion of the involved villi may explain why formed stromal villi are not present in metastatic lesions or in the later stages of choriocarcinoma.

REFERENCES

1. Lurain, J. R., Brewer, J. I., Torok, E. E., and Halpern, B., Gestational trophoblastic disease: treatment results at the Brewer Trophoblastic Disease Center, Obstet. Gynecol. 60:354 (1982).
2. Lurain, J. R., Brewer, J. I., Mazur, M. T., and Torok, E. E., Fatal gestational trophoblastic disease: an analysis of treatment failures, Amer. J. Obstet. Gynecol. 144:391 (1982).
3. Mazur, M. T., Lurain, J. R., and Brewer, J. I., Fatal gestational choriocarcinoma. Clinicopathologic study of patients treated at a trophoblastic disease center, Cancer 50:1833 (1982).
4. Sand, P. K., Lurain, J. R., and Brewer, J. I., Repeat gestational trophoblastic disease, Obstet. Gynecol. 63:140 (1983).
5. Lurain, J. R., Brewer, J. I., Torok, E. E., and Halpern, B., Natural history of hydatidiform mole after primary evacuation, Amer. J. Obstet. Gynecol. 145:591 (1983).
6. Brewer, J. I., Torok, E. E., Kahan, B. D., Stanhope, C. R., and Halpern, B., Gestational trophoblastic disease: origin of choriocarcinoma, invasive mole and choriocarcinoma associated with hydatidiform mole, and some immunologic aspects, Adv. Cancer Res. 27:89 (1978).
7. Brewer, J. I., and Mazur, M. T., Gestational choriocarcinoma. Its origin in the placenta during seemingly normal pregnancy, Amer. J. Surg. Pathol. 5:267 (1981).

PITFALLS IN THE MANAGEMENT OF TROPHOBLASTIC DISEASE IN AFRICA

J. K. G. Mati and C. Sekade Kigondu

Department of Obstetrics and Gynaecology
University of Nairobi
Kenya

INTRODUCTION

A clinician managing trophoblastic disease in Africa is inevitably faced with a number of fundamental problems. Among these are inadequate data on the magnitude of trophoblastic disease as a public health problem, late diagnosis and therefore advanced nature of the disease, non-availability or restrictive costs of chemotherapeutic agents, difficulties in monitoring patients during chemotherapy, and poor patient compliance, making follow-up of cases difficult.

This discussion highlights these problems and makes a suggestion for a coordinated effort and regional approach to the management of this disease.

INCIDENCE OF TROPHOBLASTIC DISEASE

It is generally stated that trophoblastic disease in Africa occupies a midpoint between high incidence in oriental and low level in western countries. However, there has not been any good epidemiological study to establish the prevalence of the disease in the community. Most of the data have been based on referral hospital patients. In Nigeria, Ayangade (1) recorded 35 cases of trophoblastic disease in a hospital delivering 13,182 women over the same period, and he gave a ratio of 1:375 deliveries as reflecting the national average. From his paper it is not clear what proportion of these cases were hydatidiform moles and which were malignant. In most referral hospitals, only malignant cases will be sent from surrounding health institutions. In Kenyatta

National Hospital in Nairobi, choriocarcinoma ranks second to carcinoma of the cervix in the register of gynecologic cancer. Between 1973 and 1979, 64 cases of choriocarcinoma were admitted to the hospital (2). Kenyatta National Hospital has the only public gynecologic unit in Nairobi, where most of the cases would be referred for treatment. During the seven year period, approximately 28,000 deliveries took place in the hospital, for a ratio of malignant trophoblastic disease to deliveries of 1:438. Assuming that most malignant trophoblastic disease cases were treated in the hospital, the incidence of the disease for Nairobi would be 1:2734 (there were approximately 175,000 deliveries in the city during the seven year period).

Hydatidiform mole, on the other hand, was seen relatively less commonly. Taking the generally accepted formula that 50% of the malignant cases follow a molar pregnancy, one would expect a higher incidence of moles than is the impression of clinicians in Nairobi. The possibility is therefore raised that some mole cases are missed and classified as incomplete abortions. To test this hypothesis, histology on incomplete abortions admitted at Kenyatta National Hospital was performed. In a series of 600 consecutive cases studied, only one was found to be molar (Storey *et al.*, unpublished data). This differs very much from published data elsewhere. Javey and associates (3) reported an incidence of 24.4 moles per 1,000 abortions in Iran. In Nairobi, hydatidiform mole ranks third as preceding pregnancy in choriocarcinoma Table 1).

THE PROBLEM OF LATE DIAGNOSIS

In Kenya, as in most other parts of Africa, malignant trophoblastic disease is often diagnosed in advanced stage. This is one of the most important factors affecting the results of treatment. When diagnosis of hydatidiform mole is made it is standard practice to arrange follow-up and therefore be in a position to make an early diagnosis of malignant transformation. In Africa, follow-up of cases is poor and, as indicated above, the majority of the cases are preceded by either abortion or term delivery. The problem is

Table 1. Type of Preceding Pregnancy in 64 Choriocarcinoma Patients

Abortion	24
Term delivery	21
Hydatidiform mole	11
Not known	8

Table 2. Frequency of Symptoms in Choriocarcinoma Patients

Symptom	No. of patients	%
Irregular bleeding	50	77
Lower abdominal pain and backache	18	28
Chest symptoms (pain, cough, hemoptysis)	14	22
Neurological	3	4.6
Liver/renal/GIT involvement	15	24

aggravated by the many ways in which a choriocarcinoma may present. The presenting symptoms and signs may not be gynecologic in nature, as no system of the body is exempt from this disease. Quite often the diagnosis is made purely on suspicion when a woman presents with a bizarre picture of otherwise unexplained disease (Table 2). This means, therefore, that in places with inadequate medical care -- particularly laboratory facilities -- many cases are missed, and those finally diagnosed are recognized late. The leading symptoms in the Nairobi series are summarized in Table 2.

Based on Bagshawe's rating of risk, a substantial number of the cases fall into the high risk category (Table 3). This means that single agent chemotherapy is indicated in only a very small proportion of cases. Only 3 of the 64 patients managed at Kenyatta National Hospital were offered methotrexate alone.

NON-AVAILABILITY OF DRUGS

Chemotherapeutic agents are very expensive and sometimes largely unavailable in parts of Africa. The need to use several courses of multiple drugs makes the treatment of choriocarcinoma even more costly. In countries with per capita health budgets below US$10, health administrators find it very difficult to balance ethical practice against the realities of providing basic health care to the nation at large. As a result, many patients with choriocarcinoma are under-treated, contributing to a high mortality rate.

Table 3. Presence of High Risk Factor in 64 Choriocarcinoma Cases

High risk factor	No. of patients
Age over 39 years	17
Gravidity 2-5	26
Presentation after 7 month lapse from previous pregnancy	19
Choriocarcinoma preceding delivery term or abortion	45

MONITORING CHEMOTHERAPY RESPONSE

There are two aspects of monitoring a patient receiving treatment. There is need to know not only the response of the disease to chemotherapy, but also how the patient responds to the treatment. In both instances, clinicians in Africa are confronted with endless difficulties.

Chemotherapy is immunosuppressive, and the patient is at risk of succumbing to infections which she would normally resist. Indeed, in developed countries such patients have been nursed in a germ-free environment. This is not possible in most general hospitals in Africa, nor may it be easy to monitor hematological changes in the patient and therefore withold chemotherapy when there is severe bone marrow suppression. These difficulties are undoubtedly responsible for a number of otherwise avoidable deaths.

Radioimmunoassay (RIA) of β-hCG is currently available in only two or three centers in sub-Saharan Africa. Even in these places, however, the problem of importation of radioisotopes makes the test infrequent. This is particularly true if kits have to be used when it becomes necessary to accumulate samples in order to avoid wastage of the kits.

In a number of African countries, LH assay is performed regularly for the management of infertility. This offers an opportunity for using the LH assay to monitor cases of trophoblastic disease, as shown earlier by Bagshawe and associates (4).

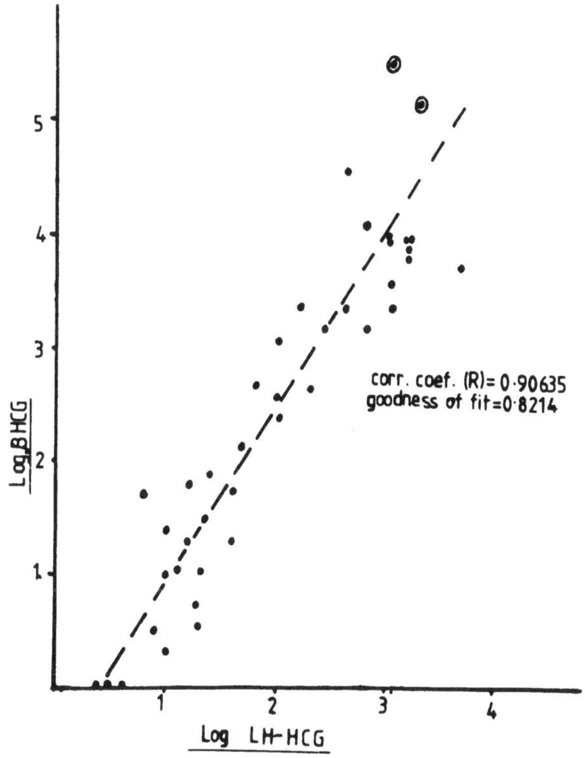

Fig. 1. Correlation between β-hCG levels and LH-hCG levels.

We have tested the correlation between LH and β-hCG assay in Nairobi (5), and have shown it to be adequately close to permit use of the LH assay to monitor patients until the physiological levels are reached, when the less frequently employed hCG assay becomes necessary.

Fig. 1 shows that there was good correlation between the levels of LH and β-hCG until the physiological range was reached (*i.e.*, log 0.5 of LH-hCG). This has made it possible to use LH results to monitor the response to chemotherapy during treatment. Levels of β-hCG are then determined after the follicular LH levels are attained.

Fig. 2 shows that LH and β-hCG run parallel during the treatment of patient AC. The routinely used pregnancy test became negative while the levels of both LH and β-hCG remained high.

Fig. 3 shows that LH levels indicate clearly the failure in the treatment of patient J. S., since the levels remained elevated throughout the treatment.

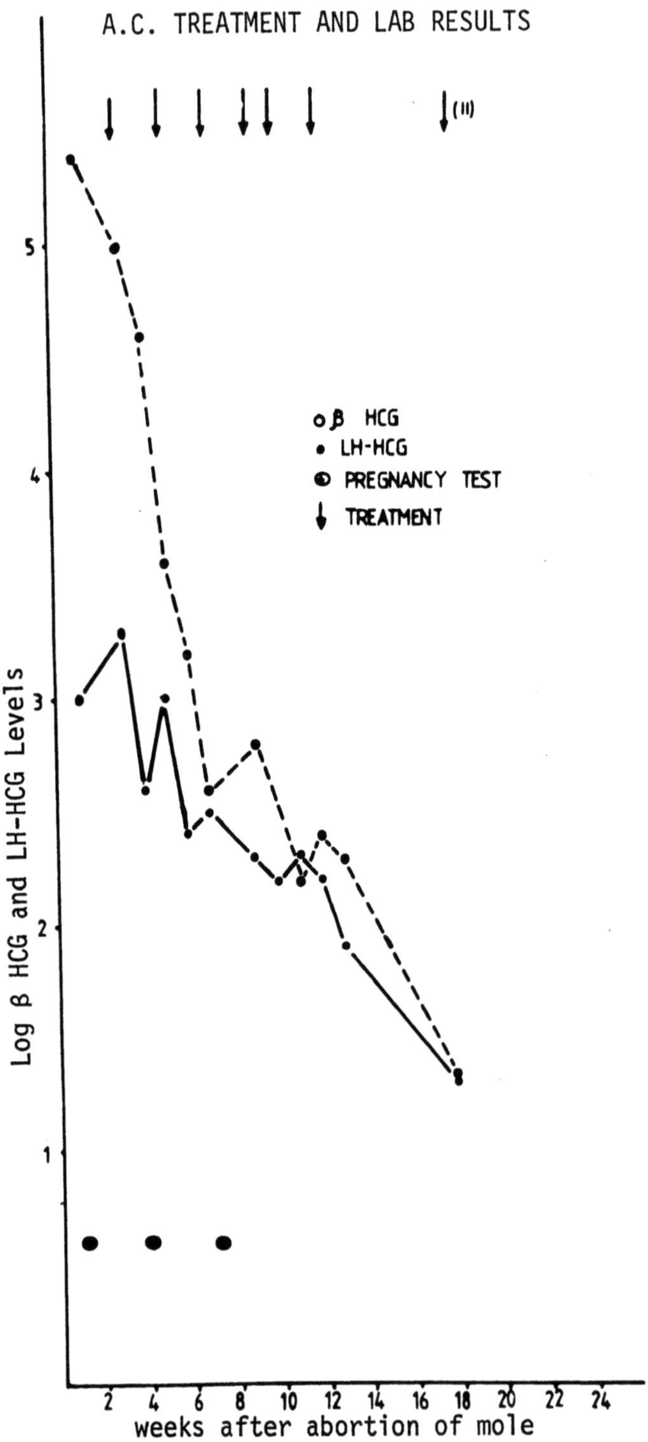

Fig. 2. Treatment summary and laboratory results on patient A. C.

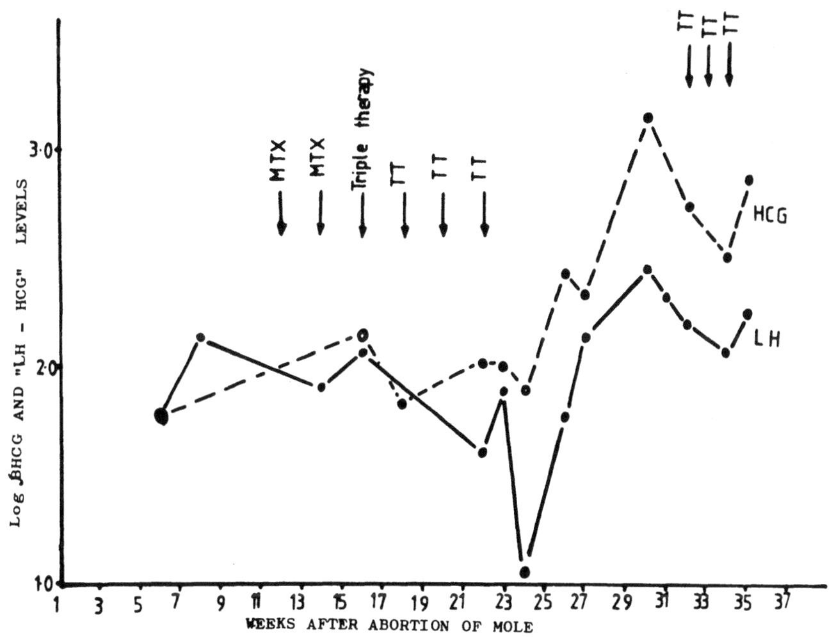

Fig. 3. Treatment summary and laboratory results on patient J. S. Abbreviations: MTX, methotrexate; TT, triple therapy.

POOR CASE FOLLOW-UP

The management of trophoblastic disease requires prolonged follow-up. This is necessary in molar pregnancy to identify any change to malignancy, and in treated choriocarcinoma to identify early recurrence. For a patient who feels well this requires a lot of motivation to return for follow-up. The requirement that these patients must defer pregnancy is in conflict with the cultural demands, particularly on young women, to have children. Consequently, contraceptive advice is not accepted, and many patients avoid the clinics. This state of affairs makes it difficult to evaluate results of treatment of trophoblastic disease in Africa.

CONCLUSION

The above discussion has shown that there has not been much advance in the management of trophoblastic disease in Africa, and some of the factors responsible have been identified. The basic constraint is inadequate resources and the high costs of therapy and monitoring of patients.

A number of proposals can be put forward for discussion and possible implementation. One of these, and perhaps the most important, is that since modern treatment of choriocarcinoma is not presently within reach of most countries in Africa, a coordinated effort is needed to establish regional centers of excellence, with facilities for modern investigation and treatment of the disease. To make this possible, input of national governments, international agencies, and other organizations will be required. Such centers should, among other things, take a lead in the study of epidemiology of trophoblastic disease in Africa and, in the long run, develop a technology that would be appropriately applied to the management of trophoblastic disease in the smaller units. There is need, for example, to investigate if central laboratories could monitor patients in provincial units using a postal service. Introduction of such an innovative program could also improve patient compliance and therefore improve case follow-up.

REFERENCES

1. Ayangade, O., Gestational trophoblastic disease in Nigeria - a 10 year review, East Afr. Med. J. 56:278 (1979).

2. Makokha, A. E. and Mati, J. K. G., Choriocarcinoma at Kenyatta National Hospital, 1973-79, J. Obstet. Gynae. East Central Afr. 1:27 (1982).

3. Javey, H. and Sajadi, H., Hydatidiform mole in Southern Iran: a statistical survey of 113 cases, Int. J. Gynaecol. Obstet. 15:390 (1978).

4. Bagshawe, K. D., Wilson, H., et al., J. Obstet. Gynaecol. Brit. Commonwlth. 80:461 (1973).

5. Sekadde-Kigondu, C. B., Fongoh, F. B., et al., The use of luteinizing hormone (LH) and beta human chorionic gonadotropin RIA in the diagnosis and treatment of choriocarcinoma at Kenyatta National Hospital, J. Obstet. Gynaecol. East Central Afr. 1:148 (1982).

THE PROBLEMS OF MANAGEMENT OF GESTATIONAL TROPHOBLASTIC NEOPLASMS AT THE UNIVERSITY OF BENIN TEACHING HOSPITAL, BENIN CITY, NIGERIA

F. M. E. Diejomaoh, A. E. Omu, E. E. Okpere,
M. Ezimokhai, O. Tabowei, and L. N. Ajabor

Department of Obstetrics and Gynaecology
College of Medical Sciences
University of Benin and
University of Benin Teaching Hospital
Benin City, Nigeria

ABSTRACT

Analysis of 31 cases of gestational trophoblastic neoplasms at the University of Benin Teaching Hospital, Benin City, over a 7½ year period (1/1/75 to 6/30/82) was carried out. The incidence of this disease was 1:656 deliveries. Although it was more prevalent in grandmultipara, it occurred in all parities and ages. The main clinical features were secondary amenorrhea, vaginal bleeding, uterine enlargement, and vaginal secondaries. The most common gestational antecedent event of gestational trophoblastic disease was a normal pregnancy. This was believed to have contributed to the high overall mortality of 35.5%. Numerous shortcomings during the management of these cases (inadequate laboratory facilities, shortage of reagents, shortage of drugs) were highlighted.

INTRODUCTION

There are different kinds of tumors of the trophoblast (1). Because of the varied behavior of the trophoblastic tumors and the progression of the disease from benign to malignant, with multiple metastases in the same patient, and the intensive follow-up after both benign and malignant disease, there is much to be said for grouping all tumors of the trophoblast together under the term, "gestational trophoblastic neoplasms," a terminology which is used in this report. Gestational trophoblastic neoplasms include all cases of benign hydatidiform mole, chorioadenoma destruens (malignant mole), and choriocarcinoma. At the University of Benin Teaching Hospital, tumors of the trophoblast are usually classified into benign and malignant trophoblastic disease.

With the varied clinical presentation, it is only with the support of modern laboratory, laparoscopy, ultrasound, and radiology services, and modern accurate estimation of hCG, that more cases of gestational trophoblastic disease will be diagnosed and treated. Although the prognosis of this disease has improved tremendously in recent times (2, 3), especially with the utilization of prognostic factors and individualization of chemotherapy (4, 5), mortality is still high in some communities because of late presentation and scarce facilities for treatment and follow-up monitoring of the patients. Hammond and associates (6) have warned that patients with long-standing and widespread disease can only expect a 20 to 25% remission rate.

We have therefore been motivated to review our experience in the management of gestational trophoblastic neoplasms at the University of Benin Teaching Hospital with the intent of identifying the mode of presentation, the management, and the prognosis of these diseases in our particular environment. In view of our limited facilities, our second objective is to make suggestions towards the further management of these neoplasms in similar settings.

MATERIALS AND METHODS

A retrospective analysis of the case reports of all patients admitted into the University of Benin Teaching Hospital, Benin City, Nigeria, from January 1, 1975, to June 30, 1982, was carried out. During this period, 31 patients were admitted with gestational trophoblastic neoplasms. The case reports of only 25 of these patients could be retrieved. These cases were then reviewed to ascertain the mode of presentation, the course of management, and the outcome of the disease in the patients.

Diagnosis of gestational trophoblastic neoplasm was based on a combination of any two or all of the following criteria: clinical diagnosis, urinary hCG estimation, and radiologic examination. Histological confirmation of the diagnosis was performed, where possible, by limited diagnostic curettage or excisional biopsy of secondaries. The mainstay of treatment in malignant cases was chemotherapy with a first-line regimen of combination oral therapy with methotrexate and 6-mercaptopurine, and a second-line regimen of intravenous actinomycin D. Surgery was usually indicated as supportive therapy and for specific conditions, such as persistent hemorrhage or resistant disease.

RESULTS

During the period under review there were 20,352 deliveries at the University of Benin Teaching Hospital. Thus, the incidence of gestational trophoblastic neoplasms at this hospital was 1:656 deliveries. The incidence of malignant trophoblastic disease (17 patients) was 1:1197 deliveries, while the incidence of hydatidiform mole (benign trophoblastic tumor) was 1:2544.

The age and parity distribution of gestational trophoblastic neoplasms are summarized in Table 1. Three patients (12%) were under 20 years while two patients (8%) were over 40 years old. The mean age of the patients was 29.4 ± 8.0 years and the age range was 16 to 52 years. The majority of the patients (17 patients, 68.0%) was in the active reproductive age group of 21 to 35 years. This age group represents the maximum reproductive age group in our community. The mean parity of the patients was 3.76 ± 3.1 with a range of 0 to 12. Five patients (20%) were primipara, and 7 (28%) were grandmultipara. Thirteen patients (52%) were in the low parity range of 1 to 4.

Table 2 shows the staging of gestational trophoblastic neoplasma, as extracted from Goldstein and Berkowitz (4). In our present series of patients, 8 cases (32%) were in Stage 0 (benign trophoblastic disease), while 17 cases (68%) were in Stages I-IV (malignant trophoblastic disease).

The staging of the disease as a prognostic index is shown in Table 3. Patients in Stage 0 all survived, whereas Stage I patients had a mortality rate of 40%. Patients in Stages II-IV had a mortality range of 66 to 100%. Therefore, it appears that staging alone cannot serve as a useful prognostic indicator for the disease.

Table 4 illustrates the variety of ways in which gestational trophoblastic neoplasms presented at the University of Benin Teaching Hospital. The most frequent symptoms were secondary amenorrhea (88%) and vaginal bleeding (84%). Abdominal swelling (indicative of an abdominal mass) was evident in 32% of the patients, hemoptysis in 20%, and dyspnea in 16%. The most frequent physical sign in these patients was uterine enlargement, which was noted in 84% of the cases (Table 5). Vaginal secondaries were noted in 28% of the patients, ovarian enlargement in 28%, and chest signs in 20%. Only 8% of the patients had symptoms of central nervous system involvement.

As shown in Table 6, the most frequent antecedent event before the occurrence of gestational trophoblastic neoplasms was a normal pregnancy (48%). The antecedent pregnancy was an abortion in 24% of the cases, and a hydatidiform mole in 20% of the cases. Only 8% of the patients had had no previous pregnancies.

Table 1. Age and Parity Distribution of 25 Patients with Gestational Trophoblastic Neoplasms at University of Benin Teaching Hospital

	Parity (Number of patients)						
Age in years	0	1-3	4-6	7-9	≥10	Total	%
19-20	3					3	12
21-25	1	3				4	16
26-30	1	4	4			9	36
31-35			4			4	16
36-40			2	1		3	12
41-50					1	1	4
52					1	1	4
Total	5	7	10	1	2	25	100
Percent	20	28	40	4	8	100	

Mean age: 29.4 years (range: 16-52).
Mean parity: 3.76 (range: 0-12).
Grandmultipara (para 5) = 7 patients (35.5%).

Table 2. Staging of Gestational Trophoblastic Neoplasms[a]

Stage	Characteristics
0[b]	Molar pregnancy
A	Low-risk
B	High-risk
I[c]	Confined to uterine corpus
II[c]	Metastases to pelvis and vagina
III[c]	Metastases to lung
IV[c]	Distant metastases (spread to liver, kidneys, spleen, brain, gastrointestinal tract)

[a]From Goldstein and Berkowitz (4).
[b]Benign trophoblastic disease (8 patients).
[c]Malignant trophoblastic disease (17 patients).

Table 3. Staging of Gestational Trophoblastic Neoplasms and its Prognostic Significance at University of Benin Teaching Hospital

Stage	No. of cases	Cases in remission	Defaulters/ refused therapy	Deaths	Mortality (%)
0	8	8			0
I	5	2	1	2	40
II	3			3	100
III	6	1	1	4	66.7
IV	3		1	2	66.7
Total	25	11	3	11[a]	

[a]Mortality rate = 11/25 x 100% = 44.0%; overall mortality rate = 11/31 x 100% = 35.5%.

Table 4. Presenting Symptoms in Gestational Trophoblastic Neoplasms at University of Benin Teaching Hospital

Symptom	No. of cases	Percent
Amenorrhea	22	88
Vaginal bleeding	21	84
Abdominal swelling	8	32
Hemoptysis	5	20
Dyspnea	4	16
Abdominal pain	2	8
Hemiparesis	2	8
Headache	2	8
Vomiting	2	8
Convulsions	2	8
Hemiplegia	1	4

Table 5. Initial Physical Signs in Gestational Trophoblastic Neoplasms at University of Benin Teaching Hospital

Physical sign	No. of cases	Percent
Uterine enlargement	21	84
Vaginal secondary	7	28
Ovarian enlargement	7	28
Chest signs	5	20
Uterus large for dates	5	20
Liver enlargement	4	16
Hypertension	3	12
Lower abdominal tenderness	3	12
Adnexal tenderness	3	12
Central nervous system signs	2	8
Fever	2	8

Table 6. Antecedent Pregnancy in Gestational Trophoblastic Neoplasms at University of Benin Teaching Hospital

Antecedent pregnancy	No. of cases	Percent
Normal pregnancy	12	48
Abortion	6	24
Hydatidiform mole	5	20
No previous pregnancy	2	8
Total	25	100

Table 7. Duration of Symptoms Prior to Hospitalization at University of Benin Teaching Hospital

Duration (Months)	No. of cases	Percent
3	11	44
4-6	9	36
7-9	3	12
10-12	1	4
More than 12	1	4
Total	25	100

The duration of symptoms before admission to hospital was 3 months or less in 44% of the cases, while 8% had symptoms for 10 months or longer before admission (Table 7). Thirty-six percent of the patients had symptoms for 4 to 6 months prior to admission. Of these, 3 had received a dilatation and curettage on 3 different occasions in private hospitals within a period of 3 months prior to admission, because of irregular vaginal bleeding.

Seven of the patients with Stage 0 disease had oxytocin induction and/or uterine evacuation with usual follow-up. The eighth patient, a 52 year-old Para 12+, received a course of combined chemotherapy with methotrexate and 6-mercaptopurine followed by a total abdominal hysterectomy and follow-up as usual.

Two of the patients with disease in Stages I-IV died before any chemotherapy could be instituted, while a third patient died within 2 days of the commencement of therapy. In all of the other 14 patients, standard chemotherapy regimens were followed, while urinary hCG estimation and ancillary blood and radiologic investigations were carried out. In three patients with resistant disease, second line chemotherapy with actinomycin D was carried out. In another patient with resistant metastatic disease, total abdominal hysterectomy was performed followed by massive intermittent combined therapy with intravenous cyclophosphamide (Endoxan) and adriamycin. The patient survived and has remained well since then.

Three patients defaulted while on chemotherapy, two because of toxic effects of the drugs and accusation of infidelity, both who were discharged against medical advice, the latter to atone for her unfaithfulness. The third patient had to be discharged because of closure of the hospital following an industrial action.

During the period under review, multiple problems were encountered. Breakdown in radiology services prevented or delayed chest X-rays and pelvic angiograms required for early diagnosis and follow-up. Lack of blood for transfusion contributed directly to many patients lying because of severe hemorrhage (6 cases, 3 who were adolescent girls). Inadequate laboratory facilities for doing blood tests hampered follow-up of chemotherapy, while lack of reagents for urinary hCG estimation delayed diagnosis and affected monitoring of the patients in many cases.

The disease ran a very rapid course in most cases. As shown in Table 7, 80% of the patients had experienced symptoms for 6 months or less prior to admission to the hospital. Three patients died before anything could really be done for them in the hospital (Table 8). Of the 11 patients who died (81.8% of the deaths), 9 had been hospitalized for 6 months or less before they died. The other two patients who died stayed in hospital for longer periods although they both had widespread disease. One of the two patients in addition had resistant disease; she might have benefited from a timely hysterectomy and more aggressive chemotherapy.

The overall mortality due to this disease was 35.5%, while the mortality rate due to Stages I-IV (malignant trophoblastic disease) was 64.7%. The remission rate of the disease (Stages I-IV) was 17.6% (3 patients), with 3 other patients defaulting from treatment. Two of these latter patients were already in the recovery phase and would have been cured, while the third patient had secondary and widespread disease and would probably have died. Thus, the probable remission rate for malignant trophoblastic disease (Stages I-IV) would have been 29.4%. Unfortunately, because of a shortage of morbid anatomists and for socio-cultural reasons, postmortem examination was not performed on any of the patients who died.

DISCUSSION

The overall incidence of gestational trophoblastic disease at the University of Benin Teaching Hospital cannot be accurately determined because of inadequate collation of data and inadequate medical services. However, the overall incidence of gestational trophoblastic disease (1:656 pregnancies) reported in this study is quite low compared to most published series, bearing in mind the reported higher incidence of this disease in Nigeria (7). It is most likely that Stage 0 cases (benign hydatidiform mole) have been grossly under-reported, thus accounting for the lower incidence of this disease as reported. It is also likely that the incidence of this disease is lower in our community when compared to Ibadan, from where the above reports emanated. The incidence of malignant trophoblastic disease (Stages I-IV) in the present study, of 1:1197 deliveries, is higher than the estimated incidence

Table 8. Gestational Trophoblastic Disease Deaths at the University of Benin Teaching Hospital

Case no.	Duration of hospitalization	Age (Years)	Parity	Causes of death
1	24 hours	23	2+0	Anemia, widespread disease
2	12 days	16	0+1	Severe hemorrhage, anemia
3	14 days	40	6+1	Anemia, hemorrhage
4	6 weeks	18	0+1	Anemia, severe sepsis
5	3 months	18	0+1	Hemorrhage, anemia
6	3 months	39	8+0	Hemorrhage, anemia, widespread disease
7	4 months	21	2+0	Hemorrhage, anemia
8	6 months	29	3+1	Widespread disease
9	7 months	32	4+0	Hemorrhage, metastasis
10	1 year	31	4+0	Widespread disease, resistant disease
11	3 months	29	3+0	Widespread disease, central nervous system complications

of 1:2518 pregnancies (8), and also higher than the incidence of choriocarcinoma of 1:4298 deliveries in Singapore (9). Our incidence, however, is much lower than the incidence of 1:197 hospital deliveries at the University College Hospital, Ibadan, a major referral center (10). This may confirm further the relative rarity of this disease in our community, although this finding needs to be further investigated.

The risk of developing choriocarcinoma is higher in elderly women of high parity (11-13). In our study, age does not appear to be a factor in the incidence of gestational trophoblastic neoplasms, although the incidence of the disease in grandmultipara (28% incidence) is higher in comparison to other parities. Since the incidence of grandmultiparity at the University of Benin Teaching Hospital is 17.4% (14), gestational trophoblastic disease appears to be more common in grandmultipara. This observation was also made previously by Onadeko and associates (15).

The clinical presentation of gestational trophoblastic neoplasms that we observed is similar to the findings of other authors (3, 7, 16). The most frequent antecedent gestational event in the present series was a normal pregnancy. Other studies found hydatidiform mole and previous abortion as more frequent antecedent events preceding the development of trophoblastic neoplasms. Adeleye and associates (10) noted that normal pregnancy was the most frequent antecedent event in deaths from malignant trophoblastic disease, hence its worse prognosis in the scoring index of Bagshawe and Begent (13) and of Goldstein and Berkowitz (4). The significance of normal pregnancy as antecedent event may be related to the rapid course and higher mortality reported in our present series.

Numerous problems were encountered in the management of our patients. Of the patients who died, some arrived too late at the hospital to be helped. Others had widespread resistant disease which did not respond to therapy. Hemorrhage was a major contributing factor to mortality, since blood transfusion facilities were inadequate. All these factors have contributed to the high mortality rate and poor remission rate in gestational trophoblastic disease at the University of Benin Teaching Hospital. In addition, the neoplasms appeared to have progressed rather repidly. Because the histology of these cases was not evaluated, the contribution of this factor cannot be assessed.

The remission rate for gestational trophoblastic disease reported by most authors ranges from 43.3% to 100% (4, 8, 13). In our community the remission rate could be improved by the adoption of the prognostic scoring index of Bagshawe and Begent (13) or of Goldstein and Berkowitz (4), such that therapy is individualized and aggressive. The improvement of our facilities and supply of a wider spectrum of drugs could help reduce the mortality and morbidity due to this disease.

CONCLUSIONS

Gestational trophoblastic neoplasms are an important cause of morbidity and mortality in women of reproductive age at the University of Benin Teaching Hospital, Benin City, Nigeria. The disease runs a rather rapid course. Numerous problems were encountered in the diagnosis and management of these cases. The problems included inadequate laboratory facilities, shortage of reagents for estimation of urinary hCG levels, shortage of blood for transfusion, inadequate radiologic facilities, and shortage of drugs. There is need for efforts to increase the awareness of physicians and patients to the mode of presentation of this disease such that it can be adequately controlled. We recommend the creation of well equipped and adequately financed regional referral centers. The centers should be manned by dedicated and knowledgeable physicians, to utilize the prognostic scoring index and institute aggressive therapy. A wider spectrum of drugs should be made available to these regional centers, where they could be utilized most efficiently and appropriately to keep gestational trophoblastic disease in check.

REFERENCES

1. Park, W. W., in: "Pathology and Classification of Trophoblastic Tumours: Gynaecologic Oncology," M. Coppleson, ed., Churchill Livingstone, London, Vol. 2 (1981), p. 745.
2. Hendrickse, J. P. de V., Willis, A. J. P., and Evans, K. T. E., J. Obstet. Gyn. Brit. Commonwealth 72:73 (1965).
3. Hendrickse, J. P. de V., Hendrickse, M., Aimakhu, V. E., Adeleye, J. A., Osinusi, B. O., and Adewunmi, O. A., Malignant trophoblastic disease: the Ibadan experience, Tropic. J. Obstet. Gyn. 2:87 (1981).
4. Goldstein, D. P. and Berkowitz, R. A., Management of gestational neoplastic neoplasm, Curr. Probl. Obstet. Gynecol. 3:6 (1980).
5. Bagshawe, K. D., Risk and prognostic factors in trophoblastic neoplasia, Cancer 38:1371 (1976).
6. Hammond, C. B., Borchert, L. G., Tyrey, L., Creasman, W. T., and Parker, R. T., Treatment of metastatic trophoblastic disease: good and poor prognosis, Amer. J. Obstet. Gynecol. 115:451 (1973).
7. Hendrickse, J. P. de V., Cockshott, W. P., Evans, K. T. E., and Barton, C. T., Pelvic angiography in the diagnosis of malignant trophoblastic disease, N. Engl. J. Med. 271:859 (1964).
8. Hendrickse, J. P. de V., Scientific meeting, Ibadan, Nigeria (1970).
9. Teoh, E. S., Dawood, M. Y., and Ratnam, S. S., Observations on choriocarcinoma in Singapore, Obstet. Gynecol. 40:519 (1972).
10. Adeleye, J. A., Osinusi, B. O., Adewunmi, O. A., and Junaid, T. A., Malignant trophoblastic disease: review of 21 deaths at the U. C. H., Ibadan, Nigeria, Singapore J. Obstet. Gynecol. 11:59 (1980).
11. Wei, P. Y, and Ouyang, D. C., Trophoblastic disease in Taiwan, Amer. J. Obstet. Gynecol. 85:844 (1963).
12. Chan, D. P. C., Chorio-epithelioma: a study of 41 cases, Brit. Med. J. 2:853 (1962).
13. Bagshawe, K. D. and Begent, R. H. J., Trophoblastic tumours: clinical features and management, in: "Gynaecologic Oncology

Fundamental Principles and Practice," M. Coppleson, ed., Livingstone, London (1981), p. 757.

14. Diejomaoh, F. M. E., Omene, J. A., Faal, M. K. B., and Omu, A. E., The problems of the grandmultipara as seen at the UBTH, in: "Obstetrics and Gynaecology in Developing Countries," Ojo, Aimakhu, and Akinla, eds., p. 182.
15. Onadeko, B. O., Awotedu, A., Aimakhu, V. E., and Adeleye, J. A., Malignant trophoblastic disease with special deference to pulmonary involvement in Ibadan, East African Med. J. 58: 303 (1981).
16. Adeleye, J. A., Soinusi, B. O., and Adewunmi, O. A., Epidemiological features of malignant trophoblastic disease in Ibadan, Nigeria, Singapore J. Obstet. Gynecol. 11: (1980).

TEN YEARS' EXPERIENCE WITH TROPHOBLASTIC TUMORS IN PORTUGAL

Luis Wandschneider, José Rueff, and João Branco

Instituto Português Oncologia, and
Faculdade Ciências Médicas
Lisbôa
Portugal

INTRODUCTION

With the introduction of cancer chemotherapy in the treatment of gestational trophoblastic tumors (1), a new era was opened in the prognosis of this group of neoplasms. Surgery was relegated to second place in the majority of cases, and, of even greater significance, not only was cure a reality rather than a possibility, but the patient was given the opportunity of additional pregnancies.

Although we do not have detailed figures of the morbidity of gestational trophoblastic tumors in Portugal, we feel safe in stating that it is comparable to the morbidity in the rest of Europe (2).

MATERIALS AND METHODS

From 1971 to 1980, 220 patients were seen and treated at our center. Diagnosis was based on the histopathological study of specimens obtained by uterine curettage, hysterectomy, or hysterectomy and biopsy of metastases.

Of the group studied, 160 patients (72.2%) had hydatidiform mole (Table 1) and 60 patients (27.3%) had choriocarcinoma (Table 2). In relation to age and previous pregnancies, mole is 13.8% and choriocarcinoma, 46.7% (Table 3). Secondary growths were localized in one or various organs, as shown in Table 4, arranged in order of frequency.

Table 1. Hydatidiform Mole Cases, in Relation to Age and Previous Pregnancies

	Previous pregnancies								
Age	0	1	2	3	4	5	6	≥7	Total
15-19	16	3							19
20-24	34	19	4						57
25-29	13	14	9	2	1	1			40
30-34		5	7	5	5	1	1	1	25
35-39		1	2	1	3		1	2	10
40-44			1		1		1		3
45-49				1		1		3	5
≥50								1	1
Total	63	42	23	9	10	3	3	7	160

Table 2. Choriocarcinoma Cases, in Relation to Age and Previous Pregnancies

	Previous pregnancies								
Age	0	1	2	3	4	5	6	≥7	Total
15-19	5	1	2						8
20-24	1	6							7
25-29	1	4	4						9
30-34		5	4	4					13
35-39		1	2	2		2		3	10
40-44			4					2	6
45-49			1		1		2	2	6
≥50								1	1
Total	7	17	17	6	1	2	2	8	60

Table 3. Proportion of Metastatic Trophoblastic Disease in Study Group

Disease	No. of patients	Histopathological diagnosis	
		Hydatidiform mole	Choriocarcinoma
No metastases	170	138 (86.2%)	32 (53.3%)
With metastases	50	22 (13.8%)	28 (46.7%)
Total	220	160	60

Table 4. Localization of Metastases

Solitary metastasis (33 patients)
- Lung 23 (69.6%)
- Vagina 10 (30.4%)

Multiple metastases (17 patients)
- Lung 17 (100%)
- Vagina 12 (70.5%)
- Liver 7 (41.1%)
- Brain 4 (23.5%)
- Kidney 1 (15.8%)

Table 5. Absence of Ovarian Metastases

Disease	No.	Ovarian metastasis
Choriocarcinoma	35	0
Hydatidiform mole	15	0
Total	50	0

Table 6. Summary of Clinical Results

Diagnosis	No.	Favorable diagnosis	Reserved diagnosis	Remission No.	Remission %	Resistant (deaths)
Choriocarcinoma						
No metastasis	32			32	100	
With metastasis	28	12	16	21	75	7 (25%)
Hydatidiform mole						
No metastasis	138			138	100	
With metastasis	22	13	9	22	100	
Total	220	25	25	213		7

Forty-eight patients were submitted to hysterectomy and bilateral oophorectomy. In addition, we have added the autopsy reports of another two patients. None of the 50 patients had ovarian metastases (Table 5).

Since gestational trophoblastic tumors secrete hCG, basic as a specific marker in the diagnosis and treatment of these neoplasms (3), the utilization of radioimmunoassay in measuring the levels of hCG is fundamental. The authors have employed the hCG radioimmunoassay since 1976 (4).

RESULTS

The clinical results of our study are summarized in Table 6. In our group of patients, the common factor for treatment of resistant cases was delay in establishing diagnosis. This delay averaged 20 months.

Ninety-five patients (43.1%) had later pregnancies. Of these, 66 (69.4%) had received chemotherapy (Table 7). Eight patients (8.4%) had spontaneous abortions. All eight of these patients were in the hydatidiform mole group. Of the 87 full term births, 2 of the offspring (2.2%) had congenital cardiac defects; the mothers had not been treated with chemotherapy.

DISCUSSION

It has been firmly established that early diagnosis is

Table 7. Subsequent Pregnancies, Spontaneous Abortions, Term Births, and Congenital Defects of Offspring in Trophoblastic Disease Patients of Study

	Choriocarcinoma		Hydatidiform mole		
	No mets[a]	Mets	No mets	Mets	Total
Chemotherapy					
Yes	14	8	36	8	66
No	4		25		29
Pregnancies	18	8	61	8	95 (43.1%)
Spontaneous abortions			8		8 (8.4%)
Deliveries	18	8	53	8	87 (91.6%)
Birth defects					
Yes			2		2 (2.2%)
No	18	8	51	8	85

[a]Abbreviation: mets, metastases.

essential for an effective cure rate of gestational trophoblastic tumors. The use of sonography as a routine procedure in every pregnancy, and more especially as an obligatory test in threatened abortion, is, in the majority of cases, the main key to correct diagnosis, and avoids much unnecessary hospitalization and unnecessary treatment.

Hysterectomy was performed on some of our patients in order to empty the uterine cavity. We believe that this procedure should be abandoned, since chemotherapy was still needed in all of these cases. Furthermore, there was greater drug resistance in these patients.

Surgical intervention in this group of tumors has already been defined, but needs to be reviewed in some situations. Though subject to further discussion, our experience leads us to believe that bilateral oophorectomy at the time of hysterectomy is unnecessary in the younger woman. Furthermore, these patients are very responsive to chemotherapy.

Retrospective analysis of metastatic spread of gestational trophoblastic tumors in our cases confirms our opinion that the lung is the first organ to be affected by secondary growths, and that all other metastases arise from this secondary lesion.

Because of the rarity of choriocarcinoma, we point out that in five of our patients the first signs of disease appeared after the normal delivery of full term, healthy offspring. In all these cases, the histopathological diagnosis of secondary growths was choriocarcinoma. Therefore, we are of the opinion that in unexplained postpartum bleeding, hCG values should be obtained, for these may provide a valuable clue to the diagnosis and treatment of the bleeding.

SUMMARY

Between 1971 and 1980, 220 patients were observed and treated. The patients were classified according to various parameters: age, previous pregnancies, pathology reports of specimens obtained from the uterus, and site of metastasis. The study stressed the possibility of 100% cure in patients with hydatidiform mole, while in choriocarcinoma, late diagnosis was responsible for the failure in effective treatment.

ACKNOWLEDGEMENTS

The authors wish to acknowledge manuscript review by Mrs. M. Gentil Martins, R. N., and charts by A. Ventura.

REFERENCES

1. Min, L., The historical background of successful chemotherapy for advanced gestational trophoblastic tumors, Amer. J. Obstet. Gynecol. 135:266 (1979).
2. Park, W. W., "Choriocarcinoma. A Study of Its Pathology," William Heinemann Medical Books (Publishers) Ltd., London, (1971).
3. Bagshawe, K. D., Marker proteins as indicators of tumour response to therapy, Brit. J. Cancer 41:186 (1980).
4. Wandschneider, L., Doseamento da gonadotrofina corionica pelo método radioimunológico, Bol. Soc. Port. Ginecol. 1:189 (1976).

ABSTRACTS

FIRST WORLD CONGRESS ON TROPHOBLAST NEOPLASMS

October 25-27, 1982
University of Nairobi Medical School
Nairobi, Kenya
Africa

CIRCULATING IMMUNE COMPLEX LEVELS IN PATIENTS WITH MOLAR PREGNANCIES

R. S. Berkowitz, S. J. Lahey, G. Steele, Jr., A. A. Rayner, M. L. Rodrick, and D. P. Goldstein

New England Trophoblastic Disease Center
Departments of Obstetrics and Gynecology and Surgery
Brigham and Women's Hospital
Harvard Medical School
Boston, Massachusetts, USA

Circulating immune complex (CIC) levels were measured by a polyethylene glycol turbidity assay in patients with molar pregnancy to investigate the relationship between CIC and trophoblastic tumor burden. At the time of presentation, CIC values were in normal range in 27 (87%) of 31 patients with molar pregnancy. Three of the four patients who presented with elevated CIC levels had concurrent medical illness (toxemia, hepatitis, and renovascular hypertension). Eighteen patients were followed with serial CIC measurements until they achieved gonadotropin remission and all 18 patients developed increased levels as they entered remission ($P<0.001$). As patients approach gonadotropin remission, a decreasing antigen load may provide a more favorable antigen-antibody ratio for the formation and detection of CIC. CIC values remained elevated during remission from 6 to 16 weeks (mean = 11.5 weeks) and then declined to presentation levels. In one patient, serum obtained at the time of peak CIC levels was concentrated, fractionated and characterized to identify the antigen components in the immune complexes. Importantly, this patient had only conceived two prior molar pregnancies and had received no blood product transfusions. One of the paternal HLA haplotypes (AW32) was demonstrated to be an antigen component in the maternal immune complexes. Further investigation should be undertaken to evaluate possible interactions between CIC and host immune defenses.

HYDATIDIFORM MOLE

R. Harahap

University of Indonesia
Jakarta
Indonesia

Sixty-seven cases of hydatidiform mole over 30 years of age were evaluated for the development of malignant trophoblastic disease. Without checking data from conceptus, maternal blood group O was more prone to the development of malignant trophoblastic disease. The number of previous pregnancies, parity, or gestational age had no significant influence on the development of malignant trophoblastic disease. There was a higher risk for developing malignant trophoblastic disease in women older than 34, but the type of malignant disease that developed did not differ significantly between different age groups. Follow-up for hydatidiform mole should be performed every week in the first 3 months after evacuation of the uterine cavity by using a sensitive test for low hCG levels. Although hysterectomy on hydatidiform mole patients could not prevent significantly the development of malignant trophoblastic disease, the procedure is still advocated to establish an earlier diagnosis.

GENESIS OF 46,XY HYDATIDIFORM MOLE

R. A. Pattillo, S. Sasaki, K. P. Katayama, M. Roesler, and R. F. Mattingly

The Medical College of Wisconsin
Department of Gynecology and Obstetrics
Milwaukee, Wisconsin, USA

Approximately 3 to 13% of hydatidiform moles have 46,XY karyotype. The mechanism of the genesis of this type of hydatidiform mole is not clear. A Q-band karyotype analysis of a case with 46,XY hydatidiform mole led us to conclude that this hydatidiform mole originated from fertilization by two spermatozoa of an ovum without maternal chromosomes.

The patient was a 21 year-old white woman, gravida 1, para 0000 (last menstrual period, December 15, 1980), whose uterus was found to be larger than gestational age. Human chorionic gonadotropin was 439,000 mIU/ml. Suction curettage, carried out in February, 1981, disclosed a complete hydatidiform mole both grossly and microscopically. Tissue culture was successful, and on the twenty-second day the primary culture was harvested. Lymphocytes of the patient and her husband were also analyzed by Q-band technique. The karyotype of this hydatidiform mole disclosed 46,XY, with only one of the husband's chromosomes 3 and 22 identified in duplicate.

Conceivably, there are three mechanisms that may explain the genesis of 46,XY hydatidiform mole. These are: (1) normal conception; (2) diploid spermatozoan due to nondisjunction of all the chromosomes in a cell in meiosis I, fertilizing an ovum devoid of maternal chromosomal complement; and (3) two spermatozoa fertilizing an ovum devoid of maternal chromosomal complement.

Kajii and Ohama thought that 46,XY hydatidiform mole may result from nondisjunction in meiosis I in spermatogenesis, but evidence for that theory is lacking. Jacobs and associates were not able to distinguish between the possibility of a normal conceptus and the entrance of two spermatozoa into an ovum without maternal chromosomes. Surti and associates could not distinguish between the possibility of nondisjunction in meiosis I in spermatogenesis and two spermatozoa entering an ovum devoid of maternal chromosomes.

In our case, chromosomes 3 and 22 from the hydatidiform mole were devoid of any maternal chromosomal contributions. Thus, normal conception was ruled out. Total nondisjunction in meiosis I could also be ruled out by the fact that only one of the husband's 3 and 22 was transmitted to the hydatidiform mole, which does not happen if nondisjunction takes place in all the chromosomes at the metaphase of meiosis I in sparmatogenesis. Therefore, the conclusion in our case is that the 46,XY complete hydatidiform mole derived from fertilization of an ovum by two spermatozoa. No maternal chromosomal contribution was identified.

CLINICAL FEATURES OF PARTIAL MOLAR PREGNANCY

D. P. Goldstein, R. S. Berkowitz, P. K. Zucker, and M. R. Bernstein

New England Trophoblastic Disease Center
Division of Gynecologic Oncology
Department of Obstetrics and Gynecology
Harvard Medical School
Brigham and Women's Hospital
Boston, Massachusetts, USA

Between June 1, 1967, and January 1, 1982, 33 patients were diagnosed as having partial molar pregnancy at the New England Trophoblastic Disease Center. Partial mole was characterized by the following histologic features: (1) varying sized chorionic villi with foci of hydropic swelling and cavitation, (2) embryonic or fetal tissues, (3) foci of trophoblastic hyperplasia with or without atypia, (4) marked villous scalloping, and (5) prominent stromal trophoblastic inclusions. The patients' ages ranged from 15 to 39 years (mean, 27.0 years), and 18 patients (54.5%) were older than 25 years. Gravidity ranged from 1 to 4, and 11 (33.3%) patients were primigravidas. The presenting sign or symptom was vaginal bleeding in 23 (69.7%) patients, absent fetal heart in 5 (15.1%) patients, excessive uterine size in 3 (9.1%) patients, and pre-eclampsia in 2 (6.1%) patients. The presenting clinical diagnosis was threatened or incomplete abortion in 10 (30.3%) patients, missed abortion in 18 (54.6%) patients, and molar pregnancy in 5 (15.1%) patients. The uterine size was small for dates in 16 (48.5%) patients, appropriate for dates in 13 (39.4%) patients, and large for dates in 4 (12.1%) patients. Ultrasonography was performed in 14 patients and suggested mole in 10 (71.4%) patients. Preevacuation hCG levels were measured in 14 patients and exceeded 100,000 mIU/ml in 3 patients. The 3 patients with preevacuation hCG levels greater than 100,000 mIU/ml were the only patients with pre-eclampsia. Only one (3%) patient developed post-molar gestational trophoblastic disease and required chemotherapy to attain remission. Two cases were characterized by moderate trophoblastic proliferation; one of these patients developed persistent gestational trophoblastic disease.

THE FATE OF HYDATIDIFORM MOLE IN PATIENTS OVER 40 AND UNDER 20 YEARS OLD

H. Salari and V. Partovie

Ghem Medical Center
Meshed University
Meshed, Iran

A study was conducted to analyze patients older than 40 and younger than 20 with hydatidiform mole, who were admitted and diagnosed at the Ghaem Medical Center, Meshed, Iran, for the 9-year period from 1972 to 1981. During this period, we had a total of 357 cases of hydatidiform mole, of which 52 cases were 40-54 years old and 114 cases were less than 20 years old. The 52 patients older than 40 had a minimum of 5 and a miximum of 16 deliveries before developing hydatidiform mole. Six of these patients (11.5%) had invasive mole, and 5 (9.6%) developed choriocarcinoma. Three of the patients died because of bleeding after operation, extensive metastasis to the pelvic organs, and metastasis to the central nervous system.

For the 114 cases of hydatidiform mole in patients 20 or younger, the age distribution was as follows: 13 years, 1; 14 years, 1; 15 years, 5; 16 years, 15; 17 years, 8; 18 years, 23; 19 years, 14; and 20 years, 47. Four out of the 114 cases developed choriocarcinoma, of which one had ovarian metastasis. Two cases were diagnosed as doubtful by the pathologist, and two had invasive mole. From these 8 cases, one patient died, but autopsy was denied. In this presentation, there will be detailed discussion and comparison with other age groups, and treatment of the hydatidiform mole cases will be discussed.

CLINICAL, EPIDEMIOLOGICAL AND THERAPEUTIC ANALYSIS IN MOLAR PREGNANCY

M. W. Shin

Department of Obstetrics and Gynecology
College of Medicine
Seoul National University
Seoul, Korea

This report deals with 124 patients with primary hydatidiform mole, studied from January, 1975, to June, 1982, at the Department of Obstetrics and Gynecology, Seoul National University Hospital. The frequency of molar pregnancy was one per 96.9 deliveries. There was an annual trend of increased incidence. The major symptom and sign was abnormal vaginal bleeding. Frequent use of sensitive hCG assays was the main tool for proper follow-up. Twenty of the 124 patients (16%) with hydatidiform mole developed subsequent malignant sequelae. Twelve patients (9.7%) developed nonmetastatic disease (Stage I), three patients (2.4%) had metastatic disease (Stage II), and five patients (4.0%) developed metastatic disease (Stage III). Molar pregnancies with markedly exuberant trophoblastic growth such as excessive uterine enlargement (large for dates) and markedly elevated hCG titer were at increased risk for later development of locally invasive or metastatic disease. Several drugs were administered prophylactically by various routes to 52 patients with molar pregnancy at the time of, or within one week after, evacuation. A comparable group of 29 patients with molar pregnancy untreated at the time of evacuation was used as control. Proliferative sequelae occurred in 7 patients (13.5%) in the treated group, in contrast to 7 patients (24.1%)in the control group. Three cases (5.8%) of metastatic trophoblastic disease were encountered in the treated group, but three cases (10%) of metastatic trophoblastic disease developed in untreated patients. Despite the safety and effectiveness of prophylactic chemotherapy, its use should be limited to special situations, such as over 17 weeks of gestation and high-risk molar pregnancy. But the risk of developing trophoblastic disease is greater than in other countries, and since adequate hCG follow-up is available, in most patients the use of prophylactic chemotherapy may not always be advantageous in Korea. Safe methods of evacuation include suction curettage and abdominal hysterectomy. The time interval for normal involution varies at each gestational age. Eleven cases of subsequent pregnancies were experienced, including five cases of term delivery.

STABILITY OF HUMAN CHORIONIC GONADOTROPIN (hCG) AND ALPHA-SUBUNIT IN HUMAN BLOOD

Ch. V. Rao, R. O. Hussa*, F. R. Carman, Jr.,
M. L. Rinke*, C. L. Cook, and M. A. Yussman

Department of Obstetrics and Gynecology
Midcontinental Institute for Trophoblastic Disease
University of Louisville, Louisville, Kentucky, USA
and *Department of Gynecology and Obstetrics
Medical College of Wisconsin
Milwaukee, Wisconsin, USA

The stability of hCG and glycoprotein α-subunit was evaluated in blood serum and plasma samples under handling and storage conditions commonly encountered in clinics, hospital wards, and physicians' offices. Blood samples from pregnant subjects were used for these experiments. Storage of whole blood for at least 5 days at either 4° or 22° C before separation of the serum or plasma did not affect hCG or α-subunit levels as measured by either radioimmunoassay (RIA) or radioreceptorassay (RRA). When whole blood was frozen for 24 hr, then thawed and centrifuged to separate plasma or serum, the resultant hCG and α-subunit levels were decreased by approximately 30% in both RRA and RIA. Serum or plasma could be stored frozen for at least 6 months with no significant loss in hCG or α-subunit concentration. Addition of ^{125}I-hCG to pregnancy plasma and subsequent incubation for 24 hr at 4° or 22° C did not affect the degree of acid precipitability or bindability to receptors. When ^{125}I-hCG was added to heparinized blood, 4-7% of the radioactivity was found trapped in the red blood cell pellet following centrifugation. Loss from trapping did not change for at least 24 hr of storage.

Our results clearly demonstrate that hCG and α-subunit are remarkably stable in human plasma and serum. Immediate separation of plasma or serum from the blood cell pellet is not required, although whole blood should not be frozen. Whole blood, plasma, or serum from pregnant subjects can be kept for at least 5 days at either 4° or 22° without affecting hCG or α-subunit levels. In frozen serum or plasma samples, hCG and α-subunit levels are stable for at least 6 months.

AN UNUSUAL CASE OF β-hCG PRODUCTION

H. Zakut and A. Ludomirsky

Department of Obstetrics and Gynecology
The Edith Wolfson Hospital
Sackler School of Medicine
Tel-Aviv University
Holon, Israel

A 34 year-old woman, gravida 2, para 0, was admitted to the Edith Wolfson Hospital for interruption of her third pregnancy at the sixth week of gestation (her two previous pregnancies had also been interrupted). Physical examination and laboratory tests were without pathological findings. Her past history and family history were noncontributory. Although no trophoblast cells were found in the histological examination of the small amount of tissue removed during curettage, the patient had a serum hCG level, measured by the β-subunit radioimmunoassay, of 35 mIU/ml.

The patient underwent pelviscopy and re-curettage. With the exception of a slightly enlarged uterus with an eminence in the posterior wall of the uterus, there were no pathological findings. No trophoblast cells were found in the material from the second curettage.

The β-hCG levels reached values of 35 to 65 mIU/ml, and the patient was treated with methotrexate because of the reasonable diagnosis of gestational trophoblastic disease. At the same time the patient underwent thorough tests, such as X-ray, total body scan, blood tests, etc. During treatment with methotrexate, the β-hCG level rose to 60 mIU/ml. Therefore, the patient received triple therapy with methotrexate, actinomycin D, and cytophosphan. Despite four courses of triple therapy, however, the β-hCG titer climbed to 200 mIU/ml.

Selective angiography of the uterine arteries demonstrated an enlarged uterus with a pathological vascular bed. A selective injection of methotrexate into uterine arteries was performed, and the β-hCG value decreased to 34 mIU/ml. Two weeks later, however, the titer had again risen to 50 mIU/ml.

Explorative laparotomy was performed during the fifth course of triple therapy, with partial resection of the area of the eminence at the posterior wall of the uterus. Again, no trophoblast cells were found on histological examination of the specimens, but the β-hCG value became negative.

If laparotomy had been performed earlier, we could have avoided three courses of triple therapy.

DIFFERENTIATION OF PREGNANCY hCG AND hCG-LIKE MOLECULES PRODUCED BY TUMORS

L. A. Cole, S. K. Sutphen, R. O. Hussa, and R. A. Pattillo

Department of Gynecology and Obstetrics
Medical College of Wisconsin
Milwaukee, Wisconsin, USA

Trophoblastic and nontrophoblastic tumors produce modified forms of hCG and its subunits. Three examples are asialo-hCG (Birken *et al.*, Endocrinology 108:A212, 1982), β-subunit asialo-COOH-terminal peptide (Amr *et al.*, Endocrinology 110:A199, 1982), and β-subunit minus COOH-terminal peptide (Cole *et al.*, Endocrinology 110:2198, 1982). Since these forms of hCG could be used as tumor markers, a simple method was developed for differentiating them from pregnancy hCG.

Peanut lectin binds the determinant, galactose-β1,3-N-acetyl-galactosamine, found on some glycoproteins. Such a determinant is found on the *O*-linked carbohydrate units on the hCG β-subunit COOH-terminal peptide. The immobilized lectin binds desialylated hCG, desialylated hCG β-subunit, and the desialylated β-subunit COOH-terminal peptide, but not untreated hCG or β-subunit, or desialylated hCG minus its β-subunit COOH-terminal peptide. This lectin may be used to differentiate the modified forms of hCG and β-subunit produced by cancer cells.

The percentage binding of the following materials to immobilized peanut lectin were: hCG, 5.9; desialylated hCG, 93; hCGβ minus its COOH-terminal peptide and desialylated, 2.0; desialylated COOH-terminal peptide from hCGβ, 94; hCGβ, 4.9; desialylated hCGβ, 93; hLHβ, 4.2; desialylated hLHβ, 12.

LRH INJECTION TEST AS A REMISSION CRITERION IN TROPHOBLASTIC DISEASE PATIENTS

S. J. Kim, B. C. Kang, J. K. Jung, and J. W. Lee

Department of Obstetrics and Gynecology
Catholic Medical School
Seoul, Korea

There is still an argument as to whether hCG production from trophoblast cells, in placenta of normal pregnancy as well as in trophoblastic disease patients, is dependent on some type of stimulation. Since studies were recently reported that LRH had stimulatory action on hCG production from trophoblastic cells, the authors studied 24 cases of remission and 22 cases of chemotherapy with minimal resistance. LRH was administered and its reaction was observed at various time intervals compared with 20 control patients.

The results showed significant differences as follows: in remission groups, increases in β-hCG of 272, 233, 237, and 200%; in minimal resistance groups, increases of 318, 452, 395, and 396%; and in control groups, increases of 352, 235, 211, and 194%, at 30, 60, 90, and 120 minutes, respectively, after administration of 100 μg of LRH. Although there was no statistically significant difference between remission and control groups, minimal resistance groups showed statistical significance at 60, 90, and 120 minutes after LRH administration.

From the above results, it was observed that neoplastic trophoblastic cells had action dependent on LRH. These results also suggest the possibility of using LRH as a useful clinical diagnostic method in trophoblastic disease follow-up.

THE USE OF LUTEINIZING HORMONE (LH), β-HUMAN CHORIONIC GONADOTROPIN (β-hCG) RADIOIMMUNOASSAYS AND hCG URINE PREGNANCY TEST IN MONITORING FOR TREATMENT OF CHORIOCARCINOMAS

C. B. Sekadde-Kigondu, J. K. G. Mati, A. E. Mokohka,
F. B. Fongoh, and R. M. Lequin

Department of Obstetrics and Gynecology
University of Nairobi
P.O. Box 30588
Nairobi, Kenya

Measurement of curculating or urinary hCG in patients with gestational trophoblastic diseases has served as an important marker in the diagnosis and management of these conditions. Serum "LH-hCG" using World Health Organization Matched Reagents Programme was done weekly and β-hCG (Hypolab, Serono), monthly. Pregnancy test (Gravindex, Orthodiagnostic) was performed as necessary. Five patients presenting with pain and per vaginal bleeding with positive pregnancy tests were followed up during the course of treatment with methotrexate (0.4 mg/kg body weight), 6-mercaptopurine (200 mg TDS), and actinomycin D (0.5 mg i.v.) or vincristine (1 mg i.v.). The pregnancy test became negative with still high LH-hCG levels (about 100 IU/1), and 2000 mIU/ml of β-hCG. The LH-hCG dropped gradually with treatment, in parallel with β-hCG levels. The point estimate potency ratio of β-hCG to LH-hCG was 0.324 with confidence limits of 0.4316 and 0.2457. The ratio of β-hCG and LH-hCG values was dose-dependent, increasing with dose. Low levels of β-hCG could be detected in CSF as well. Some of the LH-hCG, β-hCG, and pregnancy test data are presented in Table 1 for patient G. O. The estimation of serum LH-hCG has been found useful in the monitoring of treatment of choriocarcinomas until low levels have been reached. However, β-hCG assays, although expensive, have to be performed to test for residual levels in all cases. The pregnancy test can be used for screening because of its poor sensitivity. This work received financial support from the World Health Organization, Human Reproduction Programme.

Table 1. LH-hCG, β-hCG, and Pregnancy Test Data for Patient G. O.

LH-hCG, IU/1	690	400	100	19.0	11.5	23.4	11.8
β-hCG, mIU/ml	21,900	3,386	1,864	14.8	1.0	4.6	8.2
Pregnancy test	+	+	-	-	-	-	-

A STUDY OF PROGNOSTIC FACTORS FOR CHORIOCARCINOMA

T. Tanaka, H. Ito, and T. Hosokawa

Department of Obstetrics and Gynecology
The Jikei University School of Medicine
Tokyo, Japan

Since the advent of methotrexate and actinomycin D in the chemotherapy of choriocarcinoma, the prognosis for this disease has undergone a marked improvement, but even today is still considered one of the refractory diseases. With respect to collected choriocarcinomas diagnosed histologically, we studied various clinical background factors, treatment methods, prognosis, etc., to contribute to the improvement of the prognosis for choriocarcinoma.

Patients were classified into four groups based on the prognosis: Group I, the group cured without any relapse; Group II, the group cured after relapse; Group III, the group that died after remission; and Group IV, the group that died without remission. The background factors studied in the four groups included a preceding pregnancy (whether hydatidiform mole or not), latent period within or exceeding four months, hCG value above or below 100,000 IU/1, and the presence or absence of metastases. Also, in regard to therapeutic methods, we grossly divided the patients into two groups, the post-operative chemotherapy group and the post-chemotherapy operation group.

Our results indicate that the possible presence of metastases and the hCG value are important risk factors. In addition, they suggest that initial chemotherapy is more effective than initial operative therapy.

GLYCOPROTEIN HORMONE ALPHA SUBUNIT AND HUMAN CHORIONIC GONADOTROPIN IN NORMAL PREGNANCY AND GESTATIONAL TROPHOBLASTIC DISEASE (GTD)

R. A. Elegbe, R. O. Hussa, R. A. Pattillo, I. O. Damole*, R. G. Hoffmann, and W. Finlayson

Medical College of Wisconsin
Milwaukee, Wisconsin USA
and
*University of Ibadan, Dept. of Ob/Gyn
Ibadan, Nigeria

The incidence of GTD varies widely from one part of the world to another. A high incidence of 1:294 deliveries in Japan, 1:314 pregnancies in Iran, and 1:205 pregnancies in Nigeria contrasts the much lower incidence of 1:1500 to 1:2000 in the USA. It is not known whether one or more possible etiological factors (*e.g.*, genetic, viral, dietary, hormonal, immunologic, socio-economic) are more prevalent in Nigeria than in the USA. In the search for a hormonal factor, this study was intended to test whether the serum levels of glycoprotein hormone α-subunit and hCG differ in pregnant Nigerian women compared to comparable pregnant US females.

Serum samples were collected from the patients during perinatal visits in the first, middle, and last trimesters of pregnancy. Gestational age was assessed by records of the date of last menstrual period and uterine size. Serum samples so obtained from the patients attending the University College Hospital, Ibadan, Nigeria, and those from pregnant black Americans from Milwaukee, Wisconsin, were analyzed for hCG and α-subunit using double antibody radioimmunoassay (RIA). Highly purified hCGα (NIH CR-115) and the Second International Standard hCG (World Health Organization) served as reference preparations for the homologous α-subunit and hCG RIAs, respectively. RIA results were calculated from linear logit-log regression curves.

Although the patterns of hCG secretion were similar in the two populations during normal pregnancy, the level of α-subunit was higher in the second half of pregnancy in Nigerian females than in comparable pregnant US patients. This higher level of α-subunit in pregnancy in Nigerian women may signal a population of pregnancy trophoblast at higher risk for malignancy development in the Nigerian population. The specificity of the α-subunit RIA and its clinical applications, in both trophoblast neoplasms and in normal pregnancy, in Nigerian women compared to US females, were studied. We have found in some GTD cases that α-subunit determinations have clinical utility when hCG levels have become undetectable by RIA.

This study was partly funded by a grant (1F05TW03093-01 1ARG) from Fogarty International Centre of the National Institutes of Health to RAE, and by grants from the Patrick and Anna Cudahy Fund.

LATE RECURRENCE OF GESTATIONAL TROPHOBLASTIC DISEASE

W. B. Jones, G. W. Stanimir, and J. L. Lewis, Jr.

Memorial Institute-Sloane Kettering
Columbia University
New York, New York, USA

Persistent normal hCG levels for a period of one year after treatment is considered to be a reliable criterion of complete and sustained remission in patients with gestational trophoblastic disease. This is because such patients rarely require further therapy. We present 3 patients who developed recurrent disease after being in remission for 15, 18, and 22 months. One of the patients initially had metastatic disease in the lungs, another had tumors in the lungs and brain, and the remaining patient had an invasive mole. All of the patients have remained clinically free of disease after re-treatment with follow-up ranging from 2 to 5 years. The management of the patients is presented with an emphasis on the requirement for long-term surveillance. Possible mechanisms to account for the reactivation of disease after a prolonged latency period are also considered.

PELVIC ULTRASONOGRAPHY AND THE MANAGEMENT OF GESTATIONAL TROPHOBLASTIC DISEASE

R. S. Berkowitz, D. P. Goldstein, and J. Birnholz

New England Trophoblast Disease Center
Harvard Medical School
Brigham and Women's Hospital
Boston, Massachusetts, USA

Between January, 1978, and May, 1982, pelvic ultrasonography was performed in 39 patients with persistent gestational trophoblastic disease to assess trophoblastic uterine involvement as part of the pretreatment evaluation. During the same hospitalization, the patients also underwent laparoscopy and endometrial curettage (37 patients) or hysterectomy (2 patients). Four of the patients, who were initlally evaluated by laparoscopy and endometrial curettage, were subsequently treated by hysterectomy (3 patients) or local uterine resection (1 patient). Ultrasonography indicated trophoblastic uterine involvement in 20 (51.3%) patients and the ultrasound interpretation was histologically confirmed in all 20 patients by endometrial curettage and/or hysterectomy. Among the 19 patients in whom the uterus appeared normal by ultrasound, endometrial curettings demonstrated only scanty fragments of trophoblastic tumor in 6 (31.6%) patients. Furthermore, in all 19 patients in whom the uterus appeared normal by ultrasound, laparoscopy also demonstrated no uterine abnormalities. Laparoscopy detected deep myometrial invasion in 7 (35%) of the 20 patients in whom the ultrasound indicated uterine involvement. Pelvic angiography was performed in 7 patients and consistently confirmed the ultrasound findings including one patient with a solitary resistant uterine fundal nodule. Pelvic ultrasonography, therefore, appears to be useful in detecting extensive trophoblastic uterine involvement in patients with persistent gestational trophoblastic disease.

METHOTREXATE WITH CITROVORUM FACTOR RESCUE AS PRIMARY THERAPY FOR GESTATIONAL TROPHOBLASTIC DISEASE

D. P. Goldstein, R. S. Berkowitz, and M. R. Bernstein

New England Trophoblastic Disease Center
Division of Gynecologic Oncology
Brigham and Women's Hospital
Department of Obstetrics and Gynecology
Harvard Medical School
Boston, Massachusetts, USA

Methotrexate with citrovorum factor (MTX-CF) was administered as primary treatment in 118 patients with gestational trophoblastic disease (GTD) between September 1974 and December 1981. Complete remission was achieved with MTX-CF in 104 (88.2%) patients, and 85 (81.7%) of these patients required only one course of MTX-CF to attain remission. MTX-CF induced sustained remission in 96 (91.4%) of 105 patients with nonmetastatic GTD and in 8 (61.5%) of 13 patients with low-risk metastatic GTD. Resistance to MTX-CF was more common in patients with choriocarcinoma, metastatic disease, and patients with pretreatment hCG titers of 50,000 mIU/ml or greater. While resistance to MTX-CF occurred in only 9 (8.6%) of 104 patients with histology of hydatidiform mole, 5 (35.7%) of 14 patients with choriocarcinoma were resistant to MTX-CF ($P \leq 0.05$). Resistance to MTX-CF was noted in 9 (8.6%) of 105 patients with nonmetastatic GTD and in 5 (38.5%) of 13 patients with low-risk metastatic GTD ($P \leq 0.01$). Resistance to MTX-CF was observed in 5 (55.5%) of 9 patients with pretreatment hCG titers of at least 50,000 mIU/ml and in 9 (8.2%) of 109 patients with pretreatment hCG levels less than 50,000 mIU/ml ($P \leq 0.001$).

The 14 patients who were resistant to MTX-CF subsequently achieved remission with the following treatments: actinomycin D, 10 patients (1-2 courses); MAC III (MTX-CF, actinomycin D, and cytoxan), 2 patients; local uterine resection, 1 patient; hysterectomy, 1 patient. Following MTX-CF, granulocytopenia, thrombocytopenia and hepatotoxicity occurred in only 8 (6.8%), 3 (2.5%) and 15 (12.7%) patients, respectively. No patient developed sepsis or required platelet transfusions due to myelosuppression and liver function abnormalities returned to normal in all patients. MTX-CF not only achieves an excellent therapeutic outcome in nonmetastatic and low-risk metastatic GTD but also effectively limits toxicity.

CLINICAL COURSE OF DRUG-RESISTANT CHORIOCARCINOMA: REPORT OF TWO CASES

C. T. Hsu

Taipei
Taiwan
Republic of China

Two cases of choriocarcinoma which developed drug resistance during chemotherapy are presented. One case developed drug resistance with sustaining hCGβ titer of 80-120 mIU/ml during primary chemotherapy. Without further chemotherapy she bore two more children and is now in her sixth year of survival. The other case had a larger than hen egg size vaginal and suburethral choriocarcinoma with a vacant uterine cavity. After removal of the vaginal tumor, chemotherapy was instituted but hormonal titer did not come down to normal. Enucleation of a uterine tumor resulted in normal hCG titer (<3 mIU/ml) and subsequent pregnancy was terminated by Caesarean section at full term. A relapse was noted in the lung. Chemotherapy successfully cured the pulmonary lesion; however, hCG remained between 150 and 1300 mIU/ml despite a multi-drug regimen. Despite resistance to the drug, the patient has survived more than four years in excellent general condition. This case is in sharp contrast to a case observed 15 years ago, who died from solitary, steadily growing pulmonary metastasis in spite of continuously low titer (40 IU/day, LH RIA).

Urinary hormonal electrophoretic pattern of the latter case will be compared with that of hydatidiform mole and normal pregnancy. Patho-histological findings will also be discussed.

MANAGEMENT OF HYDATIDIFORM MOLE PATIENTS WITH MASSIVE PULMONARY EMBOLI OF TROPHOBLASTIC TISSUE

M. Sarram

University of Isfahan Medical School and the
Center for Population Studies of the
University of Isfahan
Isfahan, Iran

Hydatidiform mole patients with pulmonary embolization of trophoblastic tissue are divided into four categories of minimal, moderate, severe, and massive, according to the extent of the embolization and clinical cardiovasculatory signs and symptoms. The clinical criteriae for patients in each category are outlined. Illustrative case histories for each category are presented with serial chest X-rays, electrocardiography recordings and medical management. In two patients with massive embolization, death occurred after 24 and 48 hours, in spite of rapid evacuation of uterus and extensive medical management and therapy with corticosteroids, digitalization, oxygen therapy and diuretics. At the time of admission to the hospital, the uteri of both patients were tense, tender and had the size of over 28 weeks of pregnancy. Patients had been seen weeks before by physicians. However, the diagnosis of hydatidiform mole had been missed. It is expected that these catastrophic cases are seen more often in less privileged regions of the world. Measures to prevent this complication are described.

METASTATIC GESTATIONAL TROPHOBLASTIC DISEASE - A STUDY OF INSTITUTIONAL AND NON-INSTITUTIONAL CASES AT THE NATIONAL HOSPITAL FOR WOMEN

H. Baja-Panlilio

University of the East Medical Center
Jose Fabella Memorial Hospital
Ministry of Health
Manila, Philippines

This study aims to find out the results of our management of metastatic trophoblastic disease as it occurred in our hospital from 1966 to 1975. Only those that originated from hydatidiform mole were selected (49 cases). Those that came from hydatidiform mole and were admitted as such were classified as institutional cases while those that were handled outside the institution were classified as non-institutional cases. Results showed that in institutional cases, mortality was 40% while in the non-institutional group, mortality was 65.5% with an average of 55.1% for both groups. Analysis of the former group showed that follow-up was poor in 6 out of 8 cases; in 2 cases, demise could have been prevented with chemotherapy. In the non-institutional cases, evidently the cases were diagnosed late. Causes of death were analyzed. The main cause was hemorrhage from the uterine or metastatic lesion in the genitals. The most common site of metastasis was the lungs, followed by the vulva and vagina, ovaries, kidney, pelvic peritoneum, brain, bladder, and suburethral region.

This study shows that the problem of metastatic gestational disease is a serious one. Analysis of the cases showed that many of the deaths were preventable.

MANAGEMENT OF GESTATIONAL TROPHOBLASTIC NEOPLASM AT U. S. T. CLINICAL DIVISION (CHARITY WARD)

A. M. Lopez and I. C. Huy

Childrens Medical Center
Banawe, Quezon City
Philippines

From January, 1976, to July, 1978, we had 33 cases of gestational trophoblastic neoplasm. The 26 cases of hydatidiform mole were given prophylactic methtrexate either by intensive or intermittent regimen. One dose of methotrexate is given 24 hours before any procedure is done, which is suction currettage for young patients and total abdominal hysterectomy-bilateral salpingo-oophorectomy with mole *in situ* for patients 40 years old or older.

From January, 1979, to December, 1981, along with other hospitals around the metro Manila area, were were included in research on the use of radioimmunoassay in the early detection of malignant trophoblastic neoplasms. In the 35 cases of gestational trophoblastic neoplasm that we had, the same management was followed except that after two negative pregnancy tests, radioimmunoassay for hCG was performed. Usually the hCG levels by radioimmunoassay return to normal approximately 8 weeks post-evacuation. We cannot give the results of our treatment, however, because of poor follow-up. This is the main reason why we give prophylactic methotrexate routinely to all of our cases of hydatidiform mole. Our incidence of metastatic and invasive mole is now much lower, as is our mortality.

GESTATIONAL TROPHOBLASTIC NEOPLASMS (GTN): THERAPEUTIC RESULTS

E. J. Aartsen

Netherlands Cancer Institute
Plesmanlaan 121, 1066 CX
Amsterdam
The Netherlands

From 1963 to 1982, 79 patients with GTN were treated with chemotherapy. One patient was excluded. Not responding to multi-agent chemotherapy, she underwent hysterectomy with subsequent remission of the hCG titer. Fulminant syncytial endometritis was found in the pathology specimen. In one patient, metastatic choriocarcinoma was found in a fetus maceratus. One patient was 6 years postmenopausal. The remission percentage was as follows: Stage I, 93 (18/41); Stage II, 91 (10/11); Stage III, 71 (15/21); and Stage IV, 0 (0/6). The relatively high percentage of high-risk patients was probably responsible for our poor results, especially in Stages I and IV. Twenty-four patients had been previously treated elsewhere with either surgery (12), chemotherapy (6), or both (6). Because of their poor clinical status, some Stage IV patients were subjected only to single agent chemotherapy.

Prior to 1977, multi-agent chemotherapy was only given after non-response to methotrexate. After that time the Bagshawe score was applied and multi-agent chemotherapy was immediately given to medium- and high-risk patients. We did not do any primary hysterectomy, as proposed by Hammond c.s. 1980. A patient previously treated by hysterectomy and prophylactic methotrexate was referred to us 4 weeks postoperatively with multiple pulmonary metastases, resistant to subsequent multi-agent chemotherapy. A preoperative chest film had revealed no pulmonary metastases.

Twenty patients were subjected to hysterectomy because of impending drug resistance. In 16 of these a tumor locus was found in the uterus. Ten patients of our total series had recurrences, two of them twice. Recurrences were less frequent after the introduction of the serum β-hCG assay.

Some of the Bagshawe score risk factors are open to multiple interpretations. In my opinion, the revised scoring system of Goldstein-Berkowitz is easier to handle. Following single-agent chemotherapy we had 21 full-term pregnancies and 2 which ended in spontaneous abortions. Following combination chemotherapy we had 2 full-term pregnancies. No congenital anomalies were noted.

THE EXPERIENCES OF THE CHORIOCARCINOMA GROUP OF THE NETHERLANDS, 1971-1981

F. B. Lammes and M. J. ten Kate Booy

Wilhelmina Gasthuis
Amsterdam
The Netherlands

The results are presented of the Cooperative Group-Choriocarcinoma started in the Netherlands in 1970. The Dutch gynecologists were promoted to discuss their patients together in a 3 monthly based meeting. A proposal of treatment was made on a consultation basis, not as a compulsory prescription. During the years it was possible to motivate the Dutch gynecologists to refer bad-prognosis cases to cancer centers. The results can be seen in Tables 1 and 2.

In summary, the treatment of persistent trophoblastic disease can only be done outside the centers if:

(a) there is a possibility of an open, frequent contact, and possibility of open discussion, between peripheral gynecologists and central experts;
(b) reliable β-hCG determinations can be obtained and are presented on a curve on a logarithmic scale;
(c) therapeutic propositions are documented in writing, especially after telephone consultations;
(d) the individuality of the peripheral gynecologist does not prevent him from referring the patient as soon as there is insufficient reaction to the ordinary methotrexate-folic acid rescue treatment; and
(e) referral to a center is mandatory straightaway, in cases after a normal pregnancy and cases with a long time interval after a normal mole, because of the serious life-threatening situation.

The center has the responsibility of keeping the discussion lines as open as possible.

Table 1. Choriocarcinoma Committee of The Netherlands: Summary of 141 Patients with Hydatidiform Mole

β-hCG	No.	Metastasis −	Metastasis +	Chemotherapy −	Chemotherapy +	Results: Remission	Results: Death	Results: Still on therapy
Fall	32	27	5	26	6	32		
Plateau	46	44	2	2	44	46		
Rise	63	33	30	0	63	56	2	5
Total	141	104	37	28	113	134	2	5

Table 2. Choriocarcinoma Committee of The Netherlands: Summary of 35 Patients with History Other Than Mole

History	No. Cases	
Completed term pregnancy		
Normal pregnancy	17	
Stillborn child		1
Stillborn child with kidney metastasis		1
Twins		2
Mole prior to current pregnancy	4	
Possible yet incomplete abortion	1	
Possible primary ovarian carcinoma	1	
Total	23	
Miscellaneous		
Missed abortion	3	
Incomplete abortion	4	
Pregnancy undetected	1	
Depoprovera contraception	2	
Postmenopause 8 years	1	
Possible secondary amenorrhea	1	
Total	12	

CHEMOTHERAPY IN THE TREATMENT OF GESTATIONAL TROPHOBLASTIC DISEASE

Heung Tat Ng

Veterans General Hospital
Taipei
Taiwan, Asia

The gestational trophoblastic disease is the fourth most common gynecological malignancy in Taiwan, after cervical, ovarian, and endometrial malignancies. A review of 158 cases, 75 from Tri-Service General Hospital, Taipei, and 83 from Veterans General Hospital, Taipei, Republic of China, showed a ratio of 1 mole in 549 deliveries. Of the 158 cases, 117 were hydatidiform mole. The remaining 41 cases were malignant: 13 invasive mole, 25 choriocarcinoma, and 3 unclassified.

For hydatidiform mole, prophylactic chemotherapy with single agent of either actinomycin D or methotrexate is used, followed by suction curettage. Oral contraceptive is routinely given for one year afterward.

For malignant disease, non-metastatic and low-risk metastatic disease is treated initially with single-agent chemotherapy, while the high-risk group is treated initially with multi-agent chemotherapy. Hysterectomy is the procedure of choice for treatment of benign mole and non-metastatic malignancy in patients who have completed their family, but is also justified for patients with uterine lesions which are proven by pelvic arteriography. All survivors are followed up periodically by a series of β-hCG and chest X-ray determinations.

Several cases of interest will be presented, not only for their own interest, but for discussion of the procedure we planned and the adjustments that accompanied the treatment.

FOLLOW-UP IN 367 CASES OF GESTATIONAL TROPHOBLASTIC DISEASES IN KHORASSAN, IRAN

V. Partovi, H. Salari, and G. H. Nassirai

Ghaem Medical Center
Meshed University
Meshed, Iran

Three hundred sixty-seven cases of gestational trophoblastic disease were studied continuously for the last nine years in Ghaem Medical Center, Meshed University, Iran. Of these patients, 356 had hydatidiform mole with trophoblastic activity. The youngest age for hydatidiform mole was 13, and the oldest, 54 years old. Hydatidiform mole was seen in the spring more than the other seasons. Five out of 356 cases (1.4%) of hydatidiform mole were partial mole with a dead fetus. Three patients had repeated hydatidiform mole, one case ectopic tubal pregnancy, and one case tubal choriocarcinoma. Ten out of 356 cases (2.8%) of hydatidiform mole transformed to chorioadenoma destruens and 18 cases (5%) to choriocarcinoma. We have also studied 11 cases of choriocarcinoma of which 8 were developed after abortion and 3 after normal full-term pregnancy. Death due to trophoblastic diseases were 11 cases. The sites of metastasis and the numbers of cases were as follows: lung, 19; vagina, 3; central nervous system, 3; pleural surface, 1; ovary, 1; and invasive hydatidiform mole with molar ovarian metastasis, 1. Racial, geographical, socio-economical and therapeutical relations are discussed in detail.

THE PROBLEM OF TROPHOBLASTIC DISEASE IN INDONESIA

Djamhoer Martaadisoebrata

Department of Obstetrics and Gynecology
School of Medicine
Padjadjaran University
Bandung
Indonesia

Trophoblastic disease in Indonesia is not only of academic interest, but is an actual and relevant problem. The incidence is notoriously high and is uniformly distributed all over the country. It varies between 1:50 to 1:141 pregnancies for mole, and 1:280 to 1:1035 pregnancies for choriocarcinoma. The predisposing factors such as old age, high parity, and low socio-economic conditions are still common findings. Clinical findings are identical with those found in the literature, except that our patients present in a worse condition. One complication of mole which merits closer attention is thyrotoxicosis. Its incidence is higher than what was estimated.

The prognosis of the disease is poor due to social constraints and lack of facilities. The mortality rate for mole is 4.2% and for choriocarcinoma, 45.5%. We are hoping for a joint investigation with developed countries in search of the etiology.

CONTRIBUTORS

E. J. Aartsen, Netherlands Cancer Institute, Plesmanlaan 121, 1066 CX, Amsterdam, The Netherlands

O. O. Abudu, University of Lagos, Department of Obstetrics and Gynaecology, College of Medicine, P. M. B. 12003, Lagos, Nigeria

Akin Agboola, University of Lagos, Department of Obstetrics and Gynaecology, College of Medicine, P. M. B. 12003, Lagos, Nigeria

L. N. Ajabor, Department of Obstetrics and Gynaecology, College of Medical Sciences, University of Benin, and University of Benin Teaching Hospital, Benin City, Nigeria

G. Armstrong, Departments of Medicine and Pathology, College of Physicians and Surgeons of Columbia University, 630 West 168th Street, New York, New York 10032, USA

M. Farid Aziz, Medical Faculty University of Indonesia/Dr. Cipto Mangunkusumo Hospital, Department of Obstetrics and Gynaecology, Subdivision of Oncology, Jakarta, Indonesia

K. D. Bagshawe, Department of Medical Oncology, Charing Cross Hospital, Fulham Palace Road, London, W6 8RF, United Kingdom

H. Baja-Panlilio, University of the East Medical Center, Jose Fabella Memorial Hospital, Ministry of Health, Manila, Philippines

Budianto Barnas, Medical Faculty University of Indonesia/ Dr. Cipto Mangunkusumo Hospital, Department of Obstetrics and Gynaecology, Subdivision of Oncology, Jakarta, Indonesia

Ross S. Berkowitz, New England Trophoblastic Disease Center, Division of Gynecologic Oncology, Department of Obstetrics and Gynecology, Harvard Medical School, Brigham and Women's Hospital, 75 Francis Street, Boston, Massachusetts 02115, USA

Marilyn R. Bernstein, New England Trophoblastic Disease Center, Division of Gynecologic Oncology, Department of Obstetrics and Gynecology, Harvard Medical School, Brigham and Women's Hospital, Boston, Massachusetts 02115, USA

John I. Brewer, John I. Brewer Trophoblastic Disease Center, Department of Obstetrics and Gynecology, Northwestern University Medical School, Chicago, Illinois, USA

Joseph R. Bertino, Departments of Pharmacology and Medicine, Yale University School of Medicine, 333 Cedar Street, New Haven, Connecticut 06510, USA

Steven Birken, College of Physicians and Surgeons of Columbia University, The Presbyterian Hospital, 630 West 168th Street, New York, New York 10032, USA

Irving Boime, Department of Pharmacology, Washington University School of Medicine, 660 South Euclid Avenue, St. Louis, Missouri 63110, USA

João Branco, Instituto Português Oncologia, and Faculdade Ciências Médicas, Lisbôa, Portugal

H. Marvin Camel, Department of Obstetrics and Gynecology, Washington University School of Medicine, 660 South Euclid Avenue, St. Louis, Missouri 63110, USA

Robert E. Canfield, Department of Medicine, College of Physicians and Surgeons of Columbia University, The Presbyterian Hospital, 630 West 168th Street, New York, New York 10032, USA

F. R. Carman, Jr., Department of Obstetrics and Gynecology, Midcontinental Institute for Trophoblastic Disease, University of Louisville, Louisville, Kentucky, USA

Daniel L. Clarke-Pearson, The Southeastern Regional Center for Trophoblastic Disease, Department of Obstetrics and Gynecology, Duke University Medical Center, Durham, North Carolina, USA

Laurence A. Cole, University of Michigan, Ann Arbor, Michigan, USA

C. L. Cook, Department of Obstetrics and Gynecology, Midcontinental Institute for Trophoblastic Disease, University of Louisville, Louisville, Kentucky, USA

I. O. Damole, University of Ibadan, Department of Obstetrics and Gynaecology, Ibadan, Nigeria

F. M. E. Diejomaoh, Department of Obstetrics and Gynaecology, College of Medical Sciences, University of Benin and University of Benin Teaching Hospital, Benin City, Nigeria

P. Ehrlich, College of Physicians and Surgeons of Columbia University, New York, New York 10032, USA

R. A. Elegbe, Department of Physiology, University of Ibadan, Ibadan, Nigeria

M. Ezimokhai, Department of Obstetrics and Gynaecology, College of Medical Sciences, University of Benin and University of Benin Teaching Hospital, Benin City, Nigeria

W. Finlayson, Department of Gynecology and Obstetrics, Medical College of Wisconsin, Milwaukee, Wisconsin, USA

F. B. Fongoh, Department of Obstetrics and Gynecology, University of Nairobi, P. O. Box 30588, Nairobi, Kenya

Donald P. Goldstein, New England Trophoblastic Disease Center, Division of Gynecologic Oncology, Department of Obstetrics and Gynecology, Harvard Medical School, Brigham and Women's Hospital, 75 Francis Street, Boston, Massachusetts 02115, USA

S. K. Gupta, Department of Biochemistry, All India Institute of Medical Sciences and National Institute of Immunology, New Delhi-110 029, India

Charles B. Hammond, The Southeastern Regional Center for Trophoblastic Disease, Department of Obstetrics and Gynecology, Duke University Medical Center, Durham, North Carolina, USA

Akira Hatano, Nippon Medical School, Tokyo, Japan

R. Harahap, University of Indonesia, Jakarta, Indonesia

Lawrence L. Hause, Department of Pathology, Medical College of Wisconsin, Milwaukee, Wisconsin, USA

Roy Hertz, The George Washington University Medical Center, 2300 Eye Street, NW, Washington, D. C. 20037, USA

R. G. Hoffmann, Department of Biostatistics, Medical College of Wisconsin, Milwaukee, Wisconsin, USA

Makoto Hoshina, Department of Pharmacology, Washington University School of Medicine, 660 South Euclid Avenue, St. Louis, Missouri 63110, USA

T. Hosokawa, Department of Obstetrics and Gynecology, The Jikei University School of Medicine, Tokyo, Japan

C. T. Hsu, Taipei, Taiwan, Republic of China

Robert Hussa, Department of Gynecology and Obstetrics, Medical College of Wisconsin, 8700 W. Wisconsin Avenue, Milwaukee, Wisconsin 53226, USA

I. C. Huy, Childrens Medical Center, Banawe, Quezon City, Philippines

H. Ito, Department of Obstetrics and Gynecology, The Jikei University School of Medicine, Tokyo, Japan

Walter B. Jones, Memorial Institute-Sloane Kettering, Columbia University, New York, New York, USA

T. A. Junaid, Department of Pathology, University College Hospital and College of Medicine, University of Ibadan, Ibadan, Nigeria

J. K. Jung, Department of Obstetrics and Gynecology, Catholic Medical School, Seoul, Korea

Nugroho Kampono, Medical Faculty University of Indonesia/Dr. Cipto Mangunkusumo Hospital, Department of Obstetrics and Gynaecology, Subdivision of Oncology, Jakarta, Indonesia

B. C. Kang, Department of Obstetrics and Gynecology, Catholic Medical School, Seoul, Korea

K. P. Katayama, Department of Gynecology and Obstetrics, Medical College of Wisconsin, Milwaukee, Wisconsin, USA

M. J. ten Kate Booy, Wilhelmina Gasthuis, Amsterdam, The Netherlands

S. J. Kim, Department of Obstetrics and Gynecology, Catholic Medical School, Seoul, Korea

S. J. Lahey, New England Trophoblastic Disease Center, Brigham and Women's Hospital, Harvard Medical School, Boston, Massachusetts, USA

F. B. Lammes, Wilhelmina Gasthuis, Amsterdam, The Netherlands

Sylvia D. Lawler, Section of Human Genetics, Institute of Cancer Research, Royal Marsden Hospital, Fulham Road, London, SW3 6JJ, United Kingdom

J. W. Lee, Department of Obstetrics and Gynecology, Catholic Medical School, Seoul, Korea

R. M. Lequin, Department of Obstetrics and Gynecology, University of Nairobi, P. O. Box 30588, Nairobi, Kenya

J. L. Lewis, Jr., Memorial Institute-Sloane Kettering, Columbia University, New York, New York, USA

A. M. Lopez, Childrens Medical Center, Banawe, Quezon City, Philippines

A. Ludomirsky, Department of Obstetrics and Gynecology, The Edith Wolfson Hospital, Sackler School of Medicine, Tel-Aviv University, Holon, Israel

John R. Lurain, John I. Brewer Trophoblastic Disease Center, Department of Obstetrics and Gynecology, Northwestern University Medical School, Chicago, Illinois, USA

Djamhoer Martaadisoebrata, Department of Obstetrics and Gynecology, School of Medicine, Padjadjaran University, Bandung, Indonesia

J. K. G. Mati, Department of Obstetrics and Gynaecology, University of Nairobi, Nairobi, Kenya

R. F. Mattingly, Department of Gynecology and Obstetrics, Medical College of Wisconsin, Milwaukee, Wisconsin, USA

Endy Muhardin Moegni, Medical Faculty University of Indonesia/ Dr. Cipto Mangunkusumo Hospital, Department of Obstetrics and Gynaecology, Subdivision of Oncology, Jakarta, Indonesia

A. E. Mokohka, Department of Obstetrics and Gynecology, University of Nairobi, Nairobi, Kenya

G. H. Nassirai, Ghaem Medical Center, Meshed University, Meshed, Iran

Heung Tat Ng, Veterans General Hospital, Taipei, Taiwan, Asia

Toshikatsu Ohhashi, Department of Gynecology and Obstetrics, Nippon Medical School, Tokyo, Japan

Kimiyasu Ohkawa, Department of Gynecology and Obstetrics, Nippon Medical School, Tokyo, Japan

Ryoki Ohkawa, Department of Gynecology and Obstetrics, Nippon Medical School, 1-1-5 Sendagi-cho, Bunkyo-ku, Tokyo, Japan

Tsutomu Ohkawa, Department of Biochemistry, Kanazawa University School of Medicine, 13-1 Takara-cho Kanazawa-shi, Ishikawa-ken, Japan

E. E. Okpere, Department of Obstetrics and Gynaecology, College of Medical Sciences, University of Benin and University of Benin Teaching Hospital, Benin City, Nigeria

A. E. Omu, Department of Obstetrics and Gynaecology, College of Medical Sciences, University of Benin and University of Benin Teaching Hospital, Benin City, Nigeria

Tim Parmley, Department of Gynecologic Pathology, Johns Hopkins University, Baltimore, Maryland, USA

V. Partovi, Ghaem Medical Center, Meshed University, Meshed, Iran

Roland A. Pattillo, Department of Gynecology and Obstetrics, Medical College of Wisconsin, 8700 W. Wisconsin Avenue, Milwaukee, Wisconsin 53226, USA

Ch. V. Rao, Department of Obstetrics and Gynecology, Midcontinental Institute for Trophoblastic Disease, University of Louisville, Louisville, Kentucky, USA

A. A. Rayner, Brigham and Women's Hospital, Harvard Medical School, Boston, Massachusetts, USA

Jerry M. Rice, Laboratory of Comparative Carcinogenesis, National Cancer Institute, Frederick Cancer Research Facility, Frederick, Maryland 21701, USA

M. L. Rinke, Medical College of Wisconsin, Milwaukee, Wisconsin, USA

M. L. Rodrick, Brigham and Women's Hospital, Harvard Medical School, Boston, Massachusetts, USA

M. Roesler, Medical College of Wisconsin, Milwaukee, Wisconsin, USA

José Rueff, Instituto Português Oncologia, and Faculdade Ciências Médicas, Lisbôa, Portugal

H. Salari, Ghaem Medical Center, Meshed University, Meshed, Iran

Ratna Suprapti Samil, Medical Faculty University of Indonesia/Dr. Cipto Mangunkusumo Hospital, Department of Obstetrics and Gynaecology, Subdivision of Oncology, Jakarta, Indonesia

M. Sarram, University of Isfahan Medical School and the Center for Population Studies of the University of Isfahan, Isfahan, Iran

S. Sasaki, The Medical College of Wisconsin, Milwaukee, Wisconsin, USA

C. B. Sakadde-Kigondu, Department of Obstetrics and Gynecology, University of Nairobi, Nairobi, Kenya

M. W. Shin, Department of Obstetrics and Gynecology, College of Medicine, Seoul National University, Seoul, Korea

Sjahrul Sjamsuddin, Medical Faculty University of Indonesia/ Dr. Cipto Mangunkusumo Hospital, Department of Obstetrics and Gynaecology, Subdivision of Oncology, Jakarta, Indonesia

Alberto Sobrero, Yale University School of Medicine, New Haven, Connecticut, USA

John T. Soper, The Southeastern Regional Center for Trophoblastic Disease, Department of Obstetrics and Gynecology, Duke University Medical Center, Durham, North Carolina, USA

G. W. Stanimir, Memorial Institute-Sloane Kettering, Columbia University, New York, New York, USA

G. Steele, Jr., Brigham and Women's Hospital, Harvard Medical School, Boston, Massachusetts, USA

Hung-Chao Sung, Department of Obstetrics and Gynecology, Capital Hospital, Chinese Academy of Medical Sciences, Beijing, China

Urvashi Surti, Department of Pathology, Magee-Womens Hospital and School of Medicine, University of Pittsburgh, Pittsburgh, Pennsylvania, USA

S. K. Sutphen, Medical College of Wisconsin, Milwaukee, Wisconsin, USA

A. E. Szulman, Department of Pathology, Magee-Womens Hospital and School of Medicine, University of Pittsburgh, Pittsburgh, Pennsylvania, USA

O. Tabowei, Department of Obstetrics and Gynaecology, College of Medical Sciences, University of Benin and University of Benin Teaching Hospital, Benin City, Nigeria

Shoshichi Takeuchi, Department of Obstetrics and Gynecology, School of Medicine, Niigata University, Niigata, Japan

G. P. Talwar, Department of Biochemistry, All India Institute of Medical Sciences and National Institute of Immunology, New Delhi-110 029, India

T. Tanaka, Department of Obstetrics and Gynecology, The Jikei University School of Medicine, Tokyo, Japan

Ming-Yi Tang, Department of Obstetrics and Gynecology, Capital Hospital, Chinese Academy of Medical Sciences, Beijing, China

Norio Tosaka, Medical College of Wisconsin, Milwaukee, Wisconsin, USA

Luis Wandschneider, Instituto Português Oncologia, and Faculdade Ciências Médicas, Lisbôa, Protugal

Yuan-Bh Wang, Department of Obstetrics and Gynecology, Capital Hospital, Chinese Academy of Medical Sciences, Peking, China

Yuan-E Wang, Department of Obstetrics and Gynecology, Capital Hospital, Chinese Academy of Medical Sciences, Beijing, China

Pao-Chen Wu, Department of Obstetrics and Gynecology, Capital Hospital, Chinese Academy of Medical Sciences, Beijing, China

Hsiou-Yu Yang, Department of Obstetrics and Gynecolgoy, Capital Hospital, Chinese Academy of Medical Sciences, Beijing, China

M. A. Yussman, Department of Obstetrics and Gynecology, Midcontinental Institute for Trophoblastic Disease, University of Louisville, Louisville, Kentucky, USA

H. Zakut, Department of Obstetrics and Gynecology, The Edith Wolfson Hospital, Sackler School of Medicine, Tel-Aviv University, Holon, Israel

P. K. Zucker, New England Trophoblastic Disease Center, Division of Gynecologic Oncology, Department of Obstetrics and Gynecology, Harvard Medical School, Boston, Massachusetts, USA

INDEX

A102 monoclonal antibody to hCGα, 207
A103 monoclonal antibody to hCGα, 207
Aberrant hCG detection results, 225-232
  circulating antibodies and, 225, 226
  binding proteins for hCG and, 225, 226
  anti-rabbit IgG antibodies and, 225, 226
  positive-displacement pipetting systems and, 225
  low serum protein and, 225, 226
  nephrotic syndrome and, 225, 226
  hyperlipidemia and, 225, 226
  nonspecific serum factors and, 225, 226
  different hCG reference preparations and, 225, 226
Abdominal colic, 361 (*see also* Trophoblastic disease chemotherapy, toxicity)
ABO blood groups and choriocarcinoma, 173, 181, 183, 191, 192, 347
ABO blood groups and trophoblastic disease, 173, 181, 183, 191, 192, 347, 437
ABO blood groups and B-cell testing, 74
Abortion (*see also* Trophoblastic disease, risk factors)
Abortion (continued)
  and malignant trophoblastic disease, 170, 181, 189-191, 347, 406, 410, 422, 433, 461
  immune reaction in, 8, 63, 66-68, 82-106
  trophoblast rejection in, 8, 66-68, 82-106
  and partial mole, 82-106, 140, 143, 144, 150, 151, 154-156, 158, 433, 440
  and complete (total) mole, 82-106, 139, 151-158, 433
  chromosomal anomalies and, 82-106
Abortion, clinical, 83
  early, 83
  late, 83
Abortion, habitual, 83-106
  possible causes of, 83-106
  Abortion, occult (subclinical), 83
N-Acetylglucosamine estimation, 249
β-*N*-Acetylglucosaminidase
  assay of, 248
  digestion of NRG-hCGβ, 253, 256, 261
  digestion of NRG-^{3}H-hCGβ, 259, 262
  digestion of NRG-ectopic hCGβ, 263, 266
N-Acetylhexosamine estimation, 249
α_1-Acid glycoprotein, 266
Acid phosphatase 1, 152

Acid phosphatase 1, 152
ACP, *see* Acid phosphatase 1
ACT, *see* Actinomycin D
Actinomycin D, *see* Trophoblastic disease chemotherapy
Adaptive aging, 129-131 (*see also* Placental aging)
Adenylate kinase 1, 152
Adnexal metastasis, *see* Trophoblastic disease metastasis
Adriamycin, *see* Trophoblastic disease chemotherapy
Actins of Amida, 147
Affinity chromatography
  purification of hCGβ, 220, 250
Aflatoxicosis, 42
Aflatoxin, 16, 42
Africa, 42, 177, 184, 187, 409-427, 448, 450 (*see also* Trophoblastic disease, epidemiology)
Age
  and incidence of trophoblastic disease, 166-168, 178-180, 183, 188, 190, 192, 193, 316, 419, 420, 425, 429, 430, 434, 437
Aging of placenta, *see* Placental aging
Aging pigments, 130 (*see also* Placental aging)
  formation of, 130
  detection of, 131
Agglutination
  monoclonal antibodies in, 234
AK_1, *see* Adenylate kinase 1
$Al\text{-}CH_{50}$, 115, 119-121, 123
Alkaline phosphatase
  in hCG immunoassays, 236
  placental, 313
Alkylating agents, 17-42
All India Institute of Medical Sciences, 271
Alloantigens, 93
  and stimulation of feto-maternal unit, 93
Alopecia, 360 (*see also* Trophoblastic disease chemotherapy, toxicity)
Altered forms of hCG, 224, 225
  aberrant hCG radioimmunoassay results and, 225, 226
Alternate pathway, 112, 113, 115, 117, 120, 123, 124
Amenorrhea, 421
Amethopterin, 10
AMI, *see* Antibody-mediated immunity
Amino acid sequence
  of hCGα, 201, 202
  of hCGβ, 201, 202
4-Aminobiphenyl, 14
2-Aminonaphthalene, 14
4-Aminophenazone, 275
Aminopterin, 10, 344
Amniotic fluid cultures, 136
Amsterdam, The Netherlands, 459-461
Anaphylatoxin, 115, 123, 124
Androgenetic mole, 40, 82-106, 135, 137, 138, 152-154, 158
Anencephalic, 131
Ann Arbor, Michigan, 245
Antagonistic principle, 10
Antecedent pregnancy (*see also* Previous pregnancy; Trophoblastic disease, risk factors)
  in choriocarcinoma, 179, 181, 190-193, 347, 419, 422, 426
  and origin of gestational trophoblastic disease, 4
Antennary, 251 (*see also* Oligosaccharides)
Antibiotics, 366, 377
Antibodies against chorionic gonadotropin, 271-285
  effect on BeWo choriocarcinoma cells, 271-285

Antibodies
  to HLA D/DR, 93, 96
  to HLA D locus determinants, as blocking antibodies, 93, 96
Antibodies, blocking, 82-106
  characterization, 93-99
  and immune selection mechanisms, 100-106
Antibodies, enhancing, 82
Antibody-combining site
  monoclonal antibodies in elucidation of, 206, 207, 234
Antibody-mediated immunity, 73
Anticomplement activity
  of chorion, 120
Antifertility vaccines, 202, 203
Antigen topography
  monoclonal antibodies in elucidation of, 206, 207, 234
Anti-hCG immunization, 271
Anti-IgG affinity chromatography, 93
Antimetabolites, *see* Methotrexate; 6-Mercaptopurine; 5-Fluorouracil
Anti-Pr-β-hCG-TT, 272-285
Anti-rabbit IgG antibodies
  aberrant hCG determinations and, 225, 226
Arachis hypogaea agglutinin (*see also* Oligosaccharides)
  binding of asialo-hCGβ, 223, 247, 248, 264, 446
  binding specificity, 223, 249, 265, 446
  in differentiation of pregnancy hCG and ectopic hCG, 264, 266, 446
  procedure, 249
Arachnoid arteries, 333, 334
Armadillo, 39
Arsenic, 13
Arterial metastases, 338
Arteriography, 321, 328, 331, 332, 370
Asbestos, 14
Asia, 42, 462
Asialo-CTP fragment of hCGβ, 209, 210, 224, 446
Asialo-hCG
  in choriocarcinoma urine, 209, 210, 224, 446
Asn, 247, 251, 252
Aspergillus flavus, 42
Aspergillus niger β-*N*-acetylglucosaminidase, *see* Acetylglucosaminidase
Aspergillus niger β-galactosidase, *see* β-Galactosidase
Autoantibodies for hCG
  aberrant hCG results and, 225, 226
  assay for, 228
Autocrine, 220
Autologous serum, 89
Autoradiography, 301, 302
  bright-field, 301, 302
  dark-field, 301, 302
Azocoll, 246, 247

B101 monoclonal antibody to hCGβ, 207
B102 monoclonal antibody to hCGβ, 207
B103 monoclonal antibody to hCGβ, 207
Baboon, 39, 272
Bacillus calmette-guerin, *see* BCG
Bacteria
  hCG production by, 7, 219
Bacterial flora, 365
Bagshawe score risk factors, 411, 412, 426, 459
Bagshawe regimen, 375
Ball-like shadows, 339
Baltimore, Maryland, USA, 127
Banawe, Quezon City, Philippines, 458
Bandung, Indonesia, 464
  epidemiology of trophoblastic disease in, 464

B/Bo, 254, 255
B-cell, *see* B-lymphocyte
B cell rosettes, 74
BCG, 71, 115-117
Beijing, 327 (*see also* Peking)
Benin City, Nigeria, 417-427
Benzene, 14
Benzidine, 14
Benzo[*a*]pyrene, 16, 17
$Beta_2$-microglobulin, 62-66
Beta-Tec radioimmunoassay
  characteristics of, 227, 228
  results with, 229-232
Bethesda, Maryland, USA, 200
BeWo choriocarcinoma cells, 65, 74, 221, 271-285
  resistance to anti-hCG, 272-285
  surface charge, 292-296
BeWo P cells, 278, 282
BeWo R cells, 278, 282
βhCG, *see* Human chorionic gonadotropin monitoring; Human chorionic gonadotropin β-subunit
Biantennary, 245 (*see also* Oligosaccharides)
Bidiscoidal placentation, 28
Binding proteins for hCG
  aberrant hCG results and, 225, 226
Bioassay of hCG, 7, 370, 385
Bio-Gel P10, 246, 248-250, 253 (*see also* Desalting)
Bio-Gel P100, 246, 248, 256-260 (*see also* Gel filtration)
Birth defects, 432, 433
Bis(chloromethyl) ether, 14, 17
Bladder metastasis, *see* Trophoblastic disease metastasis
Blastogenic factor, 73
Blastomere, 152
Bleomycin, *see* Trophoblastic disease chemotherapy
Blighted (pathologic) ovum, 87
Blocked ontogeny, 7, 219, 220
Blocking antibodies, *see* Antibodies, blocking
Blocking assays, mixed leucocyte reaction, 89-106
Blocking effect, 89-106
  definition of, 89
Blocking factor, 94-96, 115, 117, 121
  in pregnancy, 96
Blood-brain barrier, 9, 321
Blood group (*see also* Trophoblastic disease, risk factors)
  ABO, and trophoblastic disease, 173, 181, 183, 191, 192, 347, 437
  AB, and B cell testing, 74
Blue dextran 2000, 248, 257
B-lymphocyte, 69
Bone marrow suppression, *see* Trophoblastic disease chemotherapy, toxicity
Boston Hospital for Women, 384
Boston Lying-In Hospital, 384
Boston, Massachusetts, USA, 383, 436, 440, 453, 454
Bowel metastasis, *see* Trophoblastic disease metastasis, bowel
Bowel resection, 395
Bracken fern croziers
  carcinogens in, 42
Brain metastasis, *see* Trophoblastic disease metastasis, brain
Brain scans, 370
Brewer Trophoblastic Disease Center, 401-409
Brigham and Women's Hospital, 384, 436, 440, 453, 454
Bright-field autoradiography, 301, 302
Bursal equivalents, 72
Butterfly, 10, 11

C_3, 111-124
C_4, 112, 123, 124
CA, *see* Carbonic anhydrase
C_3-a, *see* Anaphylatoxin
C_3-activator, 114, 118, 119, 121, 124

Calcification, 128 (*see also* Placental aging)
Canada, 149, 155
Cancer à deux, 5
Candida albicans, 73, 115
Capital Hospital, Chinese Academy of Medical Sciences, Peking, China, 327, 355
Caraghenan, 115, 118
Carbohydrate on hCG, 201, 203, 245-270 (*see also* Oligosaccharides)
Carbonic anhydrase, 248, 257, 258
Carboquone, *see* Trophoblastic disease chemotherapy
Carboxyl-terminal peptide of hCGβ (*see also* Oligosaccharides)
  antisera to, 205-210, 221-223, 236, 250, 251, 254, 259, 261, 263, 264
  antiserum H100, 221-223, 250, 251, 259, 261, 263, 264
  antiserum R141, 209
  recognition by antibody IE5, 235
S-Carboxymethylation, *see* Reduction and S-carboxymethylation
Carcinogenesis, 60
Carcinogens, 13-42 (*see also* Chemical carcinogens)
Cardiovascular signs in trophoblastic disease, 456
CaSki cervical carcinoma cells, 220, 221, 245, 250
Catholic Medical School, 447
CCA, *see* Choriocarcinoma
cDNA, *see* Complementary DNA probes
Cell-cell communication, 22
Cell column cytotrophoblast, 303
Cell electrophoresis, 290, 291, 293-295
Cell-mediated immunity, 65-75, 88-106, 111-124
Cell-mediated lymphocyte, 72
Cell surface charge, 289-296
Center for Population Research, National Institutes of Health, Bethesda, Maryland, 200
Center for Population Studies of the University of Isfahan, 456
Central nervous system metastasis, 349, 350 (*see also* Trophoblastic disease metastasis)
Cerebral metastasis, *see* Trophoblastic disease metastasis, brain
Cerebrospinal fluid, 350 (*see also* Central nervous system; Trophoblastic disease chemotherapy, in central nervous system metastasis)
Ceruloplasmin, 266
Cervical carcinoma, 245
  production of hCGβ in, *see* Ectopic hCGβ
CH_{50}, 115, 119-121, 123
CHAMOCA, *see* Trophoblastic disease chemotherapy
Charing Cross Hospital, London, 313
Cheek pouch, hamster, 271
Chemical carcinogens, 13-42
  in bracken fern, 42
  cooking and, 41, 42
  in cycad nuts, 41, 42
  definition, 17
  direct-acting, 15, 17
  fungal, 42
  in origin of gestational choriocarcinoma, 40-42
Chemotherapy of malignant trophoblastic disease, *see* Trophoblastic disease chemotherapy
Chicago, Illinois, USA, 401
Chick oviduct, 344
China, 327, 355
Chinese Academy of Medical Sciences, 327, 355
Chitobiose, 247
Chlorambucil, *see* Trophoblastic

Chlorambucil (continued)
disease chemotherapy
Chlornaphthazine, 14
Chlorooxirane, 20
Chorioadenoma destruens, Complete mole; Invasive mole
Choriocarcinoma (*see also* Trophoblastic disease)
carcinogenesis and, 32-42
chemotherapy of, *see* Trophoblastic disease chemotherapy
epidemiology of, *see* Trophoblastic disease epidemiology
etiology of, 40-42, 407
histology of, 303, 309
incidence of, *see* Trophoblastic disease epidemiology
prognostic factors of, *see* Trophoblastic disease, prognostic factors
risk factors, 166-168, 172, 173, 177-184, 188, 190-193, 299, 316, 346, 347, 374, 376, 377, 389, 402, 420-426, 429, 430, 434, 437, 449 (*see also* Trophoblastic disease, risk factors)
testicular, 59, 234, 345
Choriocarcinoma chemotherapy, *see* Trophoblastic disease chemotherapy
Choriocarcinoma management, *see* Trophoblastic disease treatment
Choriocarcinoma outcome, *see* Trophoblastic disease outcome
Chorionic somatomammotropin, 129
Chromium, 13, 14
Chromosomal anomalies
blighted ova and, 87
and habitual abortion, 83
in spontaneous abortion, 82-106
Chromosomal anomalies (continued)
translocation type, 83
Chromosome
banding, 136, 138, 139, 152, 438
enzyme polymorphisms, 136-138, 153-156
esterase, 54
glucose-6-phosphate dehydrogenase, 54
paternal, in hydatidiform moles, 53, 82-106, 137, 138, 147-158
Chronic renal failure
elevated α-subunit levels and, 17
and habitual abortion, 83
CIC, 436
Cipto (Dr.) Mangunkusumo Hospital, Jakarta, Indonesia, 165
Circulating antibodies for hCG
aberrant hCG results and, 225, 226
assay for, 228
Circulating immune complexes, 436
Cis-platinum, *see* Trophoblastic disease chemotherapy
Citrovorum factor rescue, *see* Trophoblastic disease chemotherapy
Clara cells, 24
Class 1 MHC antigens, 92, 93, 96
Class 2 MHC antigens, 92, 96, 97
Classical mole, 152 (*see also* Complete mole)
Classification of trophoblastic disease, *see* Trophoblastic disease, staging
Clearance
of hCG, 7, 233
of hCGα, 233
Clinical abortion, *see* Abortion, clinical, early; Abortion, clinical, late
Clinical applications of hCG, 313
Clinical staging of malignant trophoblastic neoplasms, 327-340 (*see also* Trophoblastic disease, staging)

Clomomycin, *see* Trophoblastic disease chemotherapy
Clones
  bearing cDNAs, 300
Cloning
  in production of monoclonal antibodies, 234
Clostridium perfringens neuraminidase, *see* Neuraminidase
CML, *see* Cell-mediated lymphocyte
Coagulation defects
  and habitual abortion, 83
Co-enzyme Q, 116
Cohnheim, 7
Colic, 361 (*see also* Trophoblastic disease chemotherapy, toxicity)
Colitis, 361, 365 (*see also* Trophoblastic disease chemotherapy, toxicity)
Collagenase, 293
College of Physicians and Surgeons of Columbia University, 199
Columbia University, 199, 452
Combination chemotherapy, Trophoblastic disease chemotherapy
Complement, 73, 111-124, 272-285
Complement-dependent cytotoxicity reaction, 65, 111-124, 273-285
Complenent profiles in pregnancy, 111-124
Complement system, 111-124
  in trophoblastic disease, 111-124
Complementary DNA probes, 300-310
Complete mole, 5, 40, 53, 81-106, 135-145, 151-158, 187, 388 (*see also* Invasive mole)
  distinction from partial mole, 103, 136-145, 155-158, 230
  embolization to lungs, 144
Complete mole (continued)
  46,XX karyotype in, 87-106, 137, 138, 140, 151, 152
  46,XY karyotype in, 53, 84, 135-140
  necrobiosis of mesenchymal cells in, 139, 141
  persistent trophoblastic disease and, 5, 156-158
Complex *N*-linked oligosaccharides, 247 (*see also* Oligosaccharides)
Complex oligosaccharides, 247, 262, 266 (*see also* Oligosaccharides)
Computerized axial tomography, 370
Con A, 73, 118, 245, 247, 249, 261-266 (*see also* Oligosaccharides; Con A-Sepharose)
  binding to hCG from normal and neoplastic tissues, 246
  binding site on *N*-linked oligosaccharides, 247, 249, 261
  nonbinding oligosaccharides, 265
  procedure for binding of hCGβ, 249, 261-263
Con A-blocking β-GlcNAc, 265
Concanavalin A, *see* Con A; Con A-Sepharose
Con A-Sepharose, 208, 246, 249, 261-263 (*see also* Con A; Oligosaccharides)
  binding procedure, 249, 261-263
Concep-7-β-hCG radioimmunoassay
  characteristics of, 227-228
  results with, 229-232
Conformation of a protein
  antibodies and, 204-207
Conglutinin, 112
Connecticut, USA, 343
Control of fertility, 271
Conversion stage of tumor promotion, 21, 22

COOH-terminal region of hCGβ, *see* Carboxyl-terminal peptide of hCGβ
Cooperative Group-Choriocarcinoma, 460-461
Core β-Man, 266
Core-directed antisera to hCGβ, *see* H1a antiserum; H2 antiserum; IE5 antiserum; SB6 antiserum; Human chorionic gonadotropin β-subunit, antisera to
Countess Margaret of Cracow, 147
Countess Margaret of Flanders, 147
CPA Y-digested hCGβ, 235
Counterimmunoelectrophoresis
  monoclonal antibodies in, 234
C_3-proactivator, 114, 115, 117, 120, 123, 124
CR-123 hCGβ, 245
Craniotomy, 395
Croton oil, 115, 118
Croton tiglium, 21
Croziers, 42
C_3-shunt pathway, 112
CT scanning, 320, 321
CTP, *see* Carboxyl-terminal peptide of hCGβ
Cycad nuts, 41, 42
Cycasin, 16, 20, 41, 42
Cyclophosphamide, *see* Trophoblastic disease chemotherapy
Cytochrome c, 248, 257
Cytogenetic aspects of hydatidiform moles, 7, 82-106, 135-145, 152-154
Cytological distribution of hCGα, hCGβ, and hPL mRNAs, 300-310
Cytophosphan, *see* Trophoblastic disease chemotherapy
Cytotoxic antibody anti-Pr-β-hCG-TT, 272-285
Cytotoxicity assay, 75, 272-279
Cytotrophoblast/syncytium conversion, 302-310
Cytoxan, *see* Trophoblastic disease chemotherapy

DAB, *see* 3',3'-Diaminobenzidine hydrochloride
Dark-field optics, 293
DEAE-Sepharose chromatography, 221-223, 249
  of ectopic hCGβ-I, 221-223
  of ectopic hCGβ-II, 221-223
  procedure, 249
  of standard hCGβ, 221-223
Deaths, *see* Trophoblastic disease, mortality
Delayed hypersensitivity, 112, 115, 117, 121, 123
Denmark, 155
Depoprovera, 461
DES, *see* Diethylstilbestrol
Desalting, 248, 250
Desialylated COOH-terminal peptide from hCGβ, 224, 446
Desialylated hCG, 446
Desialylated hCGβ, 224, 446
Desialylated RCM hCGβ, 235
Development of malignant trophoblastic neoplasms, and clinical staging, 327-340
Dextran sulfate, 117
Diabetic pregnancy
  elevated α-subunit levels in, 233
Di-*N*-Acetylchitobiose, 247
3',3'-Diaminobenzidine hydrochloride, 275
Diandry, 85, 97, 105, 106, 140, 154
Diarrhea, 361, 365, 366 (*see also* Trophoblastic disease chemotherapy, toxicity)
Diethylstilbestrol (DES), 14, 17, 27
Diethyl sulfate, 15
Differentiation and aging, 129, 130 (*see also* Placental aging)

Differentiation
of cytotrophoblast, 299-310, 318, 319
of pregnancy hCG from nontroblastic hCG, 446
Digyny, 85, 105, 154, 155
7,12-Dimethylbenz[*a*]anthracene (DMBA), 16, 26
Dimethyl sulfate, 15
Dinitrochlorobenzene sensitization, 73
Diptheria antigen, 74
Direct-acting carcinogens, *see* Chemical carcinogens
Discordant hCG detection results, 226-232
Discordant hCG results in different assays, 226-232
Dispermic moles, 84, 105, 137-140, 152-154, 158
Distribution coefficient (Kd), 257
Dithiothreitol, 248
Dizygotic twins, 156
DMBA, *see* 7,12-Dimethylbenz[*a*]-anthracene
DMN, *see* *N*-Nitrosodimethylamine
DNA polymerase I, 300
DNA probes, *see* Complementary DNA probes
DNA recombination, 219, 220
DNA repair, 130
DNAse I, 300
DNA-to-RNA transfer, 56-58
DNCB, 73, 115, 118
DoT cervical carcinoma cells, 220, 221, 245, 250, 267, 292-296
Double-stranded complementary DNA probes, 300
Dundee, United Kingdom, 316
Dr. Cipto Mangunkusumo Hospital, Jakarta, Indonesia, 165
Drug resistance, *see* Trophoblastic disease chemotherapy, resistance to drugs
Duke University Medical Center, 369-379
Durham, North Carolina, USA, 369
Dutch, 3

EA, *see* Ovalbumin
Early pregnancy factors, 96
Eclampsia
elevated α-subunit levels in, 233
Ectopic hCG
in nontrophoblastic cancers, 58-60, 203, 446
differentiation from pregnancy hCG, 446
Ectopic hCGα from cervical carcinoma, 246
Ectopic hCGβ from cervical carcinoma, 220-224, 245-270
binding to *Arachis hypogaea* agglutinin, 223, 264-266
carbohydrate structure, 265
characterization, 220-224, 263-267
Con A binding, 263-266
gel filtration, 223, 267
glycosidase digestion, 263-267
hCGβ-I, 221-223
hCGβ-II, 221-223
immunoreactivity to CTP antisera, 221-223, 263, 264
ion-exchange chromatography, 221-223
purification, 220-223, 250
radioimmunoassay of, 221-223, 246, 250, 251, 263, 264
Ricinus communis binding, 264, 266, 267
thermolysin digestion, 223
Ectopic pregnancy (*see also* Trophoblastic disease, risk factors)
and choriocarcinoma, 170, 193, 347
elevated α-subunit levels in, 233
ED_{50}, 259
Edith Wolfson Hospital, 444
Effector T cells, 72
Einhorn regimen, 375

ElCo breast carcinoma cells, 221, 292-296
Electrophoretic mobility, 293-296
Electrophysiology, 291
Elson-Morgan reaction, 249
Elution volume (Ve), 257
Embryonal demise
  and clinical early spontaneous abortion, 83-106
Empty egg, 138, 154
Embryotoxicity, 344, 345
Endo(glycosidase) D, 247, 248, 251, 253, 256, 259, 261-263, 266 (*see also* Oligosaccharides)
  cleavage site, 247, 266
  digestion conditions, 248, 251
  digestion of hCGβ derivatives, 253, 261
  digestion of ^{3}H-hCGβ derivatives, 259, 262
  digestion of ectopic-hCGβ derivatives, 263, 266
  specificity, 247, 266
Endoxan, *see* Trophoblastic disease chemotherapy; Cyclophosphamide
Enhancing antibodies, 82
ENU, *see* *N*-Nitrosoethylurea
Enzyme assays for sugars, 249
Enzyme immunoassay, 232, 236, 314 (*see also* Immunoenzymetric assay)
  alkaline phosphatase in, 236
  fluorogenic substrates in, 236
  β-galactosidase in, 236
  horseradish peroxidase in, 236
  penicillinase in, 236
Epidemiology, *see* Trophoblastic disease epidemiology
Epidermoid carcinoma of the cervix, *see* Cervical carcinoma
Epigenetic, 21
Epithelial toxicity, *see* Trophoblastic disease chemotherapy, toxicity
Epitope, 204, 205, 207
Epstein-Barr virus
  and gestational trophoblastic disease, 182, 184
Erythrocebus patas, *see* Patas monkey
Erythrocytes (nucleated)
  presence in partial mole, 136
  absence in complete mole, 139
Erythromycin, 366
Esquinon, *see* Trophoblastic disease chemotherapy
Esterase
  in chromosome analysis, 54
Estrogens, 129, 130
Estrogen-induced growth, 344
Ethylurea, 15
Etiology of a human trophoblast neoplasm, 53-58
Exoglycosidase, *see* β-Galactosidase; β-*N*-Acetylglucosaminidase; Neuraminidase; Glycosidase activity
External urethral meatus, 329

Faculdade Ciências Médicas, Lisbôa, 429
Fecal smear, 365
Fertility control, 271
Fetal placental artery thrombosis, 128 (*see also* Placental aging)
α-Fetoprotein, 96, 321
Fetuin, 252, 259, 260, 266
Fetus in partial mole, 142-144, 151, 158
Fibrin plaques, 127 (*see also* Placental aging)
Fibrinoid coat, 60, 61
Fibroblasts, 130 (*see also* Placental aging)
FIGO Cancer Committee, 388
First World Congress of Trophoblastic Disease, 3, 13, 435
Flow cytology, 290

Fluorescence microscopy, 131
Fluorogenic substrates
in hCG immunoassays, 236
5-Fluorouracil (*see also* Trophoblastic disease chemotherapy)
administration of
intra-arterial infusion, 364-367
intracavitary instillation, 364, 365
intratumor injection, 364, 365
oral, 364, 365
slow intravenous drip infusion, 355, 356, 364-366
toxicity, 359-366
Folia, 9
Folic acid, *see* Trophoblastic disease chemotherapy
structure of, 11
Folinic acid, *see* Trophoblastic disease chemotherapy
Fractional cell kill, 318-320
France, 149, 155
Frederick Cancer Research Facility, 13
Free-flow electrophoresis, 290
FSH activity of hCGβ, 199
FSH and cystic ovarian enlargement, 8
5-FU, *see* 5-Fluorouracil
Fuc, 247, 251, 252, 267, 292
Fungal carcinogens, 42
Fungal infection, 366

Gal, *see* Galactose
Galactose, 249, 251, 252, 262, 263, 266, 292
enzyme assay for, 249
estimation of, 249
Galactose-β1,3-*N*-acetylgalactosamine, 446 (*see also Arachis hypogaea* agglutinin, binding specificity; Galβ1-3-GalNAc
β-Galactosidase
digestion of N-hCGβ, 253, 256, 261
digestion of N-^{3}H-hCGβ, 259, 262
digestion of N-ectopic-hCGβ, 263, 266
in hCG immunoassays, 236
purification and assay of, 248
Gal-β1,3-GlcNAc, 249, 265 (*see also Arachis hypogaea* agglutinin, binding specificity)
GalNAc, 251, 252, 263
Gamma Dab radioimmunoassay, 227, 228-232, 236
characteristics of, 227, 228
results with, 229-232
Gastrinoma
elevated α-subunit levels in, 233
elevated gastrin levels in, 233
Gastrointestinal tract metastasis, *see* Trophoblastic disease metastasis
Gelatin, 301
Gel filtration, 200, 223, 248, 252, 256-258, 260
of cDNA, 301
of ectopic hCGβ-I from cervical carcinoma, 223
of ectopic hCGβ-II from cervical carcinoma, 223
of glycosidase-digested hCGβ derivatives, 252, 256, 257
of hCGβ, 223, 256
of tritiated hCGβ and glycosylated derivatives, 258, 260
of urinary hCG, 200
Gene for hPL, 299-310
Gene derepression, 7, 219, 220
Genes for α- and β-subunits of hCG, 201, 299-310
Genetic origin of trophoblast neoplasms, 4, 5, 53-55, 81-106, 147-158, 438

Genitourinary tract metastasis, *see* Trophoblastic disease metastasis
Genotoxic, 17, 21, 27, 40, 41
  definition of, 17
Gentamycin, 366
George Washington University Medical Center, 3
German, 7
Germany, 148, 155
Germ-cell tumors, testicular
  human chorionic gonadotropin in, 58-60
  hCGβ in, 234
Gestational trophoblastic disease (*see also* Trophoblastic disease; Trophoblastic disease chemotherapy; Trophoblastic disease epidemiology; Trophoblastic disease etiology; Trophoblastic disease metastasis)
α-Subunit in management of, 232, 233
  definition of, 344
  origin of term, 4 (*see also* Hydatidiform mole; Metastatic gestational trophoblastic disease; Choriocarcinoma; Placental site tumor; Complete mole; Partial mole; Invasive mole)
Gestational trophoblastic neoplasms, *see* Gestational trophoblastic disease; Trophoblastic disease
Ghem Medical Center, Meshed, Iran, 441
GlcNAc, 247, 251-253, 262, 265, 266
  Con A-blocking, 265
  extra residues, 267
GLO, *see* Glyoxalase 1
Glomerulus, 335, 336
Glucosamine
  enzyme assay for, 249
Glucosaminidase, *see* Acetylglucosaminidase
^{3}H-Glucose, *see* Tritiated glucose
Glucose-6-phosphate dehydrogenase
  in chromosome analysis, 54
Glutamic oxaloacetic transaminase, 153
Glycopeptides
  from choriocarcinoma hCG, 246
  from choriocarcinoma hCGα, 246
Glycophorin A, 266
Glycoprotein hormone α-subunit, *see* Human chorionic gonadotropin α-subunit
Glycosidase activity
  estimation using PNP derivatives, 247
Glycosidase digestion
  of ectopic hCGβ, 263-267
  of hCGβ, 251-253
  of ^{3}H-hCGβ, 258-263
Glyoxalase 1, 152
Goldstein-Berkowitz scoring system, 387, 420, 426, 459
"Good" prognosis metastatic disease, 369-379
  categorization, 371
GOT_2, *see* Glutamic oxaloacetic transaminase
Gowland-Hopkins, 9, 10
Graft-host relationship in gestational trophoblastic disease, 8
Gram-negative bacilli, 366
Gram-positive cocci, 366
Gram stain, 365
Grandmultipara, 419, 420, 425, 426
Granulocyte activation, 112
Gravidity
  and choriocarcinoma, 193
  and partial mole, 440
Gravindex pregnancy test, 448
GTD, *see* Trophoblast(ic) disease
GTN, *see* Trophoblast(ic) disease
Guam, 42
Guanidine hydrochloride, 220, 250

Guinea pig, 120

H1a antiserum, radioimmunoassay
characteristics of, 227, 228, 50, 252, 255
results with, 229-232
H2 antiserum, radioimmunoassay
characteristics of, 227, 228
results with, 229-232
H2 histocompatibility system, 65, 69
H7 antiserum, radioimmunoassay
characteristics of, 227-229
results with, 229-232, 450
H100 antiserum
in radioimmunoassay of ectopic hCGβ, 221-223, 246, 250, 251, 263, 264
results with, 256, 259, 261
specificity, with hCGβ derivatives, 254
Habitual abortion, 83
Hagfish, 111
Hamster, 14, 24, 26
Hamster cheek pouch, experimental choriocarcinoma in, 271, 275, 278, 282-285
Harvard Medical School, 383, 436, 440, 453, 454
Hawaii, 155, 156
hCG, *see* Human chorionic gonadotropin
hCGα, *see* Human chorionic gonadotropin α-subunit
hCGβ, *see* Human chorionic gonadotropin β-subunit
^{3}H-cDNA, 300
^{3}H-dATP, 300
^{3}H-dCTP, 300
^{3}H-dGTP, 300
^{3}H-dTTP, 300
^{3}H-hCGβ, *see* Tritiated hCGβ
hCG-like material or substance
in bacteria, 217, 219
in nontrophoblastic malignancies, 217, 219
in normal human tissues, 217, 219
Hellstrom assay, 115, 116
Helper T cells, 72
Hematoma, 340
Hematoxylin-eosin stain, 301, 303, 304
Hemocyanin, 115
Hemoglobin
and gestational trophoblastic disease, 182, 183
Hemolysis, assay of, 115
Hemoptysis, 340
Hemorrhage, 334, 335, 364, 406
Hemothorax, 340, 365
Hepatic artery catheter, 350 (*see also* Trophoblastic disease chemotherapy)
Hepatic toxicity, *see* Trophoblastic disease chemotherapy, toxicity
Hepatitis B and gestational trophoblastic disease, 182, 184
Hepatitis epidemics, 42
Hertig, Dr. Arthur T., 384
Hertig-Mansell histologic classification, 168, 174
Hha I restriction fragment, 300
Hickman catheter, 376
High-dose *cis*-platinum, *see* Trophoblastic disease chemotherapy, Platinum-HD
High-risk trophoblastic disease, 346, 349, 350, 389-399 (*see also* Trophoblastic disease chemotherapy; Trophoblastic disease, risk factors, staging)
Histocompatibility antigens, 55-75, 92, 93, 344
in trophoblast neoplasms, 135, 137, 344, 436
Histological classification of hydatidiform mole and postmolar malignancy, 135-145, 168, 171, 174
Histology of hydatidiform mole, 135-145, 171, 174
and postmolar malignancy, 171, 174
HLA antigens, 55, 61-75, 92, 93, 135, 137

HLA antigens (continued)
and circulating immune complexes, 436
HLA D locus
antibodies to, 93, 96
HLA D/DR antibodies, 93, 96
Holland, 148, 149
Holon, Israel, 444
Hong Kong, 184
Honolulu, Hawaii, USA, 154
Hormone Distribution Program, 245
Hormone-receptor combining site
monoclonal antibodies in elucidation of, 234
Hormonal disturbances and habitual abortion, 83
Horseredish peroxidase
in hCG immunoassays, 236
in hCG localization, 274
hPL, 137
Hubrecht, 3, 5
Human chorionic gonadotropin
altered forms, 7, 209, 210, 220-225, 245, 265-267
antisera to, 204-210, 228, 250, 255, 271-284, 314, 315 (*see also* Human chorionic gonadotropin α-subunit, antisera to; Human chorionic gonadotropin β-subunit, antisera to; Antibodies against chorionic gonadotropin; Hla antiserum)
asialo, in choriocarcinoma urine, 209, 210, 224
asparagine-linked sugar chains and, *see* Oligosaccharides
biological potency, 200
carbohydrate structure, 201-203, 245-270, 292
detection of, 7, 204-210, 225-236, 300, 313-316, 385-400, 412-416 (*see also* Human chorionic gonadotropin monitoring
Human chorionic gonadotropin (continued)
detection of (continued)
in trophoblastic disease; Enzyme immunoassay; Radioimmunoassay for hCG; Bioassay of hCG)
forms with limited renal clearance, 7
genes for, *see* Human chorionic gonadotropin α-subunit, genes for; Human chorionic gonadotropin β-subunit, genes for
glycosidase digestion of, *see* Glycosidase digestion of hCGβ
half-life in plasma, 200, 233
immunoenzymatic localization, 271, 274, 275, 280, 281, 292
immunologic recognition of, 204-207
incidence in cancer patients, 7, 217, 218, 245, 246
isolated from choriocarcinoma urine, 200
localization of, *see* Human chorionic gonadotropin, immunoenzymetric localization of
monitoring in trophoblastic disease, 7, 70, 143, 208-210, 227-236, 300, 313-322, 339, 344, 347, 370-378, 385-409, 412-416, 432, 434, 436-438, 440, 443-445, 447, 449, 450, 452, 454, 455, 458-462 (*see also* Human chorionic gonadotropin, detection of; Radioimmunoassay for hCG)
production of, *see* Human chorionic gonadotropin secretion
purification of, 200
radioimmunoassay of, 204-210, 227-232, 274, 300, 313-315,

Human chorionic gonadotropin (continued)
  radioimmunoassay of (continued)
    385, 386, 412-416 (*see also* Human chorionic gonadotropin monitoring in trophoblastic disease; Human chorionic gonadotropin, detection of; Radioimmunoassay of hCG)
  secretion of, *see* Human chorionic gonadotropin secretion
  stability in blood, 443
  standard preparations, 200
Human chorionic gonadotropin α-subunit
  amino acid sequence of, 201, 202
  antibody A102, 207
  antibody A103, 207
  antisera to, 207, 228, 450
  antiserum H7, 228, 229, 450
  elevated levels of
    in diabetic pregnancy, 233
    in ectopic pregnancy, 233
    in inevitable abortion, 233
    in metastatic gastrinoma, 233
    in nontrophoblastic malignancies, 233
    in Nigerians, 450, 451
    in postmenopausal women, 233
    in preeclampsia and eclampsia, 233
  free, in circulation, 224, 232-234
  gene for, 201, 299-310
  gene structure, 201
  gestational trophoblastic disease management and, 233, 313, 450, 451
  half-life in plasma, 233
  hyperglycosylated, 224
  precursor form, 201
  radioimmunoassay of, 228-232, 450
Human chorionic gonadotropin α-subunit (continued)
  stability in blood, 443
  unbalanced production of, 232
  utility of, 232-234, 450, 451
Human chorionic gonadotropin β-subunit
  amino acid sequence of, 201, 202
  antibodies B101, B102, and B103, 207
  antisera to, 204-210, 221-224, 228, 229, 235, 250, 255, 259, 263, 264, 271-285, 315
  antiserum H1a, 250, 251
  antiserum H2, 227, 228
  antiserum H100, 221-223, 250, 251, 259, 261, 263, 264
  antiserum IE5, 228, 229, 235
  antiserum Pr-β-hCG-TT, 271-285
  antiserum R141, 209, 210
  antiserum R529, 209
  antiserum SB6, 204, 205, 208, 227, 228, 274
  antiserum to partially reduced and alkylated β-subunit, 205, 207
  asialo-CTP fragment of, 209, 210, 224, 446
  asparagine-linked sugar chains and, 245-266 (*see also* Oligosaccharides, *N*-linked)
  carbohydrate structure, 201, 203, 245-270 (*see also* Oligosaccharides)
  core-directed antisera to, 204, 205, 208, 221-224, 227-229, 235, 250, 255
  core peptide, 235, 446
  free, in circulation, 224, 233, 234
    in testicular tumors, 234
  genes for, 201, 299-310
  gene structure, 202
  glycosidase-digested derivatives, 256-267 (*see also* Glycosidase digestion of hCGβ)

Human chorionic gonadotropin β-subunit (continued)
  glycosidase-digested derivatives, 251-262
  glycosidase digestion, *see* Glycosidase digestion of hCGβ
  hyperglycosylated, 224
  linked to tetanus toxoid, 271
  minus CTP, 221-224, 446
  multiple genes for, 201, 224, 225
  precursor form, 201
  radioimmunoassay of, 221, 222, 227-233, 250-255, 259-264 (*see also* Human chorionic gonadotropin β-subunit, antisera to)
  in testicular tumors, 234
  unbalanced production of, 232
Human chorionic gonadotropin-like material or substance, 217, 219 (*see also* hCG-like material or substance)
Human chorionic gonadotropin secretion
  by nontrophoblastic tissues, 7, 58-60, 217-224, 245, 317, 446
    differentiation from pregnancy hCG, 446
    hypotheses for, 219, 220
  placental aging and, 128, 129
  regulation of, 283
Human chorionic gonadotropin subunits α and β of, *see* Human chorionic gonadotropin α-subunit, β-subunit
Human chorionic thyrotropin, 59
Human placental lactogen, 299-310, 313
  genes for, 299-310
Humoral immunity, 88
Hybridization
  multiple genes for hCGβ and, 224, 225
Hybridization (continued)
  of mRNAs for hCGα, hCGβ, and hPL, 300-310
Hydatid, 147
Hydatidiform mole
  α-subunit in management of, 232, 233
  chemotherapy of, *see* Trophoblastic disease chemotherapy
  circulating immune complexes in, 436
  complete, *see* Complete mole
  cystic ovarian enlargement and, 7, 8
  epidemiology of, *see* Trophoblastic disease epidemiology
  fate of, in patients over 40 and under 20, 441 (*see also* Trophoblastic disease, outcome)
  follow-up, 190, 387, 388, 407, 441 (*see also* Trophoblastic disease, treatment)
  histology, 7, 135-145, 171, 174, 308, 309
  incidence, *see* Trophoblastic disease epidemiology
  invasive, *see* Complete mole
  malignant transformation of, 115, 117, 124, 309
  management of, *see* Trophoblastic disease, treatment
  microscopic, 86, 87, 103-106
  morphology, 104-106, 135-145, 308, 309
  partial, *see* Partial mole
  paternal chromosome in, 5, 53, 82-106, 137-140, 147-158
  total, *see* Complete mole
  treatment of, *see* Trophoblastic disease, treatment; Trophoblastic disease chemotherapy
  with twin, 156
Hydrophobic polypeptide extension, pre-hCGα and pre-hCGβ, 200

Hydropic villi, 5, 86-88, 136, 139-143, 151
Hydroxyurea, *see* Trophoblastic disease chemotherapy
Hyperalimentation, 116, 376
Hyperglycosylated α- or β-subunit, 224
Hyperlipidemia
  aberrant hCG results and, 225, 226
Hypersensitivity, *see* Delayed hypersensitivity
Hypertrophy, 129 (*see also* Placental aging)
Hypolab β-hCG test, 448
Hysterectomy in treatment of trophoblastic disease, 343, 348, 349, 369-379, 424, 429, 432, 434 (*see also* Trophoblastic disease, treatment)
Ibadan, Nigeria, 177, 184, 425, 450
IE5 antibody to hCGβ, radioimmunoassay
  characteristics of, 228, 229, 235
  results with, 229-232
  specificity of, 235
IgA, 266
IgG, 89, 93-106, 266
  blocking effect, 93-106
  and HLA D locus determinants, 93
  placenta-bound, 89
  preparation of, 89
  removal from serum, 93
IgM in spontaneous abortion, 89
Illinois, 401
Immune adherence tests, 89
Immune complex disease, 203
Immune response locus, 69
Immune response to hCG, 204
Immune selection mechanism for abortion and mole, 100-106
Immunity, *see* Cell-mediated immunity; Humoral immunity
Immunization with anti-hCG, *see* Anti-hCG immunization
Immunization with hCG, 202
Immunoassays (*see also* Radioimmunoassay; Enzyme immunoassay; Immunoradiometric assay; Immunoenzymetric assay; Two-site immunometric assay)
  monoclonal antibodies in, 234
  enzymes in, 236
Immunobiology of trophoblast neoplasms, 53-74, 344
Immunochemistry of hCG, 199-210
Immunoenzymatic localization of hCG, *see* Human chorionic gonadotropin, immunoenzymatic localization
Immunoenzymatic quantitation of anti-hCG-reacting antigens, 275, 281
Immunoglobulins, circulating, and aberrant hCG results, 225, 226
Immunologic monitoring of trophoblast tumor patients, 74
Immunologic recognition of hCG, 204-207
Immunologic surface mapping, 204-207
Immunology in genesis of mole, 81-106
Immunometric assays (*see also* Immunoradiometric assay; Immunoenzymetric assay)
  monoclonal antibodies in, 234
  enzymes in, 236
Immunoperoxidase localization of hCG, *see* Human chorionic gonadotropin, immunoenzymatic localization
Immunopurification, monoclonal antibodies in, 234
Immunoradiometric assay
  description of, 235, 236
  monoclonal antibodies and, 234-236
  polystyrene bead and, 236
  Tandem-R hCG, characteristics of

Immunoradiometric assay (continued)
  Tandem-R hCG, characteristics of (continued) 228
  Tandem-R hCG, results with, 229
  two-site, 235, 236
Immunoscintigraphy, monoclonal antibodies in, 234, 321, 322
Immunosurveillance, 71
Immunotherapy, 111-124, 234
  BCG and, 115-117
  blocking factor and, 115, 117, 121
  chemotherapy and, 111, 115-117, 121, 123, 124
  dextran sulfate and, 112, 116, 117
  enhancement of complement activity and, 113, 115, 117, 121, 123
  monoclonal antibodies in, 234
  OK432 and, 115, 117
  TGDS and, 113-117, 120, 121
Incidence, *see* Trophoblastic disease epidemiology
Incomplete abortion and trophoblastic disease, 440, 461
Imcomplete mole, 152 (*see also* Partial mole)
Incomplete suppression of hCG genome, 219, 220
India, 9, 42, 271
Indonesia, 165, 437
Inevitable abortion, elevated α-subunit levels in, 233
Infections
  and gestational trophoblastic disease, 182, 184
  and habitual abortion, 83
Inferior vena cava, 337
Inner cell mass, 82-106
In situ hybridization, 300, 301
Institute of Cancer Research, Royal Marsden Hosp., 147
Instituto Português de Oncologia, Lisbôa, 429
International Agency for Research on Cancer, 13
Interstitial tissue, 301, 303, 306
Intervillous space, 303, 306, 307
Intervillous thrombi, 127, 128 (*see also* Placental aging)
  fetal red blood cells and, 127
  Rhesus isoimmunization and, 128
Intestinal flora, 366
Intestinal metastasis, Trophoblastic disease metastasis
Intramural syndrome, 7
Intrathecal administration of methotrexate, 350
Intravenous drip infusion of 5-fluorouracil, 355, 356, 364-366
Intravenous pyelography, 363, 370
Invasive mole, 81-106, 299, 316, 318-321, 370, 407 (*see also* Complete mole)
Invasive mole, chemotherapy of, *see* Trophoblastic disease chemotherapy
Iodoacetic acid, 248
Ion-exchange chromatography
  of ectopic hCGβ, 221-223
  of hCG, 200
  of hCGβ, 221-223
Ionizing radiation, 13
Ir, *see* Immune response locus
Iran, 441, 456, 463
IRMA, *see* Immunoradiometric assay
Ischemic infarcts, 128 (*see also* Placental aging)
Isfahan, Iran, 456
Isocrine, 220
Israel, 444

Jakarta, Indonesia, 165, 437
Japan, 6, 42, 81, 111, 149, 155, 310, 449

JAr choriocarcinoma cells, 74, 221
Jikei University School of Medicine, 449
John I. Brewer Trophoblastic Disease Center, 401-409
Johns Hopkins University, 127
Jose Fabella Memorial Hospital, 457

Kanamycin, 366
Kanazawa University School of Medicine, 111
Kaolin, 208, 232, 236
  in urine assay for hCG, 208, 232, 236
Karyotype
  of hydatidiform mole, 53, 82-106, 135-145, 438, 439
  and MHC antigenicity, 97
Kd, 257
Kengshengmycin, 365, 366
Kentucky, 443
Kenya, 42, 193, 409, 448
Kenyatta National Hospital, 409, 410
Khorassan, Iran, 463
Kidney metastasis, *see* Trophoblastic disease metastasis
Klinefelter mouse uterine weight assay, 370
Kobe, Japan, 310
Kobe University, 310
Kodak NTB-2, 310
Korea, 442, 447
Krebs, Hans, 10
KSM, *see* Kengshengmycin
Kuala Lumpur, 148
Kuru-like syndrome, 26

Laboratory of Comparative Carcinogenesis, 13
Lactobacillus, 366
Lactoperoxidase, 250
Lactose, 249
Lagos, Nigeria, 187
Lagos University Teaching Hospital, 187
Langhan cell cytotrophoblast, 301, 309
Laparotomy, 339
LAP-digested hCGβ, 235
Laser doppler spectroscopy, 290
Law of Biogenesis, 7
LD, *see* Lymphocyte-defined locus
Leafy vegetables, 9
Lectin affinity chromatography procedure, 249 (*see also* Con A; *Arachis hypogaea* agglutinin; *Ricinus communis*-120 lectin)
Lentinan, 117
Leucovorin, *see* Citrovorum factor; Trophoblastic disease chemotherapy
Leukocyte
  antigen typing, 63
  migration inhibition, 74
  transfusions, 377
Leukopenia, 377
LH, *see* Luteinizing hormone
Li, Min Chiu, 3, 4
Lipid peroxidation, 51, 130 (*see also* Placental aging)
Lipofuchsin, 51, 52, 130 (*see also* Placental aging)
  detection of, 131
  in human myocardium, 130
Lipopolysaccharides of bacteria, 112
Lisbôa, Portugal, 429
Lithium carbonate, 377
  as prophylaxis for leukopenia, 377
Liver function tests, 348, 360
Liver metastasis, *see* Trophoblastic disease metastasis
Liver scan, 339, 370
LMI, *see* Leukocyte migration inhibition
Localization of human chorionic gonadotropin, *see* Human chorionic gonadotropin, immunoenzymatic localization
Logit-log calculation, 250

London, United Kingdom, 147, 313
Louisville, Kentucky, USA, 443
Low-risk trophoblastic disease, 346, 389-399 (*see also* Trophoblastic disease chemotherapy; Trophoblastic disease, staging, risk factors)
Low serum protein, aberrant hCG results and, 225, 226
LRH injection test, 447
Lung metastasis, *see* Trophoblastic disease metastasis
Lung tomography, 371
Luteinizing hormone
 aberrant results in hCG assays and, 225, 226
 denatured forms in urine, 208
 elevated blood levels, 225, 226
 immobilized, for immunosorption of anti-hCG, 205
 immunoreactivity of, 204, 205, 225
 radioimmunoassay of, in choriocarcinoma treatment, 383, 412-416, 448, 455
 receptor assays and, 205, 208
Lymph node metastasis, *see* Trophoblastic disease metastasis
Lymphocyte activation, 111, 112, 114, 122, 124
Lymphocyte-defined locus, 69, 73
Lymphokines, 73
Lysosome labilizer, 116

MAC, *see* Trophoblastic disease chemotherapy
MAC-III, *see* Trophoblastic disease chemotherapy
Macaca mulatta, *see* Rhesus monkey
Macaque, 39
Machakos district of Kenya, 42
Macrophage
 activation, 112, 122, 124
Macrophage (continued)
 aggregation factor, 73
 inhibitory factor, 74
Madagascar, 177
Magee-Women's Hospital, 135
Malagasy, 177
Malaya, 148
Malic acid, 10
Malignant trophoblast(ic) disease, *see* Choriocarcinoma; Trophoblastic disease; Trophoblastic disease metastasis
 chemotherapy of, *see* Trophoblastic disease, treatment; Trophoblastic disease chemotherapy
 epidemiology of, *see* Trophoblastic disease epidemiology
 incidence of, *see* Trophoblastic disease epidemiology
 outcome, *see* Trophoblastic disease, outcome
Malignant trophoblast(ic) neoplasms, *see* Malignant trophoblastic disease; Choriocarcinoma; Trophoblastic disease; Trophoblastic disease metastasis
Malpighian bodies, 335
Man, *see* Mannose
Manα1-6(Manα1-3)Manβ1-4GlcNAc, 247, 249 (*see also* Con A binding determinant)
Management of trophoblastic disease, *see* Trophoblastic disease, treatment
Manila, Philippines, 457
Mannose, 249, 251-253, 261-263, 266, 292, 296
 enzyme assay for, 249
 estimation, 249
Maryland, 13, 127
Mask of pregnancy, 361 (*see also* Trophoblastic disease chemotherapy)
Massachusetts, 383, 436, 440, 454

Maternal anatomical defects
in habitual abortion
83
Maternal meiosis-I error, 138, 155
Materno-fetal relationship, 8
as an allograft, 8
in rejection of trophoblast, 8
Mazy cistern formation in villi, 87
Measurement of hCG, *see* Human chorionic gonadotropin, detection of
Medical College of Wisconsin, 53, 217, 245, 267, 289, 299, 438, 443, 446, 450
Megaloblastic anemia, 9
Meiosis error, 84-87, 137, 138, 153-155
Memorial Institute-Sloane Kettering, 452
6-Mercaptopurine (*see also* Troblastic disease chemotherapy)
resistance to, 355-360
toxicity, 359, 360
Mesenchymal necrobiosis in complete mole, 139, 140
Mesenteric arteries, 335
Meshed University, Meshed, Iran, 441, 463
Mesosalpingeal vein, 331
Mesosalpinx, 331
Messenger RNAs, *see* mRNAs
Metabolism-dependent carcinogens, *see* Chemical carcinogens
Metastatic gastrinoma
elevated α-subunit levels in, 233
elevated gastrin levels in, 233
Metastatic gestational trophoblastic disease (*see also* Trophoblastic disease metastasis; Choriocarcinoma; Trophoblastic disease; etc.)
Metastatic gestational trophoblastic disease (continued)
α-subunit in management of, 232, 233
chemotherapy of, *see* Trophoblastic disease, treatment; Trophoblastic disease chemotherapy
Metastatic trophoblastic disease, *see* Trophoblastic disease metastasis; Choriocarcinoma; Metastatic gestational trophoblastic disease
Methicillin, 366
Methotrexate (*see also* Trophoblastic disease chemotherapy)
prophylactic use, 349, 350, 387
resistance, *see* Trophoblastic disease chemotherapy, resistance to drugs
toxicity, *see* Trophoblastic disease chemotherapy, toxicity
Methylazoxymethanol, 20
Methylcholanthrene, 16
α-Methylglucopyranoside, 249
Methyl methanesulfonate, 15
MFO, *see* Mixed-function oxidase
MHC antigens, 92-106
class 1 (HLA A, B, or C), 92, 93
class 2, 92
MHC antigenicity
of conceptuses, 92
of trophoblastic cells, 92, 93
Microelectrode penetration, 291
Microelectrophoresis, 290
Microscopic mole, *see* Hydatidiform mole, microscopic
Microvilli, 294
Midcontinental Institute for Trophoblastic Disease, 443
MIF, *see* Macrophage inhibitory factor
Migration inhibitory factor, 73
Milwaukee, Wisconsin, USA, 53, 217, 299, 438, 446, 450

Missouri, 299
Mitochondrial DNA, 154
Mitomycin C, 73 (*see also* Trophoblastic disease chemotherapy)
Mixed function oxidase, 19, 20, 25, 42
Mixed leucocyte reaction (MLR), 89-106
  in determination of blocking effect, 89
Mixed leucocyte (leukocyte) culture, 55, 90, 91
Mixed lymphocyte culture, 62, 68
MLC, *see* Mixed lymphocyte culture; Mixed leukocyte culture
MLR, *see* Mixed leucocyte reaction
Mobility (electrophoretic), 293-296
Molar mass concomitant with normal placenta, 156
Molar pregnancy, *see* Hydatidiform mole; Trophoblastic disease, staging
Mole with twin, 156
Mollusca, 111
Monoclonal antibodies (*see also* Immunoassays; Immunometric assays; Radioimmunoassay)
  advantages of, 206, 207, 234
  A102, A103 antibodies to hCGα, 207
  B101, B102, B103 antibodies to hCGβ, 207
  IE5 antibody, specificity of, 235
  in immunoradiometric assay, 206, 207, 232
  mixed, 206, 207, 232, 234
  production of, 206, 234
  in radioimmunoassay, 206, 207, 232
  single, 206, 232
  specificity of, 206, 207, 234, 235
  in topographical mapping, 206,
Monoclonal antibodies (continued)
  in topographical mapping (continued)
    207
  uses of, 206, 207, 234
Monosomy, *see* Chromosomal anomalies
Morphological features associated with genesis of hydatidiform mole, 103-105
Morphology of hydatidiform mole, *see* Hydatidiform mole, morphology
Mortality, *see* Trophoblastic disease, mortality; Trophoblastic disease, outcome
Mouse, 14, 24, 28, 30, 32
Mouse uterine weight assay, 370
6-MP, *see* 6-Mercaptopurine
mRNAs for hCGα, hCGβ, and hPL, 300-310
  cytological distribution of, 300-310
  in situ hybridization of, 300-310
MTD, *see* Malignant trophoblastic disease; Metastatic trophoblastic disease; Trophoblastic metastasis
mtDNA, *see* Mitochondrial DNA
MTX, *see* Methotrexate
MTX-CF, *see* Trophoblastic disease chemotherapy
Multi-agent chemotherapy, *see* Trophoblastic disease chemotherapy
Multiple forms of pre-hCGβ, 224
Multiple genes for hCGβ, 201, 224, 225
Mumps, 73
Murine labyrinthine trophoblastic cells, 92
Mutagen, 17
Mycotoxins, 42
Myleran, 14, 17
Myoglobin, 248, 257

NaB^3H_4, 246, 250
NADPH, 17
Nairobi, Kenya, 42, 409-416, 448

National Cancer Institute,
13, 28, 345, 383-385
National Institutes of Health,
200, 369
National Pituitary Agency, 200
Nature's experimental system for elucidation of immune dependency of trophoblastic cell growth, 87-99
Necrobiosis of mesenchymal cells in complete mole, 139, 141
N-Ectopic hCGβ, 263
Nephelometry
  monoclonal antibodies in, 234
Nephrotic syndrome
  aberrant hCG results and, 225, 226
Netherlands, 5, 148, 459-461
Netherlands Cancer Institute, 459
NeuAc, 251, 252, 262, 267
Neuraminidase
  digestion conditions, 248, 252
  digestion of ectopic-hCGβ, 263, 264, 266
  digestion of hCGβ, 221-223, 252, 253, 256, 261, 264
  digestion of ^{3}H-hCGβ, 259, 262
  specificity of, 247
  surface glycoproteins and, 289, 290
New Delhi, India, 271
New England Trophoblastic Disease Center, 383-400, 436, 440, 453, 454
New Haven, Connecticut, USA, 343
New horizons in hCG detection, 217-243
New York, 199, 452
N-hCGβ, 251, 253-257, 261
N-^{3}H-hCGβ, 258-260, 262
NIAMDD, 246
NICHD (NICHHD), 200, 246
Nick-translation, 300
Nigeria, 177, 184, 187, 417-427, 450
Niigata, Japan, 81
Niigata University, Niigata, Japan, 81
Nippon Medical School, 111
Nitrocaphane, 365, 366
N-Nitrosoalkylureas, 17, 41
N-Nitrosodialkylamines, 16-42
N-Nitrosodiethylamine, 16, 19, 26
N-Nitrosodimethylamine (DMN), 16, 17, 19, 20, 25, 26
N-Nitrosoethylurea (ENU), 15, 17, 18, 22-24, 26, 28-34, 39, 41
N-Nitrosomethylurea, 15
N-Linked biantennary oligosaccharides, 245 (*see also* Oligosaccharides)
N-Linked carbohydrate, Oligosaccharides
N-Linked triantennary oligosaccharides, 266 (*see also* Oligosaccharides)
3'-Noncoding region, 300
5'-Noncoding sequence, 300
Nonmetastatic trophoblastic disease, *see* Trophoblastic disease chemotherapy; Trophoblastic disease, treatment
Nonspecific binding, 254, 255
Nonspecific serum or plasma factors, aberrant hCG results and, 225, 226
Nonseminomatous testicular germ-cell tumors, human chorionic gonadotropin β-subunit in, 234
Nontrophoblastic hCG secretion, 7, 58-60, 217-224, 233, 234, 245, 446, 203
  autocrine, 220
  blocked ontogeny and, 7, 219, 220
  DNA recombination and, 219, 220
  gene derepression and, 219, 220
  hypotheses for, 219, 220
  isocrine, 220
  reactivation of embryonal foci and, 7

Nontrophoblastic hCGα secretion, 233
Nontrophoblastic hCGβ secretion, 233-235
North Carolina, 369
Northwestern Memorial Hospital, 401
Northwestern University Medical School, 401
NR-Ectopic hCGβ, 263
NRE-Ectopic hCGβ, 263
NRE-^{3}H-hCGβ, 262
NRGA-Ectopic hCGβ, 263, 264
NRGAE-Ectopic hCGβ, 263, 264
NRGAE-hCGβ, 251, 253, 254, 256, 257, 261
NRGAE-^{3}H-hCGβ, 258, 262
NRGA-hCGβ, 251, 253, 256, 257, 261, 262
NRGA-^{3}H-hCGβ, 251, 258-260, 262
NRG-Ectopic hCGβ, 263
NRG-hCGβ, 251, 253, 261
NRG-^{3}H-hCGβ, 259
NR-hCGβ, 251-257, 261
NR-^{3}H-hCGβ, 258-260, 262, 263
NSB, 249
Nuclear track emulsion, 301
Nucleated fetal red blood cells, 127 (*see also* Erythrocytes; Placental aging)
Nude mice, 144

Occult abortion, *see* Abortion, occult
ODP, *see* Onco-developmental proteins
OK432, 115, 117
Oligodendrocytes, 24
Oligosaccharides
  β-*N*-Acetylglucosaminidase digestion conditions, 248 (*see also* Acetylglucosaminidase)
  antennary, 251
  Arachis hypogaea (*see also* *Arachis hypogaea* agglutinin)
    binding specificity, 247, 249, 265, 266
    procedure, 249

Oligosaccharides (continued)
  biantennary, 245
  complex, 262, 266
  Con A binding (*see also* Con A)
    determinant, 247, 261, 294
    procedure, 249, 261-266
  Endo D cleavage site, 247, 266 (*see also* Endo D)
  β-galactosidase digestion conditions, 248 (*see also* Galactosidase)
  N-linked, 201, 203, 245, 247 249, 261, 265-267
  neuraminidase digestion (*see also* Neuraminidase)
    conditions, 247, 252
    specificity, 247
  O-linked, 201, 203, 205, 223, 245, 252, 265, 267, 446
  Ricinus communis lectin (*see also* *Ricinus communis*-120 lectin)
    binding specificity, 249, 266
    procedure, 249
  triantennary, 266
O-Linked carbohydrate, *see* Oligosaccarides
O-Linked oligosaccharides, *see* Oligosaccharides
Onco-developmental proteins, 94, 96
Oncovin, *see* Trophoblastic disease chemotherapy
One-way mixed leucocyte reaction (MLR), 89-106
  definition, 89
One-way MLC, 90, 91
Ontogenetic development, 7
Ontogeny repeats Phylogeny, 7
Oophorectomy, 432, 434
Opossum, 25
Oral contraceptive, 461, 462
Organizer substance, 56
Ovalbumin, 248, 256-258, 266
Oviduct, 344
Oxygen free radicals, 130 (*see also* Placental aging)

Padjadjaran University, Bandung, Indonesia, 464
Pancytopenia, *see* Trophoblastic disease chemotherapy, toxicity
Papio cynocephalis, 272
Paradoxical effect of anti-β-hCG antibodies on BeWo cells, 271-285
Parametrial metastasis, *see* Trophoblastic disease metastasis
Para-nitrophenol, 247
Parity
  and incidence of choriocarcinoma, 168, 172, 178, 180, 190, 193, 419, 420
  and incidence of hydatidiform mole, 168, 172, 178, 180, 188, 192, 419, 420
  and post-molar malignancy, 168, 172, 419, 420, 425
Parkway Hospital, 385
Parthenogenone, 137
Partial molar pregnancy, *see* Partial mole
Partial mole, 5, 81-106, 135-145, 151, 154-156, 158, 440
  distinction from complete mole, 5, 103, 136-145, 151-158
  frequency of, 156
  increased hCG in, 143, 144
  69,XXX karyotype in, 135, 149
  69,XXY karyotype in, 135, 139, 149
  69,XYY karyotype in, 135
  origin of, 100-106, 154-156
  triploidy in, 135, 139
PAS stain, 33
Patas monkey, 14, 27-42
  characteristics of, 28
Paternal chromosomes
  in hydatidiform mole, 5, 53-55, 82-106, 137-140, 147-158, 438, 439
  in choriocarcinoma, 54, 55
Paternal meiosis I error, 84, 138, 154,155
Paternal meiosis II error, 84, 137, 153-155
pBR322 clones, 300
PBS, 249
Peanut lectin, 223, 446
Pectin gum tragacanth, 113
PEG, *see* Polyethylene glycol
Peking, 327, 355
Pelvic metastasis, *see* Trophoblastic disease metastasis
Penicillinase, in hCG immunoassays, 236
Pennsylavania, 135
Periodate-lysine-paraformaldehyde fixative, 274
Persistent low-positive hCG levels
  discordant hCG results and, 226-232
Persistent trophoblastic disease, 5, 7, 8, 156-158, 226-232, 344, 440, 452, 453, 460
  complete mole and, 5, 156-158
  definition of, 344
  ectopic pregnancy and, 344
  hysterectomy in, 344
  late recurrence of, 452
  pelvic ultrasonography in, 453
  treatment of, 344, 453, 460
PGM_1, *see* Phosphoglucomutase 1
PGM_3, *see* Phosphoglucomutase 3
PGP_1, *see* Phophoglycolate phosphatase
PHA, 73, 115, 118, 296
PHA receptor, 292-296
Penobarbital, 21
Philippines, 457, 458
Phorbol, 21
Phosphate-buffered saline, 249
Phosphoglucomutase 1, 152, 153
Phosphoglucomutase 3, 153
Phosphoglycolate phosphatase, 152
Phylogeny, 7
Phytohemagglutinin, 73, 115, 118, 296
Pig, 14
Pigmentation, 361 (*see also* Trophoblastic disease chemotherapy, toxicity)

Pittsburgh, Pennsylvania, USA, 135
PL, *see* Placental alkaline phosphatase
Placenta-associated glycoprotein, 96
Placenta (and fetus) associated with separate molar mass, 156
Placenta-bound IgG, *see* IgG, placenta-bound
Placenta specific protein, 313
Placental aging, 127-131
  adaptive, 129-131
  calcification and, 128
  cell differentiation and, 129, 130
  DNA repair and, 130
  experiments, 130
  fetal placental artery thrombosis and, 128
  fibroblasts and, 130
  free radical oxygen in, 130, 135
  hormone production and, 128, 129, 135, 136
  host immune response and, 136
  initiation of labor and, 129
  intervillous thrombi and, 127, 128
  ischemic infarcts and, 128
  lipid peroxidation in, 130-135
  lipofuchsin and, 130
  and neoplasis, 135
  senescent nuclei in, 130
  transport function and, 128-130
Placental alkaline phosphatase, 153, 313
Placental lactogen (human), 313
Placental site tumor, 316-318
  cytotrophoblast predominance in, 317
  drug resistance and, 317
  treatment of, 317
PLAP, 313
Platelets
  5-fluorouracil and, 359, 360
  6-mercaptopurine and, 359, 360
Platelets (continued)
  methotrexate and, 359, 360
Plat-HD, *see* Trophoblastic disease chemotherapy
Pluripotential germ cells, 59
PNP, 247
PNP-α-*N*-acetylgalactosamine, 247
PNP-*N*-acetylneuraminyl lactose, 247
PNP-α-mannose, 247
PNP-β-*N*-acetylglucosamine, 247
PNP-β-gal, 247
PNP-β-mannose, 247
Pokeweed mitogen, 118
Pollutants and habitual abortion, 83
Polyethylene glycol (PEG)
  detection of autoantibodies for hCG and, 228-232
  precipitation agent and aberrant radioimmunoassay results, 225
  turbidity assay, 436
Polystyrene bead, in immunoradiometric assay, 236
"Poor" prognosis metastatic disease, 369-379
  categorization, 371
Population, and incidence of gestational trophoblastic disease, 182, 183 (*see also* Trophoblastic disease, prognostic factors; Trophoblastic disease, risk factors; Trophoblastic disease epidemiology)
Portugal, 429
Postmenopausal women, elevated α-subunit levels in, 233
Post-molar malignancy, in Indonesia, 166-174 (*see also* Choriocarcinoma)
PPD reaction, 72, 115, 118
Pr-β-hCG-TT, 272
Preeclampsia
  elevated α-subunit levels in, 233
  immune reactions in, 63
  and partial mole, 440

Pregnancy following trophoblastic disease, 396-398
Pregnancy levels of hCG and hCGα, 450, 451
Pre-hCGβ, multiple forms of, 224
Prenatal diagnosis, 136
Prepotential, 291, 295
Previous pregnancy, and malignant trophoblastic disease, 168, 347, 419, 422, 426, 429, 430, 434 (*see also* Antecedent pregnancy; Trophoblastic disease, risk factors)
Probes, *see* Complementary DNA probes
Procarbazine, 16
Progesterone, 129
Prognostic score, 347, 419-421, 425, 427 (*see also* Trophoblastic disease, prognostic factors)
Prognostic scoring system, 389
Pronucleus, 54, 84
Propagation stage of tumor promotion, 21
Propane sultone, 15
Prophylactic chemotherapy, Trophoblastic disease chemotherapy, prophylactic chemotherapy
α_1-Protease inhibitor, 266
Protein A, linked to horseradish peroxidase, 274, 275
Protoderm, 58
Protogerm DNA, 58
Protosome DNA, 58
Protovirus, 58
90th Psalm, 131
Pseudomembranous colitis, 361, 365 (*see also* Trophoclastic disease chemotherapy, toxicity)
Pst I restriction fragment, 300
Pteridins, 10
Pteroylglutamic acid, 10, 11
Pterygium, 10
Pulmonary emboli of trophoblastic tissue, 144, 456
Pulmonary insufficiency, 406
Pulmonary metastasis, *see* Trophoblastic disease metastasis, lung
Purification of ectopic hCGβ, *see* Ectopic hCGβ, purification
PWM, 118

Q-band karyotype analysis, 438 (*see also* Quinacrine banding)
Quezon City, Philippines, 458
Quinacrine banding, 136, 137, 139

R141 antiserum to desialylated hCGβ-CTP, 209, 210
R529 antiserum to CTP of hCGβ, 209
Rabbit, 14, 24
Radiation therapy of trophoblastic disease. 350, 376, 378, 392, 395, 401, 404
Radioimmunoassays
  for hCG, 227, 228, 274, 314, 315, 385, 386
  for hCGα, 228, 232, 233, 313
  for hCGβ, 221, 222, 227, 228, 232, 233, 250, 251, 252, 254, 255, 259, 261, 263, 264, 314, 315
Radioimmunolocalization of tumors, 234, 321, 322
Radioreceptorassay for hCG, 443
Radiotherapy, 350
  in combination with chemotherapy, 350 (*see also* Trophoblastic disease chemotherapy, in combination with radiotherapy)
Rat, 14, 24, 25, 30, 32
Reactivation of embryonal foci, 7
Recurrence of gestational trophoblastic disease, *see* Trophoblastic disease, recurrence
Red blood cells, 290-296

Red cell thrombi, 127, 128
(*see also* Placental aging)
Reduction and S-carboxymethylation, 205, 207, 248, 251-253, 259, 261-263, 266
procedure, 248
Reductive methylation of hCGβ, 250
(*see also* Tritiated hCGβ)
Reference preparations for hCG
aberrant hCG results and, 225, 226
Regional centers for trophoblastic disease treatment, 383-400, 416
Regionalization of trophoblastic disease treatment, 379, 383-400, 416
Registration of trophoblastic disease patients in United Kingdom, 316
Remission, *see* Trophoblastic disease, outcome; Trophoblastic disease, treatment
Renal failure, elevated α-subunit levels and, 233
Replication of fibroblasts, 130
relationship to donor age, 130
Republic of China, 455, 462
Resistance (*see also* Trophoblastic disease chemotherapy, resistance to drugs)
to drugs, 365, 455
to 5-fluorouracil, 361
to 6-mercaptopurine, 356-359, 361, 365, 366
to methotrexate, 356-359, 361, 365, 366, 454
Restriction endonuclease site polymorphisms, 154
Restriction fragment, 300
Retrograde flow, 337, 338
Reverse transcriptase, 57
Rhesus isoimmunization, 128
Rhesus monkey, 14, 28, 42, 272
Rhesus monkey (continued)
characteristics, 28
RIA, *see* Radioimmunoassays
Ricinus communis-120 lectin, 246, 247, 249, 266
binding conditions, 249
specificity, 249, 266
Risk factors, *see* Choriocarcinoma, risk factors; Troblastic disease, risk factors; High-risk trophoblastic disease; Low-risk trophoblastic disease; Trophoblastic disease, staging; Trophoblastic disease, prognostic factors
RNAse, 301
RNA-to-DNA transfer, 56-58
Royal College of Obstetricians and Gynaecologists, registration scheme for trophoblastic disease, 316
Royal Marsden Hospital, London, 147
RRA, 443

Saccharin, 21
Sacculation (irregular) of arterial wall of the lung, 332
Sackler School of Medicine, 444
Safrole, 16
Salmon sperm DNA, 300
Salmonella H and O antigens, 74
Säugetierontogenese, 5
SB6 antiserum, radioimmunoassay
characteristics of, 204, 205, 208, 227, 228
results with, 204, 205, 208, 229-232
Schwann cells, 24
SD, *see* Serologically-defined locus
Seasonal variation in gestational trophoblastic disease, 180, 181
Senescence, 127-131 (*see also* Placental aging)

Senescent nuclei, 130 (*see also* Placental aging)
Seoul, Korea, 442, 447
Sephadex G-25, 250
Sephadex G50-80, 301
Sepharose 4B, 250
Sepsis, *see* Trophoblastic disease chemotherapy, toxicity
Septicemia, 361 (*see also* Trophoblastic disease chemotherapy, toxicity)
Ser, 251, 252
Serologically-defined locus, 69
Serum βhCG assay, *see* Human chorionic gonadotropin monitoring in trophoblastic disease
Serum/CSF ratio of hCG, 320
Serum glutamate-pyruvate transaminase, 360
Sex chromatin in hydatidiform mole, 148-158
SGPT, *see* Serum glutamate-pyruvate transaminase
Shark, 112
Sheffield, United Kingdom, 316
Sickle cell gene, and trophoblastic disease, 182, 183
Signal peptides, 201
Silver grains, 301-303
Singapore, 148, 425
Skin test in pregnancy, 117, 118, 121, 123
SKSD, 73
Slip plane, 291, 294
S_N1 reaction, 17-19
S_N2 reaction, 17-19
Sodium dodecyl sulfate, 301
Sodium nitrite, 15
Sodium transport, 129 (*see also* Placental aging)
Southeastern Regional Center for Trophoblastic Disease, 369
Soybean trypsin inhibitor, 248, 256-258
SP_1, 313
Sperm, hCG production by, 7
Spermatozoa
  as gene donor in human trophoblast neoplasm, 53, 54, 84, 137, 138, 438
Spleen (cells)
  in production of monoclonal antibodies, 234
Spleen metastasis, *see* Trophoblastic disease metastasis
Squamous epithelium of vagina, 130
Stability of hCG and hCGα in blood, 443
Staging, *see* Trophoblastic disease, staging
Staging of gestational trophoblastic disease, *see* Trophoblastic disease, staging
Standard hCGβ, *see* Human chorionic gonadotropin β-subunit
Staphylococcus aureus, 366
STI, *see* Soybean trypsin inhibitor
St. Louis, Missouri, USA, 299
Stokes radius, 248, 252, 257
Stomatitis, 360 (*see also* Trophoblastic disease chemotherapy, toxicity)
Structure eludication
  monoclonal antibodies in, 234
Subclinical abortion, *see* Abortion, occult
Submucous layer of the intestine, 335, 336
Succinic acid, 10
Sulphate esters, 17
Sulphonate esters, 17
Suppressor T cells, 72
Surface charge of cells, 289-296
Surgery in treatment of trophoblastic disease, 369, 373-379, 429, 433, 434
Survival, *see* Trophoblastic disease, outcome
Switzerland, 148, 155

Syncytial knots, 130
Syncytial sprout, 303
Syrian hamster, *see* Hamster

Taipei, Taiwan, Asia, 455, 462
Taiwan, Asia, 184, 455, 462
Tandem-R hCG immunoradiometric assay (IRMA), 228-232, 236
  characteristics of, 228
  results with, 229-232
T-cell, *see* T-lymphocyte
T-cell leukemia, 58
T-cell leukemia virus, 58
Tel-Aviv University, 444
Temin, Howard, 55-58
Terminator codon, 201
Testicular choriocarcinoma, 345 (*see also* Testicular tumors)
Testicular tumors
  hCG in, 59, 203
  hCGβ in, 234
Tetanus antigen, 74
Tetanus toxoid linked to hCGβ, 271
Tetradecanoyl phorbol acetate (TPA), 27
Tetraploidy, *see* Chromosomal anomalies
TGDS, 113, 115-117, 120, 121
Thermolysin digestion of ectopic hCGβ, 223
Thermolysin digestion of standard hCGβ, 223, 235
Thiobarbituric acid, 249
Thrombocytopenia, 377
Thymosin, 71
Thyroid panel, 370
Thyrotoxicosis, 464
Tisupurine, 366
T-lymphocyte, 63-75, 112, 113
  cytotoxicity, 62-75, 112, 114
Tokyo, Japan, 111, 449
Total hydatidiform mole, Complete mole
Total volume (Vt), 257
Toxemia of pregnancy, 114, 117, 119
Toxicity, *see* Trophoblastic disease chemotherapy, toxicity
Toxoplasmosis and gestational trophoblastic disease, 182, 184
Toyomycin, *see* Trophoblastic disease chemotherapy
TPA, *see* Tetradecanoyl phorbol acetate
Tragacanth gum, *see* Pectin gum tragacanth
Tragacanthic acid, *see* Pectin gum tragacanth
Transmembrane ion separation, 289-296
Transmembrane potential, 291
Transplacental carcinogenesis, 14-42
Transplantation of choriocarcinoma cells in hamster cheek pouch, 273, 274
Transplantation immunity, 71
Treatment of trophoblastic disease, *see* Trophoblastic disease chemotherapy; Trophoblastic disease, treatment
Triantennary, 266 (*see also* Oligosaccharides)
Triantennary oligosaccharides, 266 (*see also* Oligosaccharides)
Triploidy, 82-106, 136, 139, 140, 143, 154-156, 158 (*see also* Partial mole)
Trisomy, *see* Chromosomal anomalies
Tritiated glucose, 246, 248, 253
Tritiated hCGβ, 250, 252, 253, 258-260, 262
  glycosidase-digested derivatives, 259
  as internal standard, 260
  specific activity of derivatives, 259
Trophoblast
  antigenicity of, 60
    and carcinogenesis, 60, 61

Trophoblast (continued)
differentiation of, 129, 130, 299-310
rejection of, in abortions, 66-68, 87-106
Trophoblastic disease
definition of, 4, 344
development of, and clinical staging, 81-106, 327-340, 383-400
epidemiology of, *see* Trophoblastic disease epidemiology
management of, *see* Trophoblastic disease, treatment; Trophoblastic disease chemotherapy
mortality, 318, 358, 364, 377-379, 404-406, 424-426
outcome, 192, 343, 345, 348, 350, 357-359, 366, 374-379, 391-399, 401-409, 423-425, 432-434, 442, 449, 452-456, 463, 464
presenting symptoms of, 388-399, 402, 421-423
prognostic factors of, 315, 317, 318, 346, 347, 374-379, 389, 403, 419-421, 449 (*see also* Trophoblastic disease, outcome; Trophoblastic disease, staging; Trophoblastic disease, risk factors)
prognostic scoring system, 389
recurrence, 348-350, 358, 359, 373, 406, 407
registration, 316, 386, 387
risk factors, 166-168, 172, 173, 177-184, 188, 190-193, 299, 316, 346, 347, 374, 376, 377, 389, 402, 420-426, 429, 430, 434, 437
staging, 327-340, 344, 345, 358, 388-399, 420, 421, 423, 424
Trophoblastic disease (continued)
treatment of, 7-12, 111-124, 187, 190, 313-322, 343-351, 355-366, 369-379, 387-399, 401-409, 417-427, 429-434, 437, 442, 447-449, 452-462 (*see also* Trophoblastic disease chemotherapy)
vascularity as basis for effectiveness of chemotherapy, 8
Trophoblastic disease chemotherapy, 7, 111-124, 187, 318-320, 343-351, 355-366, 369-379, 389-399, 401-409, 412-416, 418, 423, 427, 440, 444, 448, 454, 455, 457-462 (*see also* Trophoblastic disease, treatment of)
actinomycin D, 7, 116, 345, 346, 348-350, 371, 372, 374-376, 389-399, 401, 418, 444, 448, 462
adriamycin, 116, 349, 350, 423
Bagshawe regimen, 375, 391-396, 404
bleomycin, 116, 349, 350, 391, 393, 395, 396, 404
in brain metastases, 320, 371, 375-377, 392-396, 401,404
carboquone, 116
in central nervous system metastasis, 320, 349, 350, 376, 377
CHAMOCA, 349, 350, 391-396, 404
chlorambucil, 345, 375
cis-platinum, 349, 350, 391, 393, 395, 396, 404
citrovorum factor rescue, 346-351, 389, 454
clomomycin, 116
combination chemotherapy, 115-117, 124, 187, 345-351, 357, 365, 366, 369-379, 390-397, 401, 404, 415, 418, 444, 454, 455, 459, 460, 462

Trophoblastic disease chemotherapy (continued)
in combination with radiotherapy, 350, 376, 378, 392, 395, 401, 404
corticosteroids, 456
cyclophosphamide, 116, 348, 350, 390-396, 401, 423
cytophosphan, 444
cytoxan, 349, 454
digitalization, 456
Einhorn regimen, 375
Endoxan, 116
Esquinon, 116
5-fluorouracil, 116, 355-366
folic acid, 9-11, 460
folinic acid, 187, 320, 372, 374
fractional cell kill, 318-320
hepatic artery catheter and, 350
Hickman catheter and, 376
high-risk patients, 320, 349, 350, 375-379, 386-397, 423
hydroxyurea, 350
intrathecal methotrexate, 320, 350
leucovorin, *see* Trophoblastic disease chemotherapy; Citrovorum factor rescue
in liver metastasis, 350, 375, 389, 395, 403
MAC, 345, 348-350, 375, 390-396, 401
MAC III, 454
6-mercaptopurine, 345, 355, 356, 359-361, 366, 418, 423, 448
methotrexate, 7, 10, 116, 320, 343-351, 356, 359-361, 366, 371, 372, 374-376, 387-396, 401, 415, 418, 423, 444, 454, 458-460, 462
Mitomycin, 116
MTX-CF, 346-351, 374, 454
multi-agent chemotherapy, *see* Trophoblastic disease chemotherapy, combination chemotherapy
oncovin, 350
oxygen, 456
phase II drugs, 376
plat-HD, 350
prophylactic chemotherapy, 349, 350, 387
resistance to drugs, 9, 345, 347, 349, 356, 357, 359, 361, 365, 366, 372-377, 389-396, 423
toxicity, 345-349, 355, 359-361, 364-366, 370-377, 389, 406
Toyomycin, 116
VBP, 391-396
VCR, 350
Velban, 375
vinblastine, 116, 348, 349, 391-396, 404
vinca leucoblastine, 348
vincristine, 116, 349, 350, 448
VP 16-213, 349, 350, 375
VP-BC, 350
Trophoblastic disease epidemiology, in
Africa, 172, 177-184, 187-195, 409-427
Alaska, 172
Asia, 172, 177, 184, 462
Europe, 183
Indonesia, 165-175, 177, 184, 464
Iran, 172, 450
Israel, 184
Japan, 450
Korea, 442
Madagascar (Malagasy), 177
Malaysia, 172
Mexico, 172
Nigeria, 172, 177-184, 417-427, 450
Southern Africa, 177, 183
Singapore, 425
Taiwan, 172, 184, 462

Trophoblastic disease epidemiology (continued)
  Uganda, 184
  United Kingdom, 184, 315
  USA, 172, 183, 450
Trophoblastic disease etiology, 13-42, 309, 407
Trophoblastic disease metastasis, in
  adnexa, 321, 331, 337, 338
  bladder, 328
  bowel, 328, 344, 405
  brain, 320-322, 333, 334, 337-339, 344, 350, 365, 371, 374-377, 389, 392, 395, 401, 403-405, 425, 431
  central nervous system, 376, 377
  gastrointestinal tract, 335, 337-339, 364, 365, 389
  genitourinary tract, 364
  gum, 363
  intestine, 328, 335, 336
  kidney, 328, 335-340, 344, 363, 389, 431
  liver, 328, 334, 337-340, 350, 365, 371, 374-377, 389, 403, 405, 431
  lung, 9, 123, 320, 331-335, 337, 338, 340, 344, 346, 356, 362, 363, 374, 375, 389, 394, 403, 405, 431, 452, 455
  lymph node, 328
  mesosalpingeal vein, 331
  myometrium, 82, 321, 328, 329, 337, 338
  ovarian vein, 329, 330, 337, 338
  parametrium, 328, 329, 337, 338, 340
  pelvis, 328, 329, 338, 340, 344, 346, 365, 389, 403, 405
  spleen, 328, 335, 337-340, 344, 389
  uterine vein, 329-331, 337
  vagina, 329-331, 337, 338, 340, 344, 346, 364,
Trophoblastic disease metastasis, in (continued)
  vagina (continued)
    374, 375, 389, 403, 405, 431
Trophoblastic disease treatment, *see* Trophoblastic disease, treatment
Trophoblast neoplasms
  histocompatibility antigens in, *see* Histocompatibility antigens; Immunologic monitoring
Trophoblast oncogenesis, 55-58
Trypan blue dye exclusion, 273, 277
Trypsin, 293
TSH activity of hCGβ, 199
Tumor-associated antigens, 344
Tumor-promoting agents, 21, 22, 27
Tumor promotion, 21, 22
Tumor-specific antigen, 116
Twinning
  and frequency of gestational trophoblastic disease, 184
  nonfamilial dizygotic, 156, 184
  in western Nigeria, 184
Two-site immunometric assay, 235, 236
  monoclonal antibodies and, 232, 235, 236
Type II pneumocytes, 24

Uganda, 184
Ultrasound, 321, 339, 370, 398, 433, 440, 454
Ultraviolet radiation, 13
Unbalanced production of α- and β-subunits of hCG, 232
Unexplained habitual abortion, 83
United Kingdom, 147-149, 156, 184, 313
University of Benin Teaching Hospital, Benin City, Nigeria, 417-427

University College Hospital, Ibadan, Nigeria, 177, 178, 180, 183, 425, 450
University of the East Medical Center, 457
University of Ibadan, 177, 450
University of Indonesia, 437
University of Isfahan Medical School, 456
University of Louisville, 443
University of Michigan, 245
University of Nairobi, 409, 448
University of Pittsburgh School of Medicine, 135
5'-Untranslated sequence, 300
Urea, 2r0, 235, 248
Urethane, 16
Urine concentrates
  high-sensitivity RIA for hCG in, 232, 236
Urine pregnancy test in monitoring of choriocarcinoma, 7, 418, 424, 426, 448
Urokinase, 116
Uterine corpus, 346, 420 (*see also* Trophoblastic disease, staging)
Uterine size
  and trophoblastic disease, 168
Uterine weight assay, 370
Utrecht, The Netherlands, 5

Vaginal metastasis, *see* Trophoblastic disease metastasis
Varidase, 118
Vascularity and chemotherapy of trophoblastic disease, 8
Vasculo-syncytial membranes, 130
VBP, *see* Trophoblastic disease chemotherapy
VCR, *see* Trophoblastic disease chemotherapy, vincristine
Ve, 257
Velban, *see* Trophoblastic disease chemotherapy
Venous metastases, 338
Vibrio cholerae, 290
Villous hydrops, 88 (*see also* Hydropic villi)
Vinblastine, *see* Trophoblastic disease chemotherapy
Vinca leucoblastine, *see* Trophoblastic disease chemotherapy
Vincristine, *see* Trophoblastic disease chemotherapy
Vinyl chloride, 14, 16-19
Vitachange, 236
  in urine assay for hCG, 232, 236
Vitamin A, 116
VLB, *see* Vinca leucoblastine
Vo, 257
Void volume (Vo), 248, 257
VP-16, *see* VP 16-213; Trophoblastic disease chemotherapy
VP 16-213, *see* Trophoblastic disease chemotherapy
VP-BC, *see* Trophoblastic disease chemotherapy
Vt, 257

Washington, D.C., USA, 3
Washington University, St. Louis, MIssouri, USA, 299
Water transport, 129 (*see also* Placental aging)
Wheat germ cell-free translation system, 224
White blood cells
  5-fluorouracil and, 359, 360
  6-mercaptopurine and, 359, 360
  methotrexate and, 359, 360
Wilhelmina Gasthuis, 460
Wills, Dr. Helen, 9
Wisconsin, 53, 217, 245, 267, 289, 299, 438, 443, 446, 450
World Health Organization Matched Reagents Programme, 448

X chromosome, 53, 84, 86, 137, 148, 152

X-ray, 331, 339, 362, 424, 444,
450, 456, 459, 462

Yale University School of Medicine, 343
Y chromosome, 53, 84, 137, 152
Yellow butterfly

Zondek, Herman, 6
Zymosan, 112

MIX
Papier aus verantwortungsvollen Quellen
Paper from responsible sources
FSC® C105338

If you have any concerns about our products,
you can contact us on
ProductSafety@springernature.com

In case Publisher is established outside the EU,
the EU authorized representative is:
Springer Nature Customer Service Center GmbH
Europaplatz 3, 69115 Heidelberg, Germany

Printed by Libri Plureos GmbH
in Hamburg, Germany